CLINICAL NEUROPHYSIOLOGY OF THE VESTIBULAR SYSTEM

CONTEMPORARY NEUROLOGY SERIES AVAILABLE:

Fred Plum, M.D., *Editor-in-Chief*
Series Editors: Sid Gilman, M.D.
Joseph B. Martin, M.D., Ph.D.
Robert B. Daroff, M.D.
Stephen G. Waxman, M.D., Ph.D.
M-Marsel Mesulam, M.D.

CLINICAL NEUROPHYSIOLOGY OF THE VESTIBULAR SYSTEM

ROBERT W. BALOH, M.D.
Professor
Department of Neurology and
Division of Head and Neck Surgery
  (Otolaryngology)
UCLA School of Medicine
Los Angeles, California

VICENTE HONRUBIA, M.D.
Professor
Director of Research
Divison of Head and Neck Surgery
  (Otolaryngology)
UCLA School of Medicine
Los Angeles, California

EDITION 2

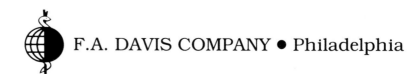

F.A. DAVIS COMPANY • Philadelphia

Printed in the United States of America

Last digit indicates print number: 10 9 8 7 6 5 4 3 2 1

Soft Cover Version

NOTE: As new scientific information becomes available through basic and clinical research, recommended treatments and drug therapies undergo changes. The author(s) and publisher have done everything possible to make this book accurate, up-to-date, and in accord with accepted standards at the time of publication. However, the reader is advised always to check product information (package inserts) for changes and new information regarding dose and contraindications before administering any drug. Caution is especially urged when using new or infrequently ordered drugs.

Library of Congress Cataloging-in-Publication Data

Baloh, Robert W. (Robert William), 1942–
    Clinical neurophysiology of the vestibular system / Robert W.
Baloh, Vicente Honrubia.—2nd ed.
        p.   cm.
        Bibliography: p.
        Includes index.
        ISBN 0-8036-0584-6
    1. Vestibular apparatus—Diseases.   2. Vestibular function tests.
    3. Neurophysiology.   I. Honrubia, Vicente, 1934–   . II. Title.
        [DNLM: 1. Neurophysiology.   2. Vestibular Apparatus.
    3. Vestibular Function Tests.]
    RF260.B25   1989
    612.8'58—dc20
    DNLM/DLC
    for Library of Congress   89-16897
                                                                          CIP

ISBN 0-8036-0584-6 Hard Cover
ISBN 0-8036-0585-4 Soft Cover

THIS BOOK IS DEDICATED
TO OUR PARENTS

PREFACE

The purpose of this book is to provide a framework for understanding the pathophysiology of diseases involving the vestibular system. The book is divided into three parts: The Vestibular System, Evaluation of the Dizzy Patient, and Diagnosis and Management of Common Neurotologic Disorders. Part I reviews the anatomy and physiology of the vestibular system, with emphasis on clinically relevant material. Part II outlines the important features in the patient's history, examination, and laboratory evaluation that determine the probable site of lesion. Part III covers the differential diagnostic points that help the clinician decide on the cause and treatment of the patient's problem.

This completely reorganized and expanded second edition covers the rapid advances that have occurred in the basic and clinical sciences in the past 10 years and includes a complete updated bibliography. It contains a detailed discussion of the differential diagnosis of dizziness of both vestibular and nonvestibular etiology as well as current treatment options for most neurotologic disorders. A balanced presentation of otologic and neurologic mechanisms is maintained, inasmuch as one cannot effectively evaluate patients complaining of dizziness without understanding both the inner ear and central nervous system aspects involved in vestibular disorders. We have added many new figures, tables, and algorithms for management as well as a new appendix that gives mathematical background for biophysics in the early chapters.

We believe that this book will be useful to all physicians who treat patients complaining of dizziness. It should be particularly helpful to those in the field of family practice, internal medicine, neurology, otolaryngology, and neurosurgery. Finally, we hope that it will encourage students (in both the clinical and basic sciences) to choose neurotology as their field of study.

ROBERT W. BALOH, M.D.
VICENTE HONRUBIA, M.D.

FOREWORD TO
THE FIRST EDITION

Extensive research on human vestibular reflexes initiated by Robert Bárány in 1907 provided the foundation for clinical analysis of pathologic processes in the labyrinth of the ear or in the pathways and centers of the vestibular system.

In the early period of clinical research, knowledge of the anatomy and physiology of the vestibular system was rudimentary and the techniques for stimulation of the labyrinth and measurement of reflexes were crude. In the past 70 years, owing to significant technologic advances and an increase in the number of investigators entering the field, there has been a spectacular change. Abundant qualitative and quantitative information is now available on the structure and function of the peripheral and central vestibular systems with numerous reports on the symptoms and diagnoses of vestibular dysfunction.

Drs. Baloh and Honrubia have met the need for a concise text that integrates the numerous advances in the field of vestibular research with clinical diagnoses. The authors have made noteworthy contributions to otoneurology and this book contains carefully prepared, concise explanations of what is known at present, and judicious treatment of areas of controversy. The simple and direct style of the first three chapters on neurophysiology will give the reader an excellent foundation for the discussion of clinical problems in later chapters. Extensive bibliographies at the end of each chapter supplement the text and are a valuable source of information on all aspects of vestibular function.

This book will be especially useful to students and residents as well as to neurologists, otologists, and ophthalmologists.

R. Lorente de Nó, M.D.

ACKNOWLEDGMENTS

Our colleagues in Neurology and Head and Neck Surgery provided inspiration. Kate Jacobson and Karl Beykirch helped prepare the figures. Gwynne Gloege made the drawings. Lyn Corum typed the manuscript. We are grateful for the continued support of our work by the National Institutes of Health.

CONTENTS

Part I
THE VESTIBULAR SYSTEM

Chapter 1

VESTIBULAR FUNCTION: AN OVERVIEW

Expressed simply, the role of the vestibular sensory organs is to transduce the forces associated with head acceleration and gravity into a biologic signal. The control centers in the brain use this signal to develop a subjective awareness of head position in relation to the environment and to produce motor reflexes for equilibrium, relating these experiences to those of other sensory systems during locomotion. This interaction of the various systems leads to orientation, a function that is different from that of all the elements acting individually. The vestibular system, by means of its receptors for the perception of linear and angular acceleration, plays a central role in orientation.

During head movement, the force (F) exerted upon the vestibular end-organs (from Newton's second principle) is equal to the product of their mass (m) and their acceleration (a): $F = ma$.* Because the mass of the end-organ is constant, the force associated with head acceleration generates a signal in the labyrinth that is proportional to the head acceleration. The mathematical operation required to convert an acceleration signal to a measure of head displacement involves two integrations: one to obtain head velocity from acceleration and the other to obtain head displacement from velocity. The overall objective of the central nervous system (CNS) is to compute head position by performing the equivalent of a mathematical integration of the labyrinthine input signals.

Modern inertial guidance systems that control the trajectory of space vehicles include the same basic components: a monitor of displacement based on sensors for linear and angular acceleration, and a central processor that integrates this information, computing the coordinates of the space position. The central processor also maintains a memory of the trajectory and can therefore make appropriate adjustments in course when necessary.[4] Here the similarities of vestibular organs to space vehicle guidance systems end, for they do not explain the complex operational capabilities of the brain in support of the sensory function of orientation. The performance of space vehicles is based upon preprogrammed strategies—that is, it is experience-based behavior—whereas the brain can resolve even the most unexpected conflicts. For example, the direction of the vestibulo-ocular reflex can be reversed (i.e., the eyes will move in the same direction as that of the head instead of in the opposite direction) if one wears glasses with reversing prisms for several days.[28] The neuroanatomic and physiologic substrate for this capability is only partially understood, but such discoveries have opened new avenues of research in the study of vestibular function in health and disease.

BIOPHYSICAL BASIS OF VESTIBULAR RECEPTOR SPECIALIZATION

The vestibular system monitors the forces associated with angular and linear

---

*If mass is in kilograms and acceleration in meters/second^2, then the unit of force is the newton (the force acting on a kilogram of mass to impart an acceleration of a meter per second per second).

accelerations of the head by means of five organs located within the labyrinthine cavities of the temporal bones on each side of the skull. The saccular and utricular maculae sense linear acceleration, and the cristae of the three semicircular canals sense angular acceleration of the head. The capacity of the maculae and cristae to function as sensors of these kinds of acceleration rests on their anatomic configurations.

Maculae

Each macula consists of a sensory membrane containing the receptor cells with a surface area less than 1 mm^2 that supports a "heavy load," the otolith (specific gravity approximately 2.7). The otolith is composed of calcareous material embedded in a gelatinous matrix and has a mean thickness of 50 μm (Fig. 1–1A). The position of the load on the receptor depends on the magnitude and direction of the force acting upon it (Fig. 1–1B, C).[15] Even when the head is at rest, the calcareous material, because of its mass, exerts a force (F_g) upon the receptor equal to the product of its

mass and the acceleration due to the gravitational pull of the earth (g), which at sea level is 9.80 m/sec^2.

The distribution of F_g acting upon the underlying sensory cells changes with different degrees of head tilt and can be represented by two vectors (Fig. 1–1B): one vector (F_t) tangential and the other (F_n) normal to the surface of the receptor. The value of the tangential vector is proportional to the sine of the angle Θ made by F_g with F_n (i.e., the angle of tilt). As will be shown later, it is this tangential force (F_t) and the resulting otolith displacement that constitute the effective stimulus to the sensory cells.

During linear head acceleration tangential to the surface of the receptor (Fig. 1–1C), the instantaneous force (F'_g) acting upon the maculae is also the result of two vector forces: one (F_t) in the direction opposite to that of head acceleration and the other (F_g) due to gravitational pull. Again, the effective force producing otolith displacement is the tangential force (F_t). In both cases, the sensory cells of the maculae transmit information on the displacement of the otolith membrane to the CNS; here, reflexes are initiated to contract mus-

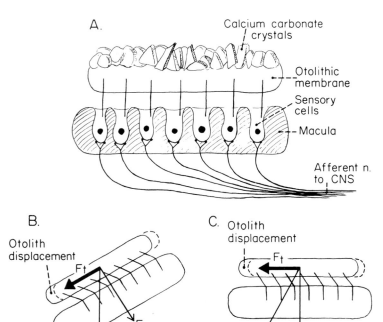

Figure 1–1. A graphic illustration of the main anatomic features of the macula (A) and the distribution of forces associated with static head tilt (B) and linear acceleration tangential to the surface (C) (for orientation of sensory cells in each macula, see Chapter 2, Figure 2–7).

hat dynamically oppose the force act-
ıpon the head and thus maintain
brium.

assic example of an otolithic reflex is
ange in eye position of fish, amphib-
and rodents when their heads and
s are tilted from the horizontal and
heia ın that position. In such a condition,
the eyes align themselves in the orbits to
maintain their normal relation parallel to
the horizon.[48, 52] To achieve this goal, the
extraocular muscles of the eyes acquire a
new level of contraction, or tone, that remains unchanged as long as the head is
held in the new position. Because of the
permanence of the muscle tone, such reflexes are classically known as the static
labyrinthine reflexes, and the maculae are
known as the static labyrinthine organs.

Cristae

Natural head movements consist of a
combination of linear and rotational vectors, the latter acting upon a different set
of sensors located in the semicircular canals.[18] The canals are small rings approximately 0.65 cm in transverse diameter
with an inner cross-sectional diameter of
0.4 mm (Fig. 1–2). They are filled with
fluid that has a density and a viscosity
slightly greater than those of water.[55] The
receptor organs, the cristae, are mounted
in the wall of the rings, where they sense
the displacement of the fluid during head
rotation. The sensory epithelium of the
cristae is covered by a bulbous, gelatinous
mass called the cupula, the specific gravity
of which is the same as that of the sur-

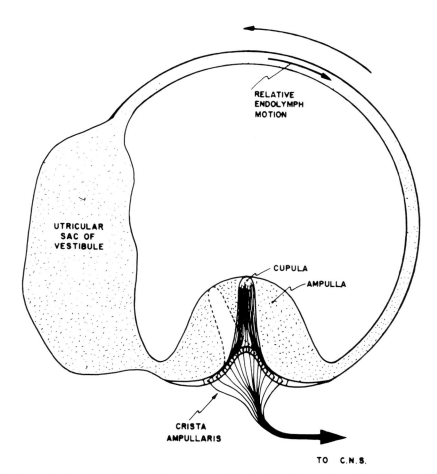

Figure 1–2. Schematic drawing of a semicircular canal illustrating the relationship between the direction of
head rotation (*large arrow*), endolymph flow (*small arrow*) and cupular deviation. (From Melvill Jones, G: Organization of neural control in the vestibulo-ocular reflex arc. In Bach-Y-Rita, P, Collins, CC, and Hyde, JE (eds):
The Control of Eye Movements. Academic Press, New York, 1971, with permission.)

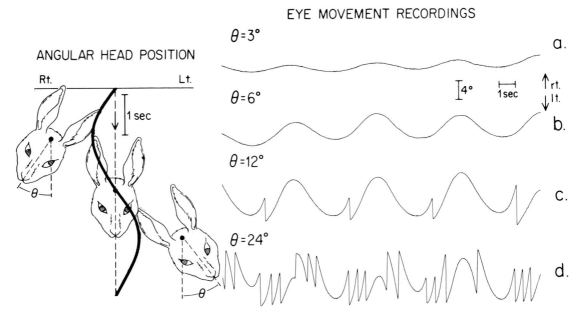

Figure 1–3. Compensatory eye movements in the rabbit produced by sinusoidal angular acceleration of the head (0.2 Hz) at four different peak angular displacements (Θ).

rounding fluid. Unlike the otolith of the maculae, therefore, the cupula does not exert a resting force on the underlying sensory epithelium. Because of the narrowness of the canals, the fluid can move only longitudinally. Angular acceleration of the head displaces the fluid relative to the wall of the canal. The cupula moves with the fluid, exerting a force on the underlying sensory epithelium.

The semicircular canal reflexes have been called phasic, or kinetic, because they are thought to be primarily responsible for muscle contractions associated with the maintenance of equilibrium during motion associated with angular head acceleration. An example of a semicircular canal reflex is the compensatory eye movement associated with head rotation (Fig. 1–3). Head rotation to one side results in eye movement in the opposite direction in order to maintain a stable gaze for clear vision.[43] If the head rotation exceeds that which can be compensated for by motion of the eye in the orbit within approximately ±20 degrees (e.g., in Fig. 1–3d), the reflex takes the form of nystagmus. This is a back-and-forth eye movement in which a slow deviation, lasting between 0.5 and 2

seconds, is interrupted by a flick in the opposite direction lasting 0.1 to 0.2 seconds. If the fast components were removed from the bottom tracings in Figure 1–3c and d and the slow components joined end to end, the resulting sinusoidal eye movement would continue to be approximately equal in magnitude and opposite in direction to the sinusoidal head movements as seen in Figure 1–3a and b.

CLASSIFICATION OF VESTIBULAR REFLEXES

The rationale for classifying the cristae of the semicircular canals as kinetic receptors and the maculae of the utriculus and sacculus as static receptors was based on a narrow view of their overall function. Both sets of receptor organs produce motor reflexes that cannot be differentiated on the basis of the resulting movement. It is more appropriate, therefore, to differentiate the reflexes by categories based on their functional role rather than on the receptor from which they originate.

At least three major functional roles for vestibular reflexes can be identified. The first is to maintain posture. Vestibular reflexes of this kind induce muscle contractions that produce negative geotropic movement or forces that compensate for steady changes in the direction of the force of gravity. If the pull of gravity on the body were unopposed by forces developed in the muscles, the body would collapse. Reflexes in this category are dependent on the function of the maculae but not on that of the semicircular canals. The second role is to produce "kinetic," or transitory, contractions of muscles for maintenance of equilibrium and ocular stability during movement. This category includes reflexes arising from both the semicircular canals during angular acceleration and the otolithic organs during linear acceleration. Most natural head movements contain both types of acceleration, and the vestibular reflexes act in combination to maintain equilibrium. A third role of vestibular reflex activity is to help maintain muscular tone,[49, 50] a role in which both the maculae and cristae participate.[51] The labyrinthine contribution to skeletal-muscular tone can be demonstrated by the change in posture that follows unilateral labyrinthectomy in normal animals.[16, 48] Tone is increased in the extensor muscles of the contralateral extremities and decreased in the ipsilateral extensor muscles. An even more striking demonstration of the vestibular role in maintenance of muscular tone is the removal of decerebrate rigidity after sectioning of both vestibular nerves or destruction of the vestibular nuclei.[3, 24] The extensor rigidity that results from transection of the nervous system at the caudal end of the mesencephalon is markedly decreased when the tonic labyrinthine input is removed.

The characteristically high spontaneous firing rate of action potentials from the primary vestibular afferents provides a constant level of neural activity to the neurons in the vestibular nuclei.[27] The peripheral vestibular influence also affects the response of the vestibular nuclei neurons to the converging inputs from other systems (vision, proprioception) and from neurons in the opposite side of the brain as well.[59] By means of commissural and reverberating circuits, an integration, in the mathematical as well as the physiologic sense,

takes place in the brainstem[25, 31] (see Chapter 3).

PHYLOGENY OF THE VESTIBULAR SYSTEM

The role of the labyrinth in maintaining orientation has remained the same from the earliest organisms in the animal kingdom. But, as with other sensory organs, some changes, both functional and morphologic, have evolved. Only the most primitive forms of life, such as Monera (bacteria and blue-green algae) and Protista, which include many unicellular organisms (flagella), have been able to adapt to the environment without specialized receptors for the detection of gravitational force. In these animals, as well as in plants, geotropic motion is probably due to the difference in density of undifferentiated parts that "detect" the pull of gravity. For example, when the stem of the plant *Bryophyllum calycinium* is placed in a horizontal position, certain chemical substances gather in greater concentration on the lower side of the stem, causing it to grow faster than the upper side. Thus the stem is forced to grow in a vertical direction.[42]

The most primitive gravity-detection organ, the statocyst, appeared more than 600 million years ago in the late Precambrian era.[29] It is present in the most developed Coelenterata, beginning with some jellyfish, allowing the animal to orient itself in relation to the horizon by sensing the direction of the gravitational force of the earth. The statocyst is a fluid-filled invagination, or sac, containing a calcareous particle—the statolith—or multiple particles—the statoconia—of a density greater than that of the fluid. Attracted by gravity, the particles rest their weight differentially over special sensory cells in the wall of the cyst. The direction of the force in the underlying sensory cells therefore depends on the position of the animal in space.

From this simple statocyst to the labyrinth of higher animals, a continuous increment in anatomic complexity occurs that accompanies the phylogenetic evolution of the taxa. Next to the statocyst of medusae, phylogenetically, is that of mollusks (e.g., octopus, sepia). In addition to a statocyst containing multiple otoconia, the first crista appears in these primitive animals. The development of this new receptor, still in the same cavity as that of the otolith, accompanies the appearance of motor responses to angular acceleration, including nystagmus.[11, 12, 17] In primitive fish (cyclostomes), the statocyst cavity, previously open to the outside, is closed and filled by an endogenous secretion (endolymph).

Two surviving cyclostomes, the hagfish and the lamprey, demonstrate an important step in the phylogenetic development of the vestibular labyrinth. In the hagfish a simple circular tube is interrupted anteriorly and posteriorly by bulbous enlargements, the ampullae, each containing a primitive crista. Between the ampullae in an intercommunicating channel lies the macula communis, the forerunner of the utricular and saccular maculae. The labyrinth of the lamprey is more complex, consisting of an anterior canal and a posterior canal communicating with a bilobulated sac containing separate utricular and saccular maculae. The predecessor of the auditory organs appears after the development of a membranous labyrinth that is divided into two cavities. In the inferior of the two cavities (the sacculus), two new re-

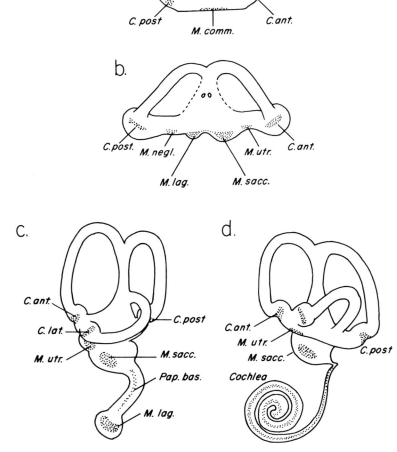

Figure 1–4. Phylogeny of the labyrinth. (*a*) myxine; (*b*) petromyzon; (*c*) bird; (*d*) mammal. *C. post.*, posterior canal; *M. comm.*, common macula; *C. ant.*, anterior canal; *M. negl.*, neglector macula; *M. lag.*, lagenar macula; *M. sacc.*, saccular macula; *M. utr.*, utricular macula; *C. lat.*, lateral or horizontal canal; *Pap. bas.*, basilar papilla. (From Wersäll, DJ and Bagger Sjöbäck, D: Morphology of the vestibular sensor organs. In Kornhuber, HH (ed): Handbook of Sensory Physiology, Vol VI, Part 2. Springer-Verlag, New York, 1974, with permission.)

ceptor areas develop, the lagenar macula and the basilar papilla. In crocodiles, however, these receptors are contained in a cavity separate from the sacculus, whereas in birds the basilar papilla is a long, uncoiled organ, the predecessor of the coiled cochlea (Fig. 1–4).[2]

With the advent of modern fish (about 100 million years ago) the vestibular labyrinth reached its peak of development, and relatively little change has taken place since that time.[29] The basic structure of the three semicircular canals, the utriculus, and the sacculus is similar in all higher vertebrates. Gray[29] considered the vestibular end-organ of modern fish to represent the "highest perfection" of the vertebrate organ of equilibrium. The utriculus and semicircular canals are relatively larger than those in other classes of vertebrates. Because fish do not have the highly developed afferent systems of proprioception, touch, and vision that higher vertebrates possess, they are apparently more dependent on the labyrinth to provide orienting information.

The membranous labyrinths of modern fish lie in the bony chamber of the skull directly behind the orbits. In its subsequent evolution in amphibians, birds, and mammals, the membranous labyrinth is completely surrounded by a bony labyrinth enclosing the periotic space. This space is filled with perilymphatic fluid and suspensory connective tissue acting as a shock absorber. The relative positions of the planes of the three semicircular canals vary from species to species, although in primates they are approximately orthogonal to each other. The shape of each semicircular canal also varies considerably from that of a triangle in reptiles to an ellipse in birds to an almost true circle in mammals.[29]

Parallel to the separation of receptor organs, afferent nerve fibers differentiate into bundles that maintain independent identity in the internal auditory canal and at the entrance to the brainstem.[44] The afferent nerve from the utriculus and horizontal and anterior semicircular canals and some of the nerve fibers from the sacculus form the superior division of the vestibular nerve, whereas most nerve fibers from the sacculus and the nerve from the

posterior semicircular canal contribute to the inferior branch (Fig. 1–5). The afferent fibers from the auditory organ form a separate nerve anterior and inferior to the vestibular nerve to innervate the organ of Corti, the auditory receptor organ. Together these two nerves constitute the eighth cranial nerve, and within them, a system of efferent fibers from the CNS gates or modulates the activity of the peripheral organs.[8, 60, 62] Phylogenetically, this neural feedback system is already present in gastropods, in which action potentials directed from the brain to the receptors have been recorded.[64]

In comparison with the vestibular sensory organs, central vestibular connections become progressively more complex in higher vertebrates. This complexity accompanies the development of other afferent systems for the maintenance of equilibrium (vision, proprioception) and pathways for interaction of these systems with the vestibular system. The vestibular nuclei are one of the first supraspinal cell groups that differentiate themselves from the reticular formation.[37] Lampreys have two discernible vestibular nuclear groups, the dorsal and ventral, composed of granular and spindle-shaped cells. Modern fish (teleosts) have four discernible vestibular nuclei, although the nuclei contain relatively few cells. This basic organization of four vestibular nuclear groups is maintained throughout the higher vertebrates, although the relative size of each nuclear group varies from species to species. In invertebrates and early vertebrates, secondary connections of the vestibular nuclei are primarily vestibulospinal, in keeping with their major role in maintaining body orientation.[53] Vestibulocerebellar connections become progressively more prominent in higher vertebrates. The development of these "modern" vestibular pathways accompanies the development of increasingly complex somatic and ocular motor skills. In primates, vestibulocerebellar and vestibulo-ocular connections form a large part of the central vestibular pathways, and vestibulospinal connections are less prominent.[39] The lateral vestibular nucleus (Deiters' nucleus), a major source of vestibulospinal fibers, is the most prominent nuclear group in lower mammals,

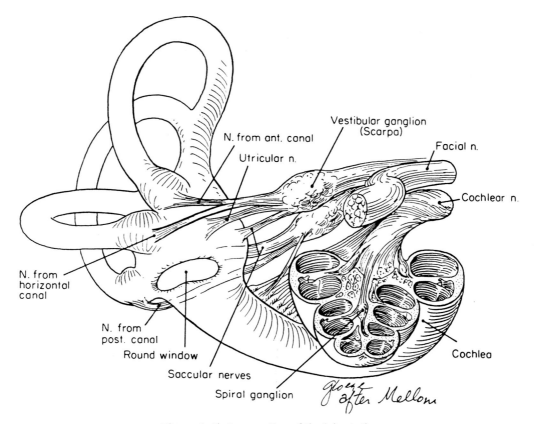

Figure 1–5. Innervation of the labyrinth.

whereas in human beings it is small and almost confined to the vestibular root entry zone. By comparison, the superior vestibular nucleus is barely detectable in lower vertebrates but is prominent in humans, where it is the major source of vestibulo-ocular fibers. It extends rostrally from the root entry zone (at the medullopontine junction) to the midpontine region.[37]

FORCE TRANSDUCTION: THE HAIR CELL

Morphologic Characteristics

The basic element of the labyrinthine receptor organs that transduces mechanical force to nerve action potentials—the hair cell (Fig. 1–6)—is already developed in the statocysts of invertebrates.[10] Transducer cells are surrounded by supporting cells in specialized epithelial areas in the walls of the statocyst. In lower vertebrates, a bundle of nonmobile cilia protrudes from the apical surface of the cylindrical hair cells. The basal portion of the cell makes contact with many terminals of afferent and efferent nerve fibers. The former carry information from the receptor to the CNS, and the latter provide feedback to the receptor cells from the CNS.

The increased complexity of the labyrinthine end-organs, from an evolutionary point of view, is not limited to changes in gross anatomic features but is also expressed in the development of new structural details in the receptor cells.[46] Two types of hair cell occur in birds and mammals (see Fig. 1–6). Type I cells are globular or flask-shaped with a single large chalicelike nerve terminal surrounding the base. The afferent fibers innervating these hair cells are among the largest in the ner-

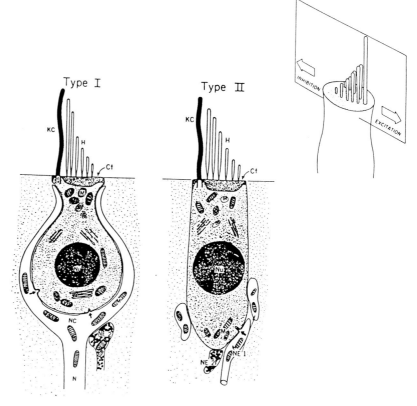

Type I   Type II

Figure 1–6. Schematic drawing of the two types of hair cells. Inset illustrates relationship between the direction of force and maximum hair cell activation. *KC*, kinocilium; *H*, hairs; *Ct*, cuticular plate; *M*, mitochondria; *Nu*, nucleus; *NC*, afferent nerve chalice; *NE 1*, afferent nerve bouton; *NE 2*, efferent nerve bouton.

vous system (up to 20 μm in diameter). Type II cells are cylindrical with multiple nerve terminals at their base (as in lower vertebrates).[63]

The stereocilia are bound together at the top to the taller neighboring kinocilium, and when experimentally a force is directly applied to them, they move together with the rigidity of glass rods.[21] Recent findings indicate that the physical properties of the stereocilia can influence the function not only of individual hair cells but of whole receptor organs. For example, the length and stiffness of the cilia in the organ of Corti influence the motion of the overlying basilar membrane.[22] The stereocilia vary in length among hair cells of different organs, and even within the same organ, depending on their location.[21, 40] In the frog crista there are two cilium patterns: the stereocilia of cells at the center are tall and thick and the kinocilia are relatively short, whereas stereocilia of the cells at the periphery are thinner and the kinocilia are very long. The former are stiffer and have, it is presumed, a higher resonance frequency than the latter. Hair cells of mammalian vestibular receptors also have at least two stereocilium patterns.[1, 41]

Relationship between the Direction of Force and Hair Cell Activation

The adequate stimulus for hair cell activation is a force acting parallel to the top of the cell, resulting in bending of the hairs (a shearing force).[61] A force applied perpendicular to the cell surface (a compressional force) is ineffective in stimulating the hair cell.[5, 20] The stimulus is maximal when the force is directed along an axis that bisects the bundle of stereocilia and passes through the kinocilium. Deflection of the hairs toward the kinocilium decreases the resting membrane potential of the sensory cells (depolarization). Bending in the opposite direction produces the reverse effect (hyperpolarization).[23] The effect is minimal when hair deflection is perpendicular to the axis of maximal excitation.

Physiologic Characteristics of Hair Cell Activation

The Davis mechanoelectric theory postulates that electric conductance of the cell membrane is modulated by mechanical deformation associated with displacement of the hairs (Fig. 1–7).[14, 32, 35] The hair-bearing surface of the cell membrane is morphologically different from the rest, being thicker and more electron dense. This part of the membrane is depolarized owing to the equal potassium concentration outside the cell in the endolymph and inside the cell protoplasm.[6] Ohmic resistance changes in proportion to the magnitude of hair deflection during physiologic stimulation cause a modulated leakage of electric currents in a local circuit between the top, from which the hairs protrude, and other areas of the cell membrane. The voltage drop produced in the vicinity of the hair cells by the changing current is known as the microphonic potential—the so-called generator potential—of these receptor organs.[35] Recent intracellular recordings from hair cells of amphibians and mammals have expanded our knowledge of the mechanoelectric transduction process.[13, 36] The basic concept of the Davis theory has been upheld by demonstration of transmembrane potential changes and associated impedance modulation during deflection of the stereocilia. Electric current seems to flow from inside of the cell to outside—or vice versa—through the lumen of the stereocilia; the field potential generated by the receptor current is maximal at the tips of the hairs.[34] The generator potential follows the frequency of the stimulus and increases almost linearly with its magnitude. In contrast to nerve action potentials, the microphonics have no refractory period (following the frequency of the stimulation above several thousand hertz), are highly resistant to anoxia, and may remain partially active after the animal's death. The electric current associated with the generator potentials acts upon the synaptic contacts between hair cells and nerve

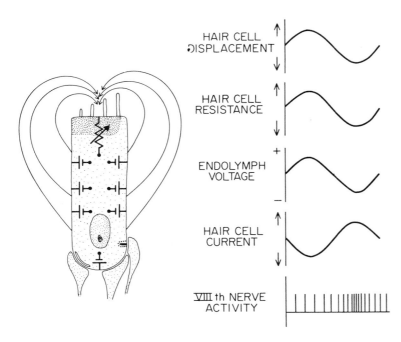

HAIR CELL DISPLACEMENT

HAIR CELL RESISTANCE

ENDOLYMPH VOLTAGE

HAIR CELL CURRENT

VIIIth NERVE ACTIVITY

Figure 1–7. Mechanism of hair cell activation. Sinusoidal displacement of the stereocilia produces a sinusoidal modulation of the vestibular nerve firing rate. See text for details.

terminals, either directly or by activating chemical transmitters, to modulate the firing of action potentials by the afferent neurons (see Fig. 1–7)

During the last 10 years, new information has been accumulated suggesting that hair cells are not passive elements but that they actively participate in the mechanotransduction process. The stereocilia of vestibular hair cells contain actin molecules and undergo an active change in stiffness if the concentration of calcium ions is experimentally changed.[58] Stereocilia of outer cochlear hair cells, which contain several contractile proteins,[22, 65] vary their length under direct electrical stimulation.[9] Thus it has been postulated that the physical properties of the stereocilia of cochlear hair cells can be influenced by the electric currents of neighboring physiologically activated cells. Likewise, their mechanical properties could be affected by postsynaptic potentials from efferent neurons innervating the receptor.[56] Physiologic properties of individual hair cells in the vestibular organs have not been investigated *in situ* at the cellular level, but it is logical to expect that anatomic differences in stereocilia reflect important differences in the process of transducing head-motion information into neural signals.

One of the most significant findings concerning hair cell function was the discovery by Hoagland in 1932 that the afferent nerves from lateral-line organs of fish generated continuous spontaneous activity.[30] This observation has subsequently been confirmed in all other hair cell systems and represents a fundamental discovery in sensory physiology. Although the mechanism responsible for the spontaneous firing of action potentials in the afferent nerves has not been identified, depolarization and hyperpolarization of the hair cells' membrane potential result in a modulation of this spontaneous activity. Bending of the hairs toward the kinocilium results in an increase of the spontaneous firing rate, and bending of the hairs away from the kinocilium results in a decrease.[47] The spontaneous firing rate varies among different animal species and among different sensory receptors. It is thought to be greatest in the afferent neurons of the semicircular canals of mammals (up to 90 spikes per second) and lowest in some of the acoustic nerve fibers innervating mammalian cochlear hair cells (1 to 2 spikes per second).[27, 38]

Basis for Stimulus Specificity of Inner Ear Receptor Organs

As suggested earlier, the density of the otolithic membrane overlying the hair cells of the macula is greater than that of the surrounding endolymph. The weight of this membrane produces a shearing force (F_t) on the underlying hair cells that is proportional to the sine of the angle between the line of resulting gravitational vector and a line perpendicular to the plane of the macula (see Fig. 1–1). The hair cell cilia in the cristae of the semicircular canals are embedded in the cupula, a jellylike substance of the same specific gravity as that of the surrounding fluids. The cupula, therefore, does not exert a force on the underlying crista and is not subject to displacement by changes in the line of gravitational force. The forces associated with angular head acceleration, however, do result in a displacement of the cupula that stimulates the hair cells of the crista in the same way that displacement of the otoliths stimulates the macular hair cells.

In the cochlea, the hair cells are mounted on the flexible basilar membrane in the organ of Corti. Covering the organ of Corti and resting over the hair cells is the tectorial membrane, a relatively rigid structure attached to the wall of the cochlea. A small, acoustically induced pressure difference across the basilar membrane causes the organ of Corti and hair cells to vibrate at the frequency of sound. When the basilar membrane moves, the hair cells are displaced in relationship to the relatively fixed tectorial membrane, which acts as a hinge.[61]

In all cases, the effective stimulus to the sensory cells is the relative displacement of the cilia produced by application of mechanical force to their surroundings. Because the mechanical properties of the "supporting and coupling" structures are different, the frequency ranges at which the cilia can be moved by the applied force are different.

ORGANIZATION OF CENTRAL VESTIBULAR PATHWAYS

Vestibular Reflexes

The basic elements of a simple vestibular reflex arc are the hair cell, an afferent bipolar neuron, an interneuron, and an effector neuron.[45] The terminal fibers of the afferent neuron make synaptic contact with the hair cell and transmit nerve signals to the nervous system where, by means of the interneuron, a connection is made with the effector neuron. The effector neuron, in turn, controls the activity in an appropriate muscle to coordinate orienting behavior. This simple three-neuron reflex arc is already developed in the phylum Mollusca, among which the class Cephalopoda has contributed to many classic anatomic and physiologic studies of gravitational reflexes.[10] An example of a three-neuron vestibular reflex in the human being is the semicircular canal–ocular reflex. Clockwise angular acceleration in the plane of the horizontal canals results in an increased firing of the afferent nerve from the ampulla of the right horizontal semicircular canal. This afferent signal is carried to the vestibular nucleus situated in the dorsolateral medulla. A neuron in the vestibular nucleus then transmits the signal to an effector neuron in the left abducens nucleus. Contraction of the left lateral rectus muscle initiates the compensatory deviation of the left eye to the left.

This simple example obviously does not provide the entire picture of the organization of the canal–ocular reflexes because it does not take into account the bilateral symmetrical canal system and the need for excitation and inhibition of four different horizontal ocular muscles. With head rotation to the right in the plane of the horizontal canals, the increase in firing of the right horizontal ampullary nerve is accompanied by a decrease in the corresponding left nerve. In addition, some of the interneurons are inhibitory, and by means of these two classes of neurons, the afferent signal arriving from the ampullary nerve exerts a dual influence on the effector system: it excites the agonist group of muscles and inhibits the antagonist group.

The control of motor responses by the labyrinth is, therefore, a four-way mechanism (Fig. 1–8). Stimulation of a receptor in the right (R) labyrinth increases the output of the afferent neurons, exerting an increased excitatory influence on the agonist ($\uparrow R^+$) and inhibitory influence on the antagonist ($\uparrow R^-$) groups of muscles. Because of the symmetry between the two labyrinths, the same receptor in the other ear simultaneously diminishes its afferent output, thereby disfacilitating the excit-

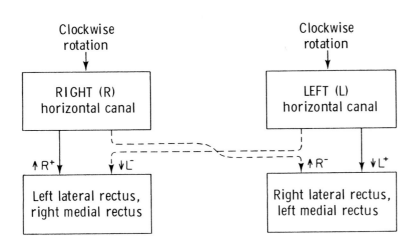

── Excitatory (+) influence
--- Inhibitory (-) influence

Figure 1–8. Organization of the horizontal semicircular canal-ocular reflex.

atory influence ($\downarrow L^+$) in the antagonist muscle and disinhibiting the agonist muscle ($\downarrow L^-$). The end result in the horizontal canal–ocular reflex is contraction of the left lateral and right medial rectus muscles and relaxation of the left medial and right lateral rectus muscles. This general plan of organization applies to all labyrinthine-mediated reflexes. We have found this simplified system to be extremely useful in the process of evaluating patients and elucidating the pathophysiologic changes associated with vestibular disorders.

Interaction with Other Systems

The maintenance of body equilibrium and posture in everyday life is a complex function involving multiple receptor organs and neural centers in addition to the labyrinths. Visual and proprioceptive reflexes, in particular, must be integrated with vestibular reflexes to insure postural stability. The prominent role of sensory interaction in orientation can already be appreciated in the behavior of gastropods. The invertebrate *Hermissenda* has only rudimentary vestibular and visual receptors, yet the two systems fully interact to control behavior.[26] Afferent signals from photoreceptors in the eye and from hair cells in the statocyst converge on interneurons in the cerebroplural ganglia, which control a putative motor neuron in each pedal ganglion. Excitation of the motor neuron produces turning of the animal's foot in the ipsilateral direction, consistent with the animal's turning behavior toward

light. In humans, during most natural head movements, gaze stabilization is achieved by a combination of vestibular, neck proprioceptive, and visual inputs; the interaction can be synergistic or antagonistic. For example, when the vestibularly induced eye movements lie in a direction opposite to that required to maintain the desired gaze position, the visual reflexes override the vestibular reflex. The kind of head rotation that would produce compensatory eye movement in the dark does not do so in the light if the subject fixates on a target moving in phase with the head (Fig. 1–9). In this simple example, failure to override the vestibular signal leads to disorientation.

The diagram in Figure 1–10 illustrates how different sensory systems—vestibular, visual, proprioceptive, auditory—provide information to a first line of individual central processors concerning orientation. These messages then converge to provide the command signals for eye movements and postural reflexes (in a common central processor). The functioning of the overall system is under adaptive control in a manner similar to that involved in other aspects of brain function and behavior.[33] The adaptive processor uses information from cross-sensory modalities in executing automated tasks, such as the repetitive execution of an athletic skill or the adjustment in eye movements to the use of magnifying or minifying lenses.[54] Adaptive mechanisms are also important in selecting orienting strategies, such as maintaining equilibrium after a shift in one's center of gravity by moving knees, hips, arms, or

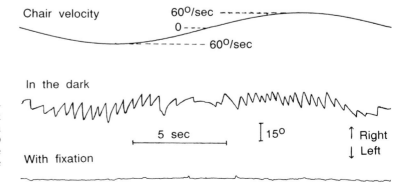

Figure 1–9. Eye movement induced in a normal human subject by sinusoidal angular acceleration (0.05 Hz, maximum velocity 60 deg/sec) in the dark and in the light with a target moving in phase with the subject.

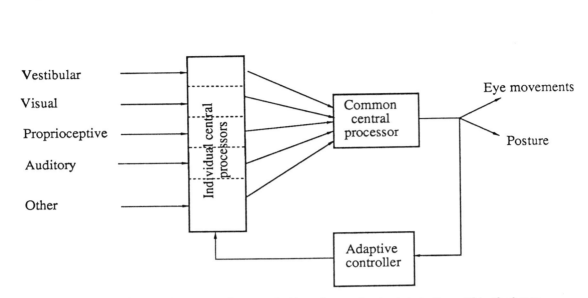

Figure 1–10. Block diagram illustrating the organization of sensorimotor integration within the brain.

all together.[57] The clinical importance of these adaptive mechanisms is just beginning to be appreciated. What are the strategies that patients use to compensate for loss of vestibular function? Why do some patients continue to complain of dizziness for months, whereas others recover rapidly? Understanding the adaptive mechanisms is fundamental to understanding patient symptoms (which can be interpreted as a reflection of the failure to develop coping strategies) and for the design of rehabilitation programs.

ABNORMAL LABYRINTHINE FUNCTION

Much of our knowledge of labyrinthine function was accumulated at the turn of the century from clinical and experimental observations in humans and animals with unilateral and bilateral lesions of the peripheral labyrinth.[7, 19, 48] At that time, a controversy existed concerning whether the symptoms associated with loss of labyrinthine function were due to irritation or paralysis of the affected labyrinth. The subsequent discovery of the continuous

flow of action potentials in the unstimulated vestibular nerve led to the present concept that symptoms are usually caused by an imbalance of the normal resting-state activity—that is, by a unilateral decrease in activity.

The magnitude of symptoms and signs following labyrinthine lesions depends on (1) whether the lesion is unilateral or bilateral, (2) the rapidity with which the functional loss occurs, and (3) the extent of the lesion. In most experimental animals, simultaneous removal of both labyrinths does not produce severe abnormalities, although vestibular reflex activity is lost and ocular and postural stability is impaired. Similarly, patients who have slowly lost vestibular function bilaterally (e.g., secondary to streptomycin treatment) may not complain of any symptoms referrable to the vestibular loss. If closely questioned, however, they report visual blurring or oscillopsia with head movements and instability when walking at night (due to loss of vestibulo-ocular and vestibulospinal reflex activity).

In contrast, animals and humans develop severe symptoms and signs following unilateral labyrinthectomy. Lower mammals are initially unable to walk and develop head torsion toward the unaffected side and decreased ipsilateral muscle tone. Nystagmus is prominent, with the slow component directed toward the damaged side and the fast component toward the intact side. These signs abate with time but may persist for months after surgery.[48]

A sudden unilateral loss of labyrinthine function in humans is a dramatic event. The patient complains of severe dizziness and nausea, is pale and perspiring, and usually vomits repeatedly. He or she prefers to lie motionlessly but can walk if forced to (deviating toward the side of the lesion). Neck torsion and changes in extremity tone rarely occur. A brisk, spontaneous nystagmus interferes with vision. These symptoms and signs are temporary, and the process of compensation starts almost immediately. Within one week of the occurrence of the labyrinthine lesion, a young patient can walk without difficulty and, with fixation, can inhibit the spontaneous nystagmus. Within one month, most patients return to work with few, if any, residual symptoms. If a patient slowly loses vestibular function unilaterally over a period of months or years (e.g., with a vestibular schwannoma), symptoms and signs may be absent.

APPROACH TO EVALUATION OF VESTIBULAR FUNCTION

Tests of vestibular function, as of other sensory system functions, may be categorized as those relying on a subjective response by the patient and those relying on objective measurements of reflex activity. Although simple in concept, evaluation of the sensation of movement derived from excitation of the vestibular receptors has been a difficult task for the clinician. With rotatory stimulation, it is often impossible for the patient to differentiate sensations that are strictly vestibular from those that are tactile and proprioceptive. Because vestibular sensations are more ambiguous than those produced by, for example, auditory or visual stimuli, the patient often has difficulty in sensing when the angular motion begins and ends and what its magnitude is. Even more important, the subjec-

tive awareness of vestibular stimulation depends on one's general state of alertness and degree of cooperation. Owing to these difficulties with tests of subjective sensation, clinicians have increasingly turned their attention to objective tests to identify and quantify the components of vestibular reflex activity.

The vestibulo-ocular reflexes, in particular, have been extensively evaluated. The neurons in this reflex arc connect the labyrinthine receptor organs with the 12 extraocular muscles of the eyes; thus, it is possible, through measurement of eye movements, to correlate vestibular lesions with impairment of reflex function. Although experimental investigations of the vestibulo-ocular reflexes were initiated in the first quarter of this century, the contribution of each receptor organ and neural connection to the production of eye movements is still not completely known. The afferent signals from different vestibular receptors to each of the eye muscles overlap, and the central neural pathways lie so close to each other that it is difficult to identify the receptor or pathway responsible for the deterioration of vestibular function.

Until recently, vestibular tests were primarily system-oriented; that is, they attempted to isolate the vestibular system from other systems. This approach had its limitations because oculomotor and postural control are complex functions that require coordinated interaction of multiple sensory and motor systems. During the last decade, new methods have been developed, based mainly on computer techniques, to analyze objectively all the systems that control eye movements. A large number of observations are being made that are producing an integrated and expanding picture of vestibular pathophysiology. This technology has created renewed interest in vestibular testing because of its importance for the evaluation not only of inner ear disorders but also of various neurologic conditions.

REFERENCES

1. Bagger-Sjöbäch, D and Takumida, M: Geometrical array of the vestibular sensory hair bundle. Acta Otolaryngol 106:393, 1988.

2. Baird, IL: Some aspects of the comparative anatomy and evolution of the inner ear in submammalian vertebrates. In Riss, W (ed): Brain, Behavior and Evolution. S Karger, Basel, 1974.

3. Bard, P: Postural coordination and locomotion and their central control. In Bard, P (ed): Medical Physiology, ed 11. CV Mosby, Philadelphia, 1961.

4. Barlow, JS: Inertial navigation as a basis for animal navigation. J Theoret Biol 6:76, 1964.

5. Bauknight, RS, Strelioff, D, and Honrubia, V: Effective stimulus for the Xenopuslaevis lateral-line hair-cell system. Laryngoscope 86:1836, 1976.

6. Bracho, H and Budelli, R: The generation of resting membrane potentials in an inner ear hair cell system. J Physiol 281:445, 1978.

7. Breuer, J: Über die Funktion der Otolithen-Apparate. Pflügers Arch Ges Physiol 48:195, 1891.

8. Brown, MC: Morphology of labeled efferent fibers in the guinea pig cochlea. J Comp Neur 260:605, 1987.

9. Brownell, WE: Microscopic observation of cochlear hair cell motility. Scand Electron Microsc 3:1401, 1984.

10. Budelmann, BU: Morphological diversity of equilibrium receptor systems in aquatic invertebrates. In Atema, J, Fay, RR, Popper, AN, Tavolga, WN (eds): Sensory Biology of Aquatic Animals. Springer-Verlag, New York, 1988.

11. Budelmann, BU: Structure and function of the angular acceleration receptor systems in the statocysts of cephalopods. Symp Zool Soc London 38:309, 1977.

12. Collewijn, H: Oculomotor reactions in cuttlefish Sepia officinalis. J Exp Biol 52:369, 1970.

13. Dallos, P: Membrane potential and response changes in mammalian cochlear hair cells during intracellular recording. J Neuroscience 5:1609, 1985.

14. Davis, H: A model for transducer action in the cochlea. Cold Spring Harbor Symp Quant Biol 30:181, 1965.

15. De Vries, H: The mechanics of labyrinth otoliths. Acta Otolaryngol 38:262, 1950.

16. Dow, RS: The effects of unilateral and bilateral labyrinthectomy in monkey, baboon and chimpanzee. Am J Physiol 121:392, 1938.

17. Dukgraaf, S: Nystagmus and related phenomena in Sepia officinalis. Experientia 19:29, 1963.

18. Egmond, AAJV, Groen, JJ, and Jongkees, LBW: The mechanism of the semicircular canal. J Physiol 110:1, 1949.

19. Ewald, J: Physiolgische Untersuchungen über das Endorgan des Nervus Octavus. Berglmann, Wiesbaden, 1892.

20. Fernández, C and Goldberg, JM: Physiology of peripheral neurons innervating otolith organs of the squirrel monkey. II. Directional selectivity and force-response relations. J Neurophysiol 39:985, 1976.

21. Flock, A and Orman, S: Micromechanical properties of sensory hairs on receptor cells of the inner ear. Hearing Res 11:249, 1983.

22. Flock, A, Flock, B, and Ulfendahl, M: Mechanisms of movement in outer hair cells and a possible structural basis. Arch Otorhinolaryngol 243:83, 1986.

23. Flock, A, Jorgensen, M, and Russell, I: The physiology of individual hair cells and their synapses. In Miller, A (ed): Basic Mechanisms in Hearing. Academic Press, New York, 1973.

24. Fulton, JF, Liddell, EGT, and Rioch, D McK: The influence of unilateral destruction of the vestibular nuclei upon posture and knee jerk. Brain 53:327, 1930.

25. Galiana, HL and Outerbridge, JS: A bilateral model for central neural pathways in vestibulo-ocular reflex. J Neurophysiol 51:210, 1984.

26. Goh, Y and Alkon, DL: Sensory, interneuronal, and motor interactions within Hermissenda visual pathway. J Neurophysiol 52:156, 1984.

27. Goldberg, JM and Fernández, C: Physiology of peripheral neurons innervating semicircular canals of the squirrel monkey. I. Resting discharge and response to constant angular accelerations. J Neurophysiol 34:635, 1971.

28. Gonshor, A and Melvill Jones, G: Extreme vestibulo-ocular adaptation induced by prolonged optical reversal of vision. J Physiol (Lond) 256:381, 1976.

29. Gray, O: A brief survey of the phylogenesis of the labyrinth. J Laryngol 69:151, 1955.

30. Hoagland, H: Impulses from sensory nerves of catfish. Proc Nat Acad Sci Washington, 18:701, 1932.

31. Honrubia, V, Jenkins, HA, Baloh, RW, and Lau, CG: Evaluation of rotatory vestibular tests in peripheral labyrinthine lesions. In Honrubia, V and Brazier, MAB (eds): Nystagmus and Vertigo: Clinical Approaches to the Patient with Dizziness. UCLA Forum in Medical Sciences, No. 24, Academic Press, New York, 1982.

32. Honrubia, V, Strelioff, D, and Sitko, ST: Physiological basis of cochlear transduction and sensitivity. Ann Otol Rhinol Laryngol 85:-697, 1976.

33. Houk, JC: Control strategies in physiological systems. Faseb J 2:97, 1988.

34. Hudspeth, AJ: Extracellular current flow and the site of transduction by vertebrate hair cells. J Neurosci 2:1, 1982.

35. Hudspeth, AJ: Mechanoelectrical transduction by hair cells in the acousticolateralis sensory system. Ann Rev Neurosci 6:187, 1983.

36. Hudspeth, AJ: The cellular basis of hearing: The biophysics of hair cells. Science 230:745, 1985.

37. Kappers, CUA, Huber, GC, and Crosby, ED: The Comparative Anatomy of the Nervous System of Vertebrates, including Man. Macmillan, New York, 1936.

38. Kiang, NYS, et al: Discharge Patterns of Single Fibers in the Cat's Auditory Nerve. Res Monograph 35, MIT Press, Cambridge, 1965.

39. Krige, WGF: Functional Neuroanatomy, ed 2. Blakiston, New York, 1953.

40. Lewis, EW: Motion sensors. In Bolis, L, Keynes, RD, and Maddrell, HP (eds): Comparative Physiology of Sensory Systems, Cambridge University, Cambridge, 1984.

41. Lim, DJ: Ultra anatomy of sensory end organs in the labyrinth and their functional implications. In Shambaugh, GE and Shea, JJ (eds): Proceedings of the Shambaugh Fifth International Workshop on Middle Ear Microsurgery and Fluctuant Hearing Loss. Strode, Huntsville, 1977.

42. Loeb, J: Forced Movements, Tropisms and Animal Conduct. JB Lippincott, Philadelphia and London, 1918.

43. Lorente De Nó, R and Berens, C: Nystagmus. In Piersol, GM and Bortz, EL (eds): Cyclopedia of Medicine, Surgery and Specialties, Vol 9. FA Davis, Philadelphia, 1959.

44. Lorente De Nó, R: Anatomy of the eighth nerve. The central projection of the nerve endings of the internal ear. Laryngoscope 43:1, 1933.

45. Lorente De Nó, R: Vestibulo-ocular reflex arc. Arch Neurol Psych 30:245, 1933.

46. Lowenstein, OE: Comparative morphology and physiology. In Kornhuber, HH (ed): Handbook of Sensory Physiology, Vol VI, Part 2. Springer-Verlag, New York, 1974.

47. Lowenstein, O and Wersall, J: A functional interpretation of the electron microscopic structure of the sensory hairs in the cristae of the elasmobranch Raja clavata in terms of directinal sensitivity. Nature 184:1807, 1959.

48. Magnus, R: Körperstellung. Springer-Verlag, Berlin, 1924.

49. Magnus, R: Some results of studies in the physiology of posture. I. Lancet 2:531, 1926.

50. Magnus, R: Some results of studies in the physiology of posture. II. Lancet 2:585, 1926.

51. Mair, IWS and Fernandez, C: Pathological and functional changes following hemisection of the lateral ampullary nerve. Acta Otolaryngol 62:513, 1966.

52. Maxwell, SS: Labyrinth and Equiilbrium. JB Lippincott, Philadelphia and London, 1923.

53. Mehler, WR: Comparative anatomy of the vestibular nuclear complex in submammalian vertebrates. In Brodal, A and Pompeiano, O (eds): Basic Aspects of Central Vestibular Mechanisms. Elsevier Publishing, New York, 1972.

54. Melvill Jones, G: Adaptive modulation of VOR parameters by vision. In Berthoz, A and Melvill Jones, G (eds): Adaptive Mechanisms in Gaze Control. Elsevier, Amsterdam, 1985.

55. Money, KE, et al: Physical properties of fluids and structures of vestibular apparatus of the pigeon. Am J Physiol 220:140, 1971.

56. Mountain, DC: Electromechanical properties of hair cells. In Altschuler, RA, Hoffman, DW, and Bobbin RP (eds): Neurobiology of Hearing: The Cochlea. Raven Press, New York, 1986.

57. Nashner, LM: Strategies for organization of human posture. In Igarashi, M and Black FO (eds): Vestibular and Visual Control on Posture and Locomotor Equilibrium. Karger, Basel, 1985.

58. Orman, S and Flock, A: Active control of sensory hair mechanics implied by susceptibility to media that induce contraction in muscle. Hearing Res 11:261, 1983.

59. Precht, W: The physiology of the vestibular nuclei. In Kornhuber, HH (ed): Handbook of Sensory Physiology. The Vestibular System, Vol VI, Part 1. Springer-Verlag, New York, 1974.

60. Rasmussen, G: The olivary peduncle and other fiber projections of the superior olivary complex. J Comp Neurol 84:141, 1946.

61. Von Békésy, G: Experimental models of cochlea with and without nerve supply. In Rasmussen, GL and Windle, WF (eds): Neural Mechanisms of the Auditory and Vestibular System. Charles C Thomas, Springfield, IL, 1960.

62. Warr, WB: Olivocochlear and vestibulocochlear efferent neurons of the feline brain stem: Their location, morphology and number determined by retrograde axonal transport and acetylcholinesterase histochemistry. J Comp Neurol 161:159, 1975.

63. Wersäll, J: Electron micrographic studies of vestibular hair cell innervation. In Rasmussen, GL and Windle, WF (eds): Neural Mechanisms of the Auditory and Vestibular System. Charles C Thomas, Springfield, 1960.

64. Wolff, HG: Efferente Aktivatät in den Statonerven einiger Landpulmonaten (Gastropoda). Z Vergl Physiol 70:401, 1970.

65. Zenner, HP: Motility of outer hair cells as an active, actin-mediated process. Acta Otolaryngol (Stockh) 105:39, 1988.

Chapter 2

THE PERIPHERAL VESTIBULAR SYSTEM

THE EAR

The ear is a compound organ sensitive to sound and the forces associated with linear and angular acceleration. It is divided into three anatomic parts: the external, middle, and inner ears. Except for the auricle and soft tissue portion of the external auditory canal, the ear is enclosed within the temporal bone of the skull.

Temporal Bone

The temporal bone contributes to the base and lateral wall of the skull and forms part of the middle and posterior fossae.[4, 24] It is divided into four parts: the squamous, tympanic, petrous, and mastoid. The squamous portion forms part of the lateral bony wall of the middle cranial fossa. The tympanic portion, the smallest, forms the anterior, inferior, and part of the posterior wall of the external auditory canal. The petrous portion, or pyramid, contains the sense organs of the inner ear. The seventh and eighth cranial nerves enter the petrous portion through the internal auditory canal; the facial nerve exits via the stylomastoid foramen of the mastoid portion (Fig. 2–1). The internal carotid artery and

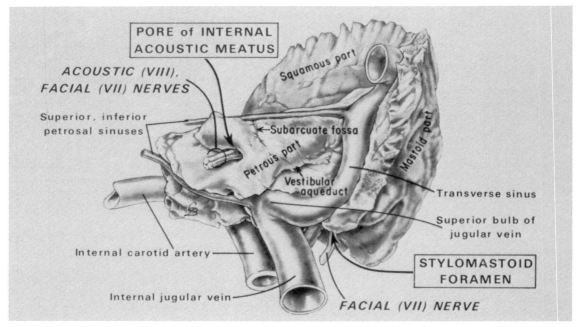

Figure 2–1. Medial view of temporal bone. (From Anson, BJ and Donaldson, JA: Surgical Anatomy of the Temporal Bone and Ear. WB Saunders, Philadelphia, 1973, with permission.)

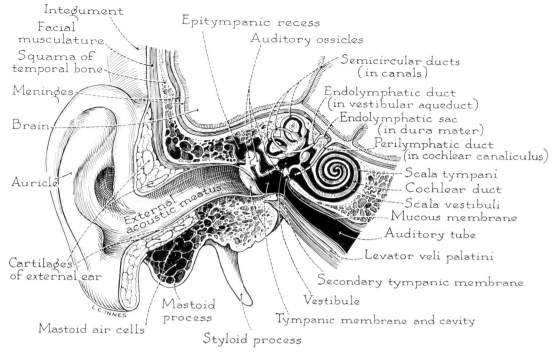

Figure 2–2. Cross section of the ear. (From Anson, BJ, and Donaldson, JA: Surgical Anatomy of the Temporal Bone and Ear. WB Saunders, Philadelphia, 1973, with permission.)

internal jugular vein enter the skull through the temporal bone, their bony canals forming part of the anteroinferior wall of the middle ear.

The cross section of the temporal bone in Figure 2–2 illustrates the relationship between the three functional parts of the ear. Although the external and middle ears are auditory organs with no direct bearing on vestibular function, a knowledge of their structure and development—particularly those of the middle ear—is important for understanding diseases involving the inner ear.[15, 56] For example, infection arising in the middle ear can spread directly through its medial wall (oval and round windows) into the inner ear, or it can enter the intracranial cavity by breaking through the roof of the epitympanic recess. The aditus ad antrum interconnects the epitympanic recess with the middle ear by means of air cells throughout the mastoid portion of the temporal bone so that infection beginning in the middle ear can spread to the vessels and nerves passing through the temporal bone.

Tympanic Membrane

The ear drum, or tympanic membrane, forms a partition between the external and middle ears. The tympanic membrane has a thickness of 0.1 mm and a diameter of 8.5 to 10 mm. It consists of three layers: an inner mucosal layer, a middle fibrous layer, and an external epidermal layer. It is attached to the tympanic ring in the external canal at a distance of 2 to 5 mm from the opposite (medial) wall of the middle ear. From the external canal, the tympanic membrane appears as a thin, semitransparent disk which normally has a glistening, pearly-gray color (see Fig. 5–1). It is concave on its external surface as if under traction from the manubrium—the long process (5.8 mm) of the malleus. The mallear stria (the manubrium shining through the tympanic membrane) passes from slightly inferior and posterior of the center (umbo) toward the superior margin of the tympanic membrane. Near the superior margin, the mallear prominence is formed by the lateral process of the malleus. From the mallear prominence, two folds stretch to the tympanic sulcus of the temporal bone, enclosing the triangular area of the pars flaccida, or Shrapnell's membrane.

Middle Ear

FUNCTIONAL ANATOMY

The middle ear, or tympanic cavity, is a flat cleft with a volume of approximately 2.0 ml, containing three tiny bones the main role of which is to provide an interface for transmitting to the inner ear the changes in atmospheric pressure produced by sound waves (Fig. 2–3).[96, 98] The manubrium is attached, like the radius of a circle, to the inner side of the tympanic membrane in a superoanterior direction.

Superiorly, the head of the malleus is bound to the incus, forming the incudomalleal articulation—a type of diarthric joint. The so-called long process of the incus (7 mm), directed down and anteriorly, is connected to the stapes—the smallest of the three middle ear ossicles. The footplate of the stapes articulates with the walls of the vestibule at the oval window to which it is attached by a ring of ligaments. The dimensions of the window are 1.2 by 3 mm, with a total area that is 1/17 that of the tympanic membrane. Sound-induced displacements of the tympanic membrane and its attached manubrium are transmitted through the medial arm of the assembly of middle ear bones, acting as a lever to the inner ear; in this fashion the middle ear functions as a mechanical transformer. Additional amplification is produced

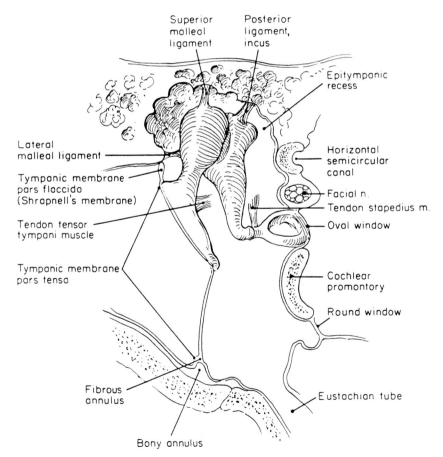

Figure 2–3. Cross section of the middle ear.

as the force applied over the surface of the tympanic membrane is funneled into the smaller area of the oval window. The middle ear compensates for the loss of energy—approximately a 99.9 percent loss—that would occur if sound were transmitted directly from air to the fluids of the inner ear.[98]

The ossicles are suspended by several ligaments and are dynamically controlled by the action of two muscles. The tensor tympani, innervated by a branch of the trigeminal nerve, is connected by a tendon to the upper part of the manubrium. Coursing in a lateral direction from the anterior part of the medial wall of the tympanic cavity, this muscle draws the manubrium medially, tensing the tympanic membrane. The stapedius muscle, innervated by the facial nerve, is attached to the posterior wall of the tympanic cavity and is directed anteriorly to anchor in the upper part of the stapes. Its contraction hinders the transmission of sound to the inner ear (see Fig. 2–3).

BOUNDARIES

For descriptive purposes, the tympanic cavity can be thought of as being bounded by six walls facing one another in pairs. The *lateral* wall, in large part, is made up of the cone-shaped tympanic membrane. The *medial,* or labyrinthine, wall is an irregular surface because of structures bulging from the inner ear: the promontory of the basal turn of the cochlea and the prominences of the facial canal and horizontal semicircular canal (see Fig. 2–3). Beneath the cochlear prominence is the membrane of the cochlea or round window, which seals the scala tympani of the cochlea and its fluid from the middle ear. It provides an outlet for equilibrium of pressure in the inner ear whenever sound displaces the stapes. Without this compliance, sound energy could not displace the basilar membrane of the cochlea because the endolymph fluid is incompressible. The vestibular, or oval, window is located just above the cochlear prominence where it is closed by the base of the stapes and the annular ligament.

The *anterior* wall of the tympanic cavity

is marked by three important structures: the eustachian tube orifice, the wall of the carotid canal, and the opening of the channel for insertion of the tensor tympani muscle. The eustachian tube connects the middle ear cavity with the nasopharynx, providing ventilation of the tympanic cavity spaces. The tubal orifice at the nasopharynx is normally closed, but during deglutition it opens owing to the contraction of palate muscles which attach to the cartilage and elastic ligaments in the opening. The most important of the muscles, the tensor veli palatini, is innervated by the trigeminal nerve. In the upper part of the *posterior* wall of the tympanic cavity is a large opening contiguous with the epitympanic recess, the aditus ad antrum. Through this opening there is communication with the mastoid antrum. The antrum is lined with mucous membrane continuous with that of both tympanic and epitympanic cavities. The antrum is a relatively large, irregular, bean-shaped cavity about 1 cm long. Many mastoid air cells open into this cavity, which is located behind and below the antrum within the mastoid process of the temporal bone. In addition to the antrum, the *posterior* wall of the tympanic cavity contains an aperture through which the tendon of the stapedius muscle passes, another through which the chorda tympani nerve enters the tympanic cavity, and a fossa where the posterior ligament of the incus is attached.

The *roof* of the tympanic cavity is formed by the tegmen tympani, a thin plate of bone separating the epitympanic recess of the tympanic cavity from the middle cranial fossa. The *floor* is composed of the jugular bulb upon which are located irregular pneumatized cells.

FACIAL NERVE

The facial nerve arises at the inferior border of the pons and proceeds to the internal auditory canal on the superior surface of the cochlear nerve. Within the temporal bone, four portions of the facial nerve can be classified: (1) the canal (meatal) segment (7 to 8 mm), (2) the labyrinthine segment (3 to 4 mm), (3) the tympanic (horizontal) segment (12 to 13 mm), and (4) the mastoid (vertical) segment (15 to 20 mm) (Fig. 2–4). The canal segment runs in close company in an anterosuperior position with the vestibular and cochlear divisions of the eighth nerve, but in its remaining segments the facial nerve lies separately within a bony canal—the facial or fallopian canal. The labyrinthine segment runs at nearly a right angle to the petrous pyramid superior to the cochlea and vestibule to reach the geniculate ganglion. At the geniculate ganglion, the nerve takes a sharp turn posteriorly, marking the beginning of the tympanic segment. The horizontal tympanic segment courses in a posterior direction along the medial wall of the tympanic cavity superior to the oval window and inferior to the horizontal semicircular canal. At the sinus tympani, the nerve bends inferiorly, marking the beginning of the vertical or mastoid segment that continues toward the stylomastoid foramen.

Three major branches of the facial nerve

lie within the temporal bone: (1) the greater superficial petrosal nerve, arising from the geniculate ganglion; (2) the nerve to the stapedius muscle, arising from the initial part of the mastoid segment; and (3) the chorda tympani, leaving the facial nerve approximately 5 mm above the stylomastoid foramen. The greater superficial petrosal nerve is composed of (1) parasympathetic efferent fibers originating in the superior salivatory nucleus for innervation of the lacrimal glands and seromucinous glands of the nasal cavity; and (2) afferent cutaneous sensory fibers from parts of the external canal, tympanic membrane, and middle ear, destined for the nucleus of the solitary tract. The nerve to the stapedius muscle and the main facial nerve trunk are motor nerves originating from the facial nucleus in the caudal pons. The chorda tympani, like the greater superficial petrosal, is a mixed nerve containing (1) parasympathetic efferent fibers from the supe-

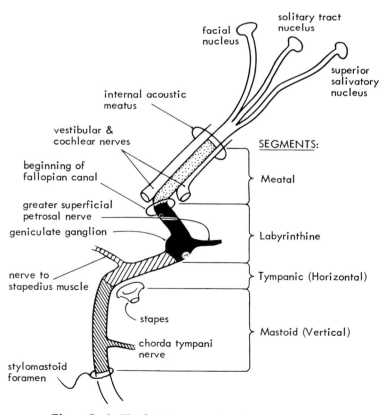

Figure 2–4. The facial nerve within the temporal bone.

rior salivatory nucleus, destined for the sublingual glands; and (2) afferent taste fibers from the anterior two thirds of the tongue, ending in the nucleus of the solitary tract.

Knowledge of the structure and function of each division of the facial nerve allows the clinician to localize disease affecting the nerve within the temporal bone. Lesions in the internal auditory canal commonly involve both the seventh and eighth cranial nerves. Lesions of the labyrinthine segment of the facial nerve above the geniculate ganglion impair ipsilateral (1) lacrimation, (2) stapedius reflex activity, (3) taste on the anterior two thirds of the tongue, and (4) facial muscular strength. A lesion of the tympanic segment central to the nerve of the stapedius muscle affects only (2), (3), and (4) above, and a lesion of the mastoid segment before the origin of the chorda tympani affects only (3) and (4). Finally, a lesion at the stylomastoid fora-

men causes only ipsilateral facial muscle weakness or paralysis.

Inner Ear

BONY LABYRINTH

Within the petrous portion of the temporal bone, a series of hollow channels—the bony labyrinth—contain the auditory and vestibular sensory organs (see Fig. 2–2). The bony labyrinth consists of an anterior cochlear part and a posterior vestibular part.[4] The vestibule is a central chamber (about 4 mm in diameter) marked by the recesses of the utriculus and sacculus. The superior and posterolateral walls contain openings for the three semicircular canals, and anteriorly the vestibule is continuous with the scala vestibuli of the snail-shaped cochlea.

Medial to the bony labyrinth is the inter-

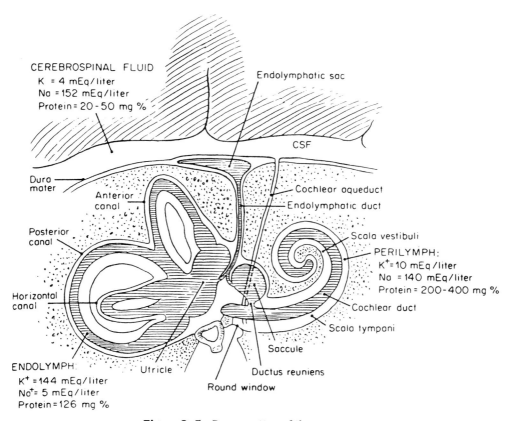

Figure 2–5. Cross section of the inner ear.

nal auditory canal, a cul-de-sac housing the seventh and eighth cranial nerves and the internal auditory artery. The aperture on the cranial side is located at approximately the center of the posterior face of the pyramid of the temporal bone (see Fig. 2–1). Two other important orifices are in this vicinity. Halfway between the canal and the sigmoid sinus, the slitlike aperture of the vestibular aqueduct contains the endolymphatic sac—a structure important in the exchange of endolymph. The second opening is that of the cochlear aqueduct, at the same level as the auditory canal but on the inferior side of the pyramid. The labyrinthine opening of this channel is located in the scala tympani, providing a connection between the subarachnoid and the perilymphatic spaces.

MEMBRANOUS LABYRINTH

The membranous labyrinth is enclosed within the channels of the bony labyrinth (Fig. 2–5). A space containing perilymphatic fluid, a supportive network of connective tissue, and blood vessels lies between the periosteum of the bony labyrinth and the membranous labyrinth; the spaces within the membranous labyrinth contain endolymphatic fluid. The endolymphatic system develops in the embryo as an invagination of the germinal ectodermal layer.[5] Starting as a simple fold, it soon becomes a closed cavity—the otocyst—isolated from the original ectoderm. By the end of the seventh week, the endolymphatic duct system is lodged in mesenchymal tissue, and by the fourteenth week, it attains the size that it will have in the adult ear. By successive infolding of the wall of the otocyst, three main areas are formed: the endolymphatic duct and sac, the utriculus and semicircular canals, and the sacculus and cochlear duct. The membranous cochlea holds the organ of Corti for the transduction of sound energy; and the utriculus, sacculus, and semicircular canals contain the receptors for sensing linear and angular motion. Together they constitute the membranous labyrinth proper. Finally, the endolymphatic duct provides a channel for the exchange of chemicals and to balance the pressure between the endolymphatic and subarachnoid spaces.

THE VESTIBULAR LABYRINTH

Structure of the Vestibular End-organs

SEMICIRCULAR CANALS

The semicircular canals are three membranous tubes with a cross-sectional diameter of 0.4 mm, each forming about two thirds of a circle with a diameter of about 6.5 mm.[76] They are aligned to form a coordinate system (Fig. 2–6).[10, 11] The plane of the horizontal semicircular canal with two openings on the lateral wall of the utriculus makes a 30-degree angle with the horizontal plane. The other two canals are in vertical positions almost orthogonal to each other. The anterior canal is directed medially and laterally over the roof of the utriculus; and the posterior, behind the utriculus, is directed downward and laterally. The two vertical canals share a common opening on the posterior side of the utriculus. Precise measurement of the planes of the canals, however, indicates that they are not aligned perfectly orthogonal. All angular movements stimulate at least two canals and often all three.

At the anterior opening of the horizontal and anterior canals and the inferior opening of the posterior canal, each tube enlarges to form the ampulla. A crestlike septum—the crista—crosses each ampulla in a perpendicular direction to the longitudinal axis of the canal (see Fig. 1–2). It rests on the bone of the canal and consists of sensory epithelium lying on a mound of connective tissue, where blood vessels and nerve fibers reach the sensory receptor area. Hair cells are located on the surface of the crista with their cilia protruding into the cupula, a gelatinous mass of the same composition as that of the otolithic membrane. The cupula extends from the surface of the crista to the ceiling of the ampulla, forming what appears to be a watertight seal.[70, 76] A higher proportion of type I hair cells are located in the ridge at the center of the crista, whereas type II hair cells predominate in the periphery.[16, 32] In the three human cristae there are about 23,000 hair cells,[78] and in the two macules, 4,000 hair cells[79]—representing a ratio of about 1.4 hair cells to af-

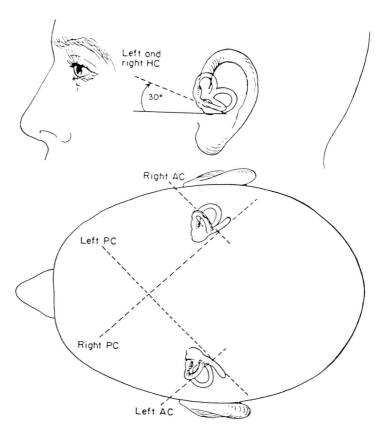

Figure 2–6. Orientation of the semi-circular canals within the head. *HC*, horizontal canal; *PC*, posterior canal; *AC*, anterior canal.

ferent fibers (see Chapter 1 for definition of hair cell types). The margins of the crista contain zones of transitional epithelium, consisting of cells rich with infoldings believed to have secretory function (the so-called dark cells).[49] Mammalian hair cells probably cannot regenerate after birth because function is permanently lost when they are damaged.[25] In quail and chickens, however, it has recently been shown that supporting cells differentiate into sensory cells following destruction of hair cells after acoustic trauma.[17, 80]

The hair cells within each crista are oriented so that all their kinocilia point in the same direction. In the vertical canals the kinocilia are directed toward the canal side of the ampulla, whereas in the horizontal canal they are directed toward the utricular side.[18] The opposing morphologic polarization is the reason for the difference in directional sensitivity between the horizontal and vertical canals.[65] The afferent nerve fibers of the horizontal canals are stimulated by endolymph movement in the utricular or ampullopetal direction, and those of the vertical canals are stimulated by ampullofugal endolymph flow.

OTOLITHS

The membranous labyrinth forms two globular cavities within the vestibule: the utriculus and the sacculus. The sacculus lies on the medial wall of the vestibule in a spherical recess inferior to the utriculus with which it is in contact but without direct connection. It communicates with the endolymphatic duct (and thus the utricular duct) by the saccular duct and with the cochlea by the ductus reuniens (see Fig. 2–5). The sensory area of the sacculus—the macula—is a differentiated patch of membrane in the medial wall, hood-shaped and predominantly in a vertical position (Fig. 2–7). The utricular cavity is oval in shape, connecting to the membranous semicircular canals via five openings. The macula of

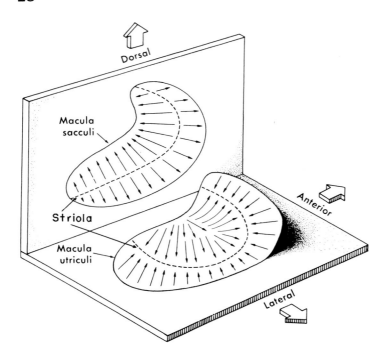

Figure 2–7. Position of the saccular and utricular maculae. *Arrows* indicate the direction of hair cell polarization on each side of the striola. (From Barber, HO and Stockwell, CW: Manual of Electronystagmography. CV Mosby, St. Louis, 1976, with permission.)

the utriculus is located next to the anterior opening of the horizontal semicircular canal and lies mostly in a horizontal position in a recess on the anterior part of the utriculus. It communicates by the utricular duct with the endolymphatic duct at the same level as but by different openings from those of the saccular duct. Thus, the endolymph in the superior or utricular part of the labyrinth is separated from that of the sacculus and cochlea by these tiny ducts. This separation may be relevant to the pathophysiology of Meniere's syndrome (see Chapter 11).

The surfaces of the utricular and saccular maculae are covered by the otolithic membrane—a structure consisting of a mesh of fibers embedded in a gel composed of acid mucopolysaccharides.[48, 54] This membrane contains a superficial calcareous deposit, the otoconia. The otoconia consist of small calcium carbonate crystals, ranging from 0.5 to 30 microns in diameter and having a density more than twice that of water.[20] As discussed in Chapter 1, the stereocilia of the macular hair cells protrude into the otolithic membrane. The striola is a distinctive curved zone running through the center of each

macula (see Fig. 2–7). A higher proportion of type I hair cells are located near the striola than in the rest of the macula.[55] The hair cells on each side of the striola are oriented so that their kinocilia point in opposite directions. In the utriculus the kinocilia face the striola, and in the sacculus they face away from it. As a consequence, displacement of the macula's otolithic membrane in one direction (as illustrated in Fig. 1–1) has an opposite physiologic influence on the set of hair cells on each side of the striola. Furthermore, because of the curvature of the striola, hair cells are oriented at different angles, making the macula multidirectionally sensitive. Because the maculae are located off center from the major axis of the head, they are subjected to tangential and centripetal forces during angular head movements.

Labyrinthine Fluids

Two separate fluid compartments exist within the inner ear: the perilymph and the endolymph. The compartments do not communicate, and each has a different chemical composition.

DYNAMICS OF FLUID FORMATION

The mechanism of formation of the inner ear fluids is still not well understood. The perilymph is, in part, a filtration of cerebrospinal fluid (CSF) and, in part, a filtration from blood vessels in the ear.[23, 81] The CSF communicates directly with the perilymphatic space through the cochlear aqueduct—a narrow channel 3 to 4 mm long with its inner-ear opening at the base of the scala tympani (see Fig. 2–5). In most instances, this channel is filled by a loose net of fibrous tissue continuous with the arachnoid. The size of the bony canal varies from individual to individual. Necropsy studies in some patients who died of subarachnoid hemorrhage or meningitis have revealed free passage of leukocytes and red blood cells into the inner ear, whereas in others the cells were blocked from passing through the aqueduct.[44, 74] Blood cells have also been found passing into the internal auditory canal and through the porous canaliculi that contain the vestibular and cochlear nerves, suggesting another route for CSF-perilymph communication.[44] Probably the most important source of perilymph, however, is filtration from blood vessels within the perilymph space, inasmuch as blocking the cochlear aqueduct does not appear to affect inner ear morphology or function.[51, 91]

The most likely site for production of endolymph is the secretory cells in the stria vascularis of the cochlea and the dark cells of the vestibular labyrinth.[49, 81] Resorption of endolymph is generally agreed to take place in the endolymphatic sac. Dye and pigment experimentally injected into the cochlea of animals accumulate in the endolymphatic sac; electron microscopic studies of the membrane that lines the sac reveal active pinocytotic activity.[1, 66]

Destruction of the epithelium lining the sac or occlusion of the duct results in an increase of endolymphatic volume in experimental animals.[50, 91] The first change is an expansion of cochlear and saccular membranes, which may completely fill the perilymphatic space. The anatomic changes resulting from this experiment are comparable to those found in the temporal bones of patients with Meniere's syndrome (either idiopathic or secondary to known inflammatory disease) (see Fig. 11–1).

FLUID CHEMISTRY

The chemical compositions of the fluids filling the inner ear are similar to those of the extracellular and intracellular fluids throughout the body. The endolymphatic system contains intracellularlike fluids with high potassium and low sodium concentrations, whereas the perilymphatic fluid resembles the extracellular fluid with low potassium and high sodium concentrations.[81, 88] Figure 2–5 shows the relationship between electrolytes and protein concentration of the different fluid compartments.[81, 86] The high protein content in the endolymphatic sac, compared with that in the rest of the endolymphatic space, is consistent with the sac's role in the resorption of endolymph. The difference in protein concentration between perilymph and CSF argues against a free communication between the compartments of these two fluids and in favor of an active process of perilymph production. The electrolyte composition of the endolymph is critical for normal functioning of the sensory organs bathed in fluid. Rupture of the membranous labyrinth in experimental animals causes destruction of the sensory and neural structures at the site of the endolymph-perilymph fistula.[84]

It is possible to sample the fluid in the vestibule by introducing a micropipette through a tiny fistula in the footplate of the stapes.[85, 87] The fluid obtained normally has the chemical composition of perilymph, given in Figure 2–5. In 29 patients with vestibular schwannomas, the protein content of the perilymph was consistently elevated, with an average value of 1800 mg percent.[87] Elevation of perilymph protein can occur when the protein content of CSF is normal or only slightly elevated. The electrolyte composition of perilymph remains normal in such patients. In patients with Meniere's syndrome, the markedly dilated sacculus or herniated cochlear duct are usually in contact with the footplate, so that endolymph rather than perilymph is obtained from tapping the vestibule. The chemical composition of perilymph obtained from other regions of the labyrinth

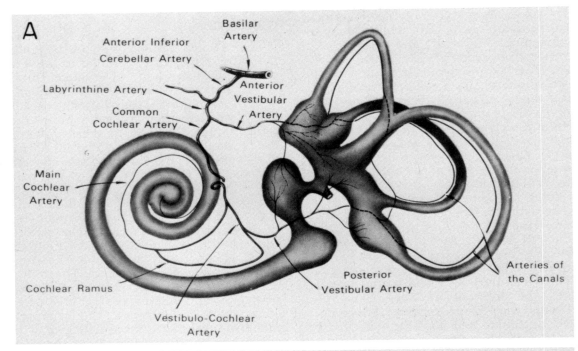

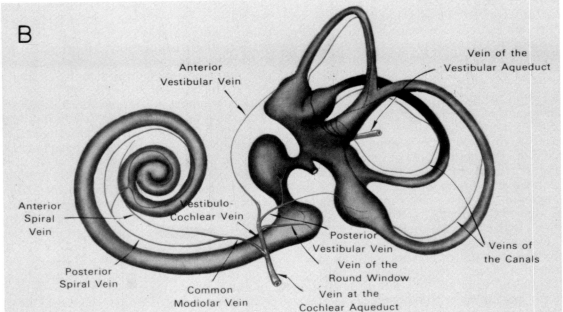

Figure 2–8. Arterial (*A*) and venous (*B*) labyrinthine circulation. (From Schuknecht, HF: Pathology of the Ear. Harvard University Press, Cambridge, 1974, with permission.)

at the time of surgery is normal in patients with Meniere's syndrome.[87]

Blood Supply

The artery that irrigates the membranous labyrinth and its neural structures is a branch of an intracranial vessel and does not communicate with arteries in the otic capsule and the tympanic cavity.[42, 69] This vessel usually originates from the anteroinferior cerebellar artery, but exceptionally it arises directly from the basilar artery or some of its branches. As it enters the temporal bone, it forms branches that irrigate the ganglion cells, nerves, dura, and arachnoidal membranes in the internal auditory canal.[6, 68] Shortly after entering the inner ear, the labyrinthine artery divides into two main branches: the common cochlear artery and the anterior vestibular artery (Fig. 2–8A). Because the arteries course independently within the canal, it is possible that alterations in one branch result in changes only in the part of the inner ear to which it provides the blood supply. The common cochlear artery forms two branches: the posterior vestibular artery and the main cochlear artery. The latter enters the central canal of the modiolus where it generates the radiating arterioles, forming a plexus within the cochlea irrigating the spiral ganglion, the structures in the basilar membrane, and the stria vascularis. The posterior vestibular artery— a branch from the common cochlear artery—is the source of blood supply to the inferior part of the sacculus and the ampulla of the posterior semicircular canal. The other primary branch of the labyrinthine artery—the anterior vestibular branch—provides irrigation to the utriculus and ampulla of the anterior and horizontal semicircular canals as well as some blood to a small portion of the sacculus. The different sources of blood supply lead to independent pathologic changes in cases of vascular abnormalities.

The anterior vestibular vein drains the utriculus and the ampullae of the anterior and horizontal canals; the posterior vestibular vein drains the sacculus, ampulla of the posterior canal, and the basal end of the cochlea (Fig. 2–8B).[6, 89] The confluence of these veins and the vein of the round window become the vestibulocochlear vein. Blood from the cochlea is carried primarily by the common modiolar vein and, when joined by the vestibulocochlear vein, becomes the vein at the cochlear aqueduct. This large venous channel enters a bony canal near the cochlear aqueduct to empty into the inferior petrosal sinus. The semicircular canals are drained by veins that pass toward the utriculus and form the vein of the vestibular aqueduct, which accompanies the endolymphatic duct and drains into the lateral venous sinus.

Interruption of the blood supply in the internal auditory artery or any of its branches seriously impairs the function of the inner ear because the labyrinthine arteries do not anastomose with any other major arterial branch.[52, 73] Within 15 seconds of blood flow interruption, the auditory nerve fibers become unexcitable, and the receptor and resting potentials in the ear abruptly diminish.[52] If the interruption lasts for a prolonged period of time, the changes are irreversible: Loss of function is followed by degenerative changes wherein ganglion cells and sensory cells undergo autolysis and new bone growth fills the ear cavity.[73]

Innervation

The internal auditory canal is a tubular excavation in the petrous portion of the temporal bone, about 15 mm in length and 6 mm in width.[2] The medial end of the tube opens into the cerebellopontine angle cistern; the lateral end is closed by a thin bony plate, the lamina cribrosa. Through tiny perforations in the lamina cribrosa, the afferent and efferent vestibular and cochlear nerve fiber endings pass into the labyrinthine cavity to contact the sensory organs. The lamina cribrosa is divided into an upper and a lower section by the crista falciformis; each of these halves is in turn divided by vertical bony cristae into an anterior and a posterior section. The auditory nerve, consisting of approximately 30,000 fibers, occupies the anteroinferior part of the internal auditory canal, and the vestibular nerve, containing approximately 20,000 fibers, occupies the posterior half (see Fig. 1–5).[77] The facial nerve is located in the remaining anterosuperior quadrant.

The afferent bipolar ganglion cells of the vestibular nerve (Scarpa's ganglion) are arranged in two cell masses in a vertical column within the internal auditory canal, the superior group forming the superior division of the vestibular nerve and the inferior forming the inferior division.[61, 82] The superior division innervates the cristae of the anterior and horizontal canals, the macula of the utriculus, and the anterosuperior part of the saccular macula. It leaves the internal auditory canal through the posterosuperior fossa of the lamina cribrosa. The inferior division innervates the crista of the posterior canal and the main portion of the macula of the sacculus and leaves the internal auditory canal through the posteroinferior area of the lamina.

Detailed study of the vestibular nerve in animals reveals a highly organized arrangement of the nerve fibers originating from the different inner ear receptors and from the two types of hair cells within each receptor.[32, 36, 45, 46, 71] Large nerve fibers arise primarily from ganglion cells in the

anterior distal part of the ganglion, and small nerve fibers arise from the posterior portion. There is a continuous unimodal distribution of primary afferent neurons with regard to axon and cell body diameter (Fig. 2–9). Classical morphologists identified three types of nerve endings in the receptors: large-diameter fibers had caliceal endings, small-diameter fibers bouton endings, and intermediate-size fibers both types of endings.[61] With recently developed techniques for labeling individual neurons and fibers by intracellular injection of horseradish peroxidase, information has been obtained in the chinchilla regarding the fiber diameters associated with different nerve endings in different parts of the crista (Fig. 2–10).[7, 32] Neurons with large axon diameters (2.81±0.58 mm) innervate one or a few hair cells with caliceal endings (type I) in the center of the crista. Neurons with intermediate axon diameters (2.26±0.57 mm) have both bouton and caliceal endings and are more or less evenly distributed throughout the crista. Neurons with small axon diameters (1.40±0.37 mm) have only bouton endings and innervate multiple type II hair

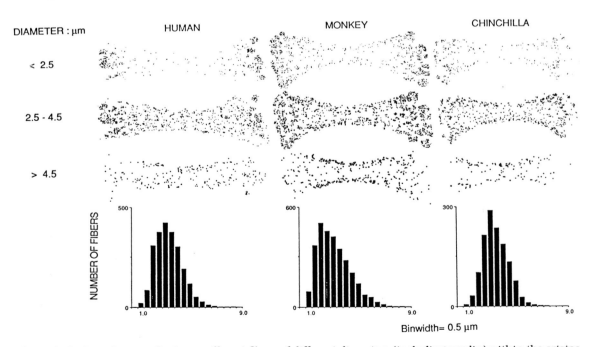

Figure 2–9. Distribution of primary afferent fibers of different diameters (including myelin) within the cristae of humans, monkeys, and chinchillas. The smallest fibers (<2.5 μm) are more numerous at the periphery while the largest fibers (>4.5μm) are concentrated at the center of the cristae. Intermediate size fibers tend to be equally distributed throughout the cristae.

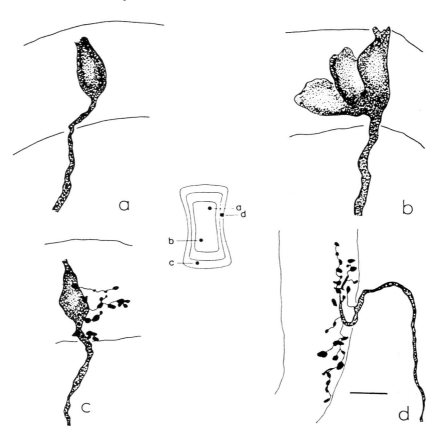

Figure 2–10. Different types of primary afferent nerve endings labeled by intracellular injection of horseradish peroxidase. Reconstructions of 2 calyx units with simple (*a*) and complex (*b*) endings, a dimorphic unit (*c*), and a bouton unit (*d*), all taken from a single horizontal canal crista. The points at which the parent axons of labeled afferents enter the sensory epithelium are indicated on a standard surface reconstruction at the center. *Bar,* 10 μm. (From Fernández, C, et al: The vestibular nerve of the chinchilla. I. Peripheral innervation patterns in the horizontal and superior semicircular canals. J Neurophysiol 1988, 60:167, with permission.)

cells predominantly in the periphery. Of a sample of 368 fibers, 40 (11.1%) were calyx units, 79 (21.5%) were bouton units and 248 (67.4%) were dimorphic units. Approximately the same distribution of fibers according to diameter is seen in the crista of the squirrel monkey and human (see Fig. 2–9). Although no comparable quantitative data exist regarding the innervation of the otolith organs, the band of type I hair cells near the striola are innervated by the largest fibers in the vestibular nerve.[61]

Peripheral vestibular efferent fibers originate from approximately 300 neurons located bilaterally ventromedial to the ventral portion of the lateral vestibular nucleus.[37] These fibers accompany the cochlear efferent fibers (the so-called olivocochlear bundle) in the vestibular nerve

trunk as far as the saccular ganglion, at which point the two efferent systems diverge almost at right angles to each other. Vestibular efferent fibers join each division of the vestibular nerve and run to each macula and crista. Here they end as vesiculated boutons containing many small homogeneous vesicles (see Fig. 1–6). One efferent fiber gives off numerous boutons that will synapse either directly on hair cells or onto their afferent nerve endings.

It is generally accepted that neurotransmission within the vestibular sensory organs (both afferent and efferent) is chemical in nature. Several chemicals have been implicated in the neurotransmission at the hair cell–afferent nerve junction. Application of monoamine-depleting drugs affects the presynaptic bar structure of the hair cell in the frog vestibule.[72] Glutamate or a glutamatelike substance increases the spontaneous and stimulus-evoked activity of vestibular neurons in the frog[3, 94] and the cat.[21] Picrotoxin, a known γ-aminobutyric acid (GABA) receptor blocker, inhibits spontaneous and evoked activity in the afferent nerve from the skate semicircular canal ampulla,[33] and iontophoretic application of GABA increases the spontaneous activity of single units in the saccular macula of the cat.[27] Acetylcholine (ACh) is the likely efferent neurotransmitter within the vertebrate vestibule.[9] Histochemical staining techniques have identified the presence of acetylcholinesterase at the vestibular receptor neural junction in the cat, and this staining is lost after vestibular nerve section.[35] Choline acetyltransferase activity in homogenates of the frog labyrinth markedly decreases after vestibular nerve transection.[60] This ACh-mediated efferent system is thought to provide a tonic inhibitory influence upon the afferent activity arising from the vestibular receptor.[14, 93]

Physiology of the Vestibular End-organs

SEMICIRCULAR CANALS

Background. The functional role of the semicircular canals was first linked to their gross anatomic features by Flourens[34] in 1842. While studying the auditory labyrinth in pigeons, he noted that opening a semicircular canal resulted in characteristic head movements in the plane of that canal. Several subsequent investigators proposed that movement of endolymphatic fluid within the canal was responsible for excitation of the cristae.[13, 18, 67] It was not until the studies of Ewald[26] in 1892, however, that a clear relationship was established between the planes of the semicircular canals, the direction of endolymph flow, and the direction of induced eye and head movements. Exposing the membranous labyrinth of the semicircular canals of pigeons, Ewald applied positive and negative pressures to each canal membrane to cause ampullopetal and ampullofugal endolymph flow. Three important observations that became known as Ewald's laws were (1) the eye and head movements always occurred in the

plane of the canal being stimulated and in the direction of endolymph flow, (2) ampullopetal endolymph flow in the horizontal canal caused a greater response (i.e., induced movements) than did ampullofugal endolymph flow, and (3) ampullofugal endolymph flow in the vertical canals caused a greater response than did ampullopetal endolymph flow.

Steinhausen[90] and later Dohlman[22] visualized the movement of the cupula during endolymph flow. By injecting India ink into the semicircular canals of fish, these investigators demonstrated that the cupula formed a seal with the ampullary wall and moved with the endolymph. Noticing the similarity between the cupular movement and that of a pendulum in a viscous medium, Steinhausen proposed a model for the description of cupular kinematics, which became known as the pendulum model. Although the large movements observed by Steinhausen were later realized to be artifactual, the basic principle has been upheld by most recent experimental[70] and theoretic studies.[99]

Physiologic verification of the model has been made by detailed study of the relationship between angular head acceleration and the flow of action potentials in isolated ampullary nerve fibers. These studies were first conducted in elasmobranches by Lowenstein and Sand,[64] later in frogs,[45, 53, 75] pigeons,[57] and mammals,[12, 19, 83, 92] and first in primates by Fernández and Goldberg.[28, 40, 41]

Mechanism of Stimulation. The pendulum model is the most useful didactic model for describing the physiologic properties of the semicircular canals and, as will be shown later, for describing the semicircular canal-induced reflexes, especially the vestibulo-oculomotor reflexes.[95, 99]

The cupula acts as the coupler between the force due to angular acceleration of the head and the hair cells (the transducer of mechanical to biological energy), leading to the production of action potentials in the vestibular afferent fibers. Because of the configuration and dimensions of the canals, the endolymph can move in only one direction along the cylindrical canalicular cavity. According to Newton's third principle, when an angular acceleration [and hence a force $M\ddot{\Theta}_h(t)$] is applied to the head, displacement of the cupula-endo-lymph system acting as a solid mass is opposed by three restraining forces: (1) an elastic force $[K\Theta_c(t)]$ due to the cupula's springlike properties (which is proportional to the magnitude of its displacement), (2) the force due to the cupula-endolymph viscosity $[C\dot{\Theta}_c(t)]$ (whose magnitude is proportional to the velocity of its displacement), and (3) an inertial force $[M\ddot{\Theta}_c(t)]$ due to the fluid's mass (proportional to the acceleration of the fluid-cupula complex). Cupular displacement can be described by the following equation, which is referred to as the equation of the pendulum model of semicircular canal function:

$$M\ddot{\Theta}_c(t) + C\dot{\Theta}_c(t) + K\Theta_c(t) = M\ddot{\Theta}_h(t) \qquad \textbf{1}$$

where Θ_c is the angular displacement of the cupula-endolymph system with respect to the wall of the canals, $\dot{\Theta}_c$ and $\ddot{\Theta}_c$ are the first (velocity) and second (acceleration) time derivatives of the cupular displacement, and $\ddot{\Theta}_h$ is the angular acceleration of the head. M is the moment of inertia; C, the moment of viscous friction; and K, the moment of elasticity. A complete description of the kinematics of the cupulo-endo-lymph system can be obtained if the values of these coefficients are known (see Appendix).

For natural to-and-fro head movements the magnitude of the elastic and inertial forces is negligible, and the following simplified equation describes the kinematics of the cupula-endolymph system.

$$C\dot{\Theta}_c(t) \approx M\ddot{\Theta}_h(t) \qquad \textbf{2}$$

The force applied to the system during angular head acceleration is opposed mostly by the viscous drag of the cupula. Integrating Equation 2 we have

$$\Theta_c(t) \approx \frac{M}{C}\dot{\Theta}_h(t) \qquad \textbf{3}$$

Thus the displacement of the cupula system during natural head movements is proportional to the velocity of head motion rather than head acceleration. The magnitude of the proportionality constant (M/C) relating angular deviation of the cupula in degrees to the velocity of the head in degrees per second has been estimated to be approximately 0.003 seconds based on the physical characteristics of the canals and endolymph.[99] Most likely, during fast head movements with velocities as great as 800 deg/sec, the deviation of the cupula does not exceed one degree of deflection.[90]

Figure 2–11 illustrates the relationship between the time course of head acceleration, head velocity, and cupular displacement as predicted by the pendulum model for three different types of angular rotation commonly used in clinical testing. The description of cupular displacement during constant angular acceleration (see Fig. 2–11a) can easily be derived from Equation 1. At the beginning of head acceleration, endolymph movement lags behind the displacement of the head and thereby that of the walls of the semicircular canals. After a few seconds, however, a balance is established between the applied and restraining forces, and the endolymph moves simultaneously with the walls of the labyrinth. At this time the position of the ring of fluid within the canal and therefore the position of the cupula $\Theta_c(t)$ differ from the initial conditions, having been displaced by a certain amount in the direction of the force. The magnitude of the displacement can easily be calculated. Once the endolymph is stationary, the cupula velocity $\dot{\Theta}_c(t)$ and its acceleration $\ddot{\Theta}_c(t)$ in relation to the walls are zero, and consequently the terms for viscous and inertial restraining forces vanish in Equation 1, which now reduces to

$$K\Theta_c(t) = M\ddot{\Theta}_h(t)$$
$$\text{or}$$
$$\Theta_c(t) = \frac{M}{K}\ddot{\Theta}_h(t) \qquad \textbf{4}$$

That is, the final displacement of the cupula depends on a proportionality constant and on the magnitude of the constant angular acceleration.

The relationships embodied in Equations 3 and 4 are two of the fundamental concepts of cupular function. To restate them: The maximum deviation of the cupula increases proportionally to the magnitude of head velocity during sinusoidal head rotations at the frequencies of natural head movements and to the magnitude of head acceleration during rotation with constant angular acceleration.

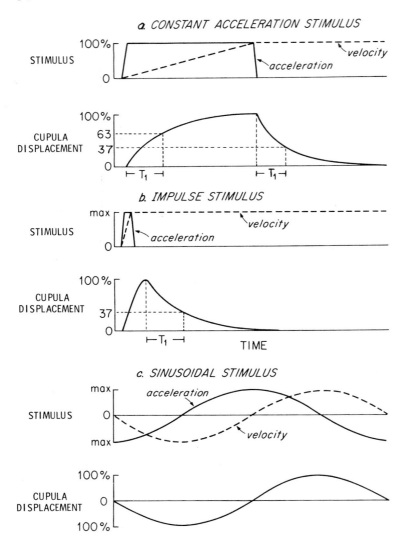

a. CONSTANT ACCELERATION STIMULUS

b. IMPULSE STIMULUS

c. SINUSOIDAL STIMULUS

Figure 2–11. Relationship between cupular displacement and three types of angular acceleration of the head as predicted by the pendulum model.

Cupula displacement after a constant angular acceleration stimulus follows an exponential time course (see Fig. 2–11a), which can be determined by a more detailed mathematical treatment of Equation 1 (see Appendix). Sixty-three percent of the total cupular deviation, regardless of its final value, always takes place after a fixed delay determined by what is known as the long time constant (T_1) of the system. The subsequent deviation of the cupula increases at the same rate (63 percent of the remainder every T_1 seconds) so that 95 percent of the final deviation will take place after approximately $3T_1$ seconds. The magnitude of the time constant depends on the viscous and elastic coefficients: $T_1 = C/K$.

That is, the time the cupula takes to reach a maximum deviation is proportional to the viscosity of the endolymph and inversely proportional to the elasticity of the cupula. T_1 cannot be measured directly, but it has been estimated to be about 7 seconds, based on the average response of primary afferent neurons in the squirrel monkey.[28, 40, 41]

According to the pendulum model, not only is the initial deviation of the cupula related to the constant acceleration stimulus, but after the stimulus is terminated the cupula returns to the resting position with the same exponential time course. It was precisely the observation by Steinhausen[90] of the slow exponential-like return of the cupula to the resting position after it had been deviated that led to the formulation of the pendulum model.

The cupular displacement following a brief impulse of angular acceleration is given in Figure 2–11b. This type of angular acceleration, although the least natural, is of great value in clinical vestibular testing. An impulse of acceleration is generated by changing the velocity of the head ($\Delta\dot\Theta_h$) with the maximum acceleration possible. The maximum deviation of the cupula takes place almost immediately and is proportional to the magnitude of the instantaneous change in head velocity $\Theta_c(t)\approx\Delta\dot\Theta_h$. Of particular note, the cupular deviation thereafter decays exponentially with the same time course as that following the constant acceleration stimulus. That is, it takes one time constant to return 63 percent of the maximum deviation.

The sinusoidal rotation in Figure 2–11c most closely resembles natural head movements because movement in one direction is followed by movement in the opposite direction. Most natural head movements can be broken down into a series of sine waves with different frequencies and amplitudes. According to Equation 3, the cupular displacement $\Theta_c(t)$ is given by $\omega A \cos \omega t$ (the differential of head displacement $A \sin \omega t$) where ω is the radian frequency ($2\pi f$) of head rotation and A is the angular head displacement. The head velocity at a given time is proportional to the value of the cosine function at that instant in the cycle of motion. Inasmuch as this value oscillates between $+1$ and -1, the head velocity ranges between $+\omega A$ and $-\omega A$. These relationships are felt to apply for sinusoidal rotations between 0.1 and 4.0 Hz and therefore cover the range of most to-and-fro head movements (see Appendix for mathematical details).[99]

Characteristics of Primary Afferent Neurons. As described in Chapter 1, the primary vestibular afferent fibers maintain a constant baseline firing rate of action potentials. Recordings from the primary afferent fibers of the cristae in mammalian and nonmammalian species reveal that physiologic stimulation producing endolymph flow toward the ampulla in the horizontal semicircular canal increases the baseline firing rate. Conversely, endo-

lymph flow away from the ampulla decreases the baseline firing rate. In the vertical canals the reverse occurs: Ampullopetal endolymph flow decreases the baseline firing rate, and ampullofugal flow increases the firing rate. Considering these observations and the previous anatomic descriptions, it is apparent that endolymph displacement that deviates the hairs of the sensory cells toward the kinocilium results in increased firing of the afferent nerve, whereas displacement away from the kinocilium results in decreased firing of the afferent nerve.

Detailed measurements of afferent nerve activity from the cristae of squirrel monkeys reveal that the firing rate associated with physiologic rotatory stimulation follows qualitatively the prediction of the pendulum model.[28] That is, the magnitude of change in frequency of action potentials is proportional to the theoretic deviation of the cupula. For example, during sinusoidal head rotation, the firing rate follows the time course of cupular displacement shown in Figure 2–11c. A sinusoidal change in firing frequency is superimposed on a rather high resting discharge (70 to 90 spikes per second). The peak firing rate occurs at the time of the peak angular head velocity. For sinusoidal rotation of small magnitude, the modulation is almost symmetrical about the baseline firing rate. For higher stimulus magnitudes, the responses become increasingly asymmetrical. For the largest magnitudes, the excitatory responses can increase up to 350 to 400 spikes per second in proportion to the stimulus magnitude, but the growth of inhibitory response is limited to the disappearance of spontaneous activity. This asymmetry in afferent nerve response to stimuli of large magnitude explains Ewald's second and third laws, because the "pneumatic hammer" that he used to apply pressure to the canals produced a massive stimulus.[26]

Just as there is a continuous spectrum in axon diameters, primary afferent neurons have a wide range of spontaneous firing rates and dynamic properties. It has proved useful to divide them, based on the regularity of their spontaneous discharge rate.[38, 39, 43] Neurons with the most irregular baseline firing rate (given by the coefficient of variation −CV− of the mean interspike interval) are the most sensitive to galvanic stimulation and have high-frequency dynamics that indicate a response to cupular velocity as well as to cupular displacement. Neurons with the most regular firing rate are the least sensitive to galvanic stimulation and have response dynamics close to those predicted by the pendulum model (Fig. 2–11). As a general rule a primary afferent's sensitivity to angular acceleration (in spikes/sec per deg/sec) is inversely related to the regularity of its baseline firing rate; that is, irregular units with high CV values have a higher sensitivity than regular units with low CV values.

How are these physiologic properties related to the anatomic features of primary afferent neurons described earlier? Recently, it has been possible to study the anatomic and physiologic properties of a single primary afferent neuron by first recording the neuron's dynamic response to angular acceleration with a micropipette and then injecting it with horseradish peroxidase to study its anatomic connections. Initial studies in the bullfrog demonstrated that "irregular" neurons had thick, rapidly conducting fibers that preferentially innervated the central ridge of the crista, whereas "regular" neurons had thin, slowly conducting fibers that predominantly innervated the periphery.[47] More recent studies in the chinchilla have correlated dynamic properties with the patterns of nerve terminals within the crista.[7] Of 56 semicircular canal units studied, 15 had caliceal endings, 1 had bouton endings, and 40 were dimorphic (caliceal and bouton endings). All caliceal units were at the center of the crista and had "irregular" dynamic properties. The single bouton unit was in the periphery and had "regular" dynamic properties (bouton units were technically difficult to study because of their thin axons). Dimorphic units were both "irregular" and "regular," with the former usually innervating the center of the crista, and the latter the periphery. Surprisingly, the caliceal units at the center of the crista had a lower rotational sensitivity than dimorphic units with similar size axons innervating the same region. Baird and associates[7] postulated that because of their lower sensitivity

these caliceal units might extend the dynamic range of vestibular reflexes; that is, they would not become saturated by the large velocities of active head movements. Dimorphic units innervating different regions of the crista varied in their dynamic properties even though they contacted similar numbers of type I and type II hair cells. Taken together, these findings indicate that the dynamic properties of a semicircular canal afferent neuron reflect multiple factors, including specific membrane features, number and type of synaptic connections, and location within the crista.

When the cristae are subjected to prolonged constant acceleration, a substantial proportion of nerve fibers undergo a slow decline in firing rate (adaptation) rather than maintain a steady state as predicted in Figure 2–11a. Because of adaptation, the firing rate does not return to baseline after cessation of acceleration but, rather, drops to a lower level before slowly returning to the resting level.[12, 40] Similar overshooting of the baseline occurs after stimulation with an impulse of acceleration. Instead of the monotonic response predicted by the pendulum model (see Fig. 2–11b), the afferent nerve firing pattern exhibits a biphasic reaction with a prolonged secondary phase that slowly returns to baseline. It is not known whether the behavior is due to anatomic or synaptic processes. Adaptation is more pronounced in "irregular" neurons. As will be shown later, the vestibulo-ocular reflex also reflects this deviation from the predicted pattern (see Fig. 7–1a).

OTOLITHS

Background. Over a century ago, Mach,[67] Crum-Brown,[18] and Breuer[13] each concluded that linear and angular acceleration must be mediated by different end-organs, and Breuer, in particular, postulated the mechanism by which the otoliths sense linear acceleration. As in the case of the semicircular canals, a gross anatomic feature of the maculae—the dense, calcified otolithic membrane—suggested the mechanisms by which they sense the direction of gravitational force. The afferent neuronal activity from the maculae associated with precise static and dynamic linear accleration forces has only recently been investigated in primates.[29-31] These studies confirm that the utricular and saccular maculae are responsive to static tilt and dynamic linear acceleration, resolving an earlier controversy as to whether the saccular macula functions as an auditory or vestibular organ. The pattern of afferent nerve response is complex, with various neurons exhibiting different resting activity, frequency response, and adaptation properties.

Mechanism of Stimulation. During head displacement, the calcified otolithic membrane is affected by the combined forces of applied linear acceleration and gravity and tends to move over the macula, which is mounted in the wall of the membranous labyrinth (see Fig. 1–2). The otolith is restrained in its motion by elastic, viscous, and inertial forces analogous to the forces associated with cupular movement. De Vries[20] measured the displacement of the large saccular otoliths of several fish and obtained estimates of the forces restraining the otoliths to the maculae. He proposed a model, analogous to the pendulum model, that described the dynamics of otolith displacement as those of a low-pass filter. Displacements due to sinusoidal linear acceleration would be greatest at low frequencies, including static head tilts. At higher frequencies, the otolith displacement would decrease by one half each time the frequency was doubled.

Characteristics of Primary Afferent Neurons. The nerve fibers innervating the maculae are activated by changes in position of the head in space.[29] Each neuron has a characteristic functional polarization vector that defines the axis of greatest sensitivity. It is as though the terminal fibers of each afferent neuron were stimulated only by hair cells with kinocilia oriented in a given direction in space, forming one functional neuronal unit. The combined polarization vectors of neurons from both maculae cover all possible positions of the head in three-dimensional space. The majority of polarization vectors, however, are near the horizontal plane for the utricular macula and the sagittal plane for the saccular macula.[29-31] Diagrams of the functional polarization vectors deter-

mined by electrophysiologic analysis in the squirrel monkey are remarkably similar to the morphologic maps that plot the polarization of hair cells within each macule (see Fig. 2–7). None of the neuronal units records a response to compressive forces, confirming previous findings in lateral line systems that displacement of hairs is the only adequate stimulus for the hair cell.[31, 63]

With the subject in the normal upright position, gravity does not stimulate most of the neuronal units of the utricular macula (because it is orthogonal to most polarization vectors). The average resting discharge of macular units in this position is approximately 65 spikes per second.[29] The macula is roughly divided into a medial and a lateral section by the striola. Because, in the utricular macula, hair cell polarization (the direction of the kinocilia) is toward the striola, ipsilateral tilt results in an increase in the baseline firing of the units medial to the striola and a decreased firing of the units lateral to the striola. Because of the curvature of the striola, many utricular macula units are also sensitive to forward and backward tilt. In contrast, the saccular macula is in a sagittal plane when a subject is in the upright position, and most of its functional polarization vectors are parallel to the gravity vector. Most neuronal units, therefore, are either excited or inhibited by the effect of 1 g of acceleration. The saccular macula exhibits less curvature, and most of its units have a preferred dorsoventral orientation. Saccular units at rest discharge at a rate essentially the same as that of the utricular units.[29]

As in the case of the cristae, their spontaneous firing rate subdivides two main classes of neuronal units in the maculae: regular and irregular.[31] The irregularly firing units adapt rapidly when stimulated with constant linear acceleration, are more sensitive to small changes in linear acceleration, and have a wider frequency response than the regular units. During stimulation with static tilts, the regular units maintain a constant ratio between the applied force and the response. During stimulation with sinusoidal linear acceleration (back-and-forth linear displacement), their sensitivity is constant up to 0.1 Hz but steadily declines at higher frequencies.

These regular units, therefore, conform to the expectations of the de Vries[20] model of otolith function. The irregular units, on the other hand, appear to respond not only to otolith displacement but also to the velocity of the displacement. Following a change in head position, they undergo an immediate increase in firing followed by a decline. This difference between the presumed displacement of the otolithic membrane and the afferent unit response may be related to the mechanical linkage between the hair cell cilia and the membrane.[54] The irregular units innervate type I hair cells, the cilia of which are not rigidly embedded in the otolithic membrane but, rather, are enclosed in fluid-filled chambers in the membrane. The cilia may sense the velocity of displacement of the otoliths by viscous coupling through the fluid. If so, the observed variation in unit response may reflect different types of coupling between different hair cells and the otolithic membrane. Another possibility is that the hair cell coupling is the same, but synaptic connections on type I (caliceal) and type II (bouton) hair cells have different transmission properties.

Functional Significance of Different Afferent Units

How different afferent units participate in different vestibular reflexes is poorly understood. Fernández and Goldberg[28] speculated that the response dynamics of primary afferent neurons could match the dynamic requirements of each reflex pathway. The vestibulo-ocular reflex (VOR) is an open-loop reflex controlling a predominantly viscous load, the eye ball, whereas the vestibulo-collic reflex (VCR) is a closed-loop reflex with a predominantly inertial load, the head; that is, the neck muscles are more sluggish than the extraocular muscles. The VOR might receive input largely from regular, more tonic, afferents, and the VCR from irregular, more phasic, afferents. Preliminary studies of secondary vestibular neurons identified as being part of the VOR or VCR in the squirrel monkey supported this hypothesis, although both reflexes received a broad range of afferent signals.[43] By contrast Lisberger and colleagues[58, 59] provided evidence for two parallel pathways from the secondary vestibular neurons to the oculomotor neurons within the VOR; one a short-latency, unmodifiable pathway and the other a longer-latency, modifiable pathway. Based on the waveforms of eye velocity records, he suggested that the former received input primarily from "irregular" phasic primary afferents and the latter from "regular" tonic afferents (see Chapter 3 for further details).

REFERENCES

1. Altmann, F, and Waltner, J.: Further investigations on the physiology of labyrinthine fluids. Ann Otol Rhinol Laryngol 59:657, 1950.
2. Anijad, AH, Scheer, AA, and Rosenthal, J: Human internal auditory canal. Arch Otolaryngol 89:709, 1969.
3. Annoni, J, Cochran, SL, and Precht, W: Glutamate or a related substance may be the transmitter at the hair cell-primary afferent synapse in the vestibular labyrinth of the frog. Experientia 39:628, 1983.
4. Anson, BJ and Donaldson, JA: Surgical Anatomy of the Temporal Bone and Ear, ed 3. WB Saunders, Philadelphia, 1981.
5. Anson, BJ: Developmental anatomy of the ear. In Paparella, MF and Shumrick, DA (eds): Otolaryngology, I. WB Saunders, Philadelphia, 1973.
6. Axelsson, A: The blood supply of the inner ear of mammals. In Keidel, WD and Neff, WD (eds): Handbook of Sensory Physiology. Auditory System, Vol. V, Part 1. Springer-Verlag, New York, 1974.
7. Baird, RA, Desmadryl, G, Fernández, C, and Goldberg, JM: The vestibular nerve in the chinchilla. II. Relation between afferent response properties and peripheral innervation patterns in the semicircular canals. J Neurophysiol 60:182, 1988.
8. Bauknight, RS, Strelioff, D, and Honrubia, V: Effective stimulus for the Xenopus laevis lateral-line hair-cell system. Laryngoscope 86:1836, 1976.
9. Bernard, C, Cochran, SL, and Precht, W: Presynaptic actions of cholinergic agents upon the hair cell-afferent fiber synapse in the vestibular labyrinth of the frog. Brain Res 338:225, 1985.
10. Blanks, RHI, Curthoys, IS, and Markham, CH: Planar relationships of the semicircular canals in man. Acta Otolaryngol 80:185, 1975.
11. Blanks, RHI, Curthoys, IS, and Markham, CH: Planar relationships of semicircular canals in the cat. Am J Physiol 223:55, 1972.
12. Blanks, RHI, Estes, MS, and Markham, CH: Physiologic characteristics of vestibular first-order canal neurons in the cat. II. Response to constant angular acceleration. J Neurophysiol 38:1250, 1975.

13. Breuer, J: Über die Funktion der Bogengänge des Ohrlabyrinthes. Wien Med Jahrb 4:72, 1874.
14. Caston, J and Rousell, H: Curare and the efferent vestibular system. Acta Otolaryngol (Stockh) 97:19, 1984.
15. Chole, RA: Petrous apicitis: Surgical anatomy. Ann Otol Rhinol Laryngol 94:251, 1985.
16. Correia, MJ, Lang, DG, and Eden, AR: A light and transmission electron microscope study of the neural processes within the pigeon anterior semicircular canal neuroepithelium. In Correia, MJ, Perachio, AA (eds): Progress in Clinical and Biological Research 176:247, Alan R Liss, New York, 1985.
17. Corwin, JT and Cotanche, DA: Regeneration of sensory hair cells after acoustic trauma. Science 240:1772, 1988.
18. Crum-Brown, A: On the sense of rotation and the anatomy and physiology of the semicircular canals of the internal ear. J Anat Physiol 8:327, 1874.
19. Curthoys, IS: The response of primary horizontal semicircular canal neurons in the rat and guinea pig to angular acceleration. Exp Brain Res 47:286, 1982.
20. de Vries, H: The mechanics of the labyrinth otoliths. Acta Otolaryngol 38:262, 1950.
21. Dechesne, C, Raymond, J, and Sans, A: Action of glutamate in the cat labyrinth. Ann Otol Rhinol Lar 93:163, 1984.
22. Dohlman, GF: Some practical and theoretical points of labyrinthology. Proc Roy Soc Med 28:1371, 1935.
23. Dohlman, GF: The mechanism of secretion and absorption of endolymph in the vestibular apparatus. Acta Otolaryngol 59:275, 1965.
24. Duckert, LG: Anatomy of the skull base, temporal bone, external ear and middle ear. In Cummings, CW, Fredrickson, JM, Harker, LA, et al (eds): Otolaryngology—Head and Neck Surgery. CV Mosby, St Louis, 1986.
25. Engstrom, H, Ades, HW, and Andersson, A: Structural pattern on the organ of corti. Williams & Wilkins, Baltimore, 1966.
26. Ewald, R: Physiologische Untersuchungen über das Endorgan des Nervous Octavus. Bergmann, Wiesbaden, 1892.
27. Felix, D and Ehrenberger, K: The action of putative neurotransmitter substances in the cat labyrinth. Acta Otolar (Stockh) 93:101, 1982.
28. Fernández, C and Goldberg, JM: Physiology of peripheral neurons innervating semi-circular canals of the squirrel monkey. II. Response to sinusoidal stimulation and dynamics of peripheral vestibular system. J Neurophysiol 34:661, 1971.
29. Fernández, C and Goldberg, JM: Physiology of peripheral neurons innervating otolith organs of the squirrel monkey. I. Response to static tilts and to long-duration centrifugal force. J Neurophysiol 39:970, 1976.
30. Fernández, C and Goldberg, JM: Physiology of peripheral neurons innervating otolith organs of the squirrel monkey. II. Directional selectivity and force-response relations. J Neurophysiol 39:985, 1976.
31. Fernández, C and Goldberg, JM: Physiology of peripheral neurons innervating otolith organs of the squirrel monkey. III. Response dynamics. J Neurophysiol 39:996, 1976.
32. Fernández, C, Baird, RA, and Goldberg, JM: The vestibular nerve of the chinchilla. I. Peripheral innervation patterns in the horizontal and superior semicircular canals. J Neurophysiol 60:167, 1988.
33. Flock, A and Lam, D: Neurotransmitter synthesis in inner ear and lateral line sense organs. Nature 249:142, 1974.
34. Flourens, P: Recherches Expérimentales sur les Propriétés et les Functions due Système Nerveux dans les Animaux Vertébrés. Crevot, Paris, 1842.
35. Gacek, RR, Nomura, Y, and Balogh, K: Acetylcholinesterase activity in the efferent fibers of the stato-acoustic nerve. Acta Otolar (Stockh) 59:541, 1965.
36. Gacek, RR: The innervation of the vestibular labyrinth. Ann Otol Rhinol Laryngol 77:676, 1968.
37. Goldberg, JM and Fernández, C: Efferent vestibular system in the squirrel monkey: Anatomical location and influence of afferent activity. J Neurophysiol 43:986, 1980.
38. Goldberg, JM, Highstein, SM, Moschovakis, A, and Fernández, C: Inputs from regularly and irregularly discharging vestibular-nerve afferents to secondary neurons in the vestibular nuclei of the squirrel monkey. I. An electrophysiological analysis. J Neurophysiol 58:700, 1987.
39. Goldberg, JM, Smith CE, and Fernández, C: Relation between discharge regularity and responses to externally applied galvanic currents in vestibular nerve afferents of the squirrel monkey. J Neurophysiol 51:1236, 1984.
40. Goldberg, J and Fernández, C: Physiology of peripheral neurons innervating semicircular canals of the squirrel monkey. I. Resting discharge and response to constant angular accelerations. J Neurophsiol 34:635, 1971.
41. Goldberg, J and Fernández, C: Physiology of peripheral neurons innervating semicircular canals of the squirrel monkey. III. Variations among units in their discharge properties. J Neurophysiol 34:676, 1971.
42. Hansen, C: Vascular anatomy of the human temporal bone: I. Anastomoses between the membranous labyrinth and its bony capsule: II. Anastomoses inside the labyrinthine capsule: III. The vascularization of the vestibulocochlear nerve. Arch Ohr Nas-Kehlk-Heilk 200:83, 1971.
43. Highstein, SM, Goldberg, JM, Moschovakis, AK, and Fernández, C: Inputs from regularly and irregularly discharging vestibular-nerve afferents to secondary neurons in the vestibular nuclei of the squirrel monkey. II. Correlation with output pathways of secondary neurons. J Neurophysiol 58:719, 1987.
44. Holden, H and Schuknecht, H: Distribution pattern of blood in the inner ear following spontaneous subarachnoid hemorrhage. J Laryngol 82:321, 1968.

45. Honrubia, V, Hoffman, LF, Sitko, S, and Schwartz, IR: Anatomic and physiological correlates in bullfrog vestibular nerve. J Neurophysiol 61:688, 1989.

46. Honrubia, V, Kuruvilla, A, Mamekunian, D, and Eichel, JE: Morphological aspects of the vestibular nerve of the squirrel monkey. Laryngoscope 97:228, 1987.

47. Honrubia, V, et al: Physiological and anatomical characteristics of primary vestibular afferent neurons in the bullfrog. Int J Neurosci 15:197, 1981.

48. Iurato, S: Submicroscopic Structure of the Inner Ear. Pergamon Press, New York, 1967.

49. Kimura, RS: Distribution, structure and function of dark cells in the vestibular labyrinth. Ann Otol Rhinol Laryngol 78:542, 1969.

50. Kimura, R and Schuknecht, H: Membranous hydrops in the inner ear of the guinea pig after obliteration of the endolymphatic sac. Pract Oto-Rhino-Laryngol 27:343, 1965.

51. Kimura, R, Schuknecht, H, and Ota, C: Blockage of the cochlear aqueduct. Acta Otolaryngol 77:1, 1974.

52. Konishi, T, Butler, RA, and Fernández, C: Effect of anoxia on cochlear potentials. J Acoust Soc Amer 33:349, 1961.

53. Ledoux, A: Les canaux semi-circulaires Etude électrophysiologique. Contribution à l'effort d'uniformisation des épreuves vestibulaires. Essai d'interprétation de la sémiologie vestibulaire. Acta Oto-Rhino-Laryngol, Belgica. 12:109, 1958.

54. Lim, DJ: Ultrastructure of the otolithic membrane and the cupula. Adv Oto-Rhino-Laryngol 19:35, 1973.

55. Lindeman, HH: Studies on the morphology of the sensory regions of the vestibular apparatus. Adv Anat Embryol Cell Biol 42:1, 1969.

56. Lindsay, JR: Petrous pyramid of the temporal bone: Pneumatization and roentgenologic appearance. Arch Otolaryngol 31:231, 1940.

57. Lipschitz, WS: Responses from the first order neurons of the horizontal semicircular canal in the pigeon. Brain Res 63:43, 1973.

58. Lisberger, SG and Pavelko, TA: Vestibular signals carried by pathways subserving plasticity of the vestibulo-ocular reflex in monkeys. J Neurosci 6:346, 1986.

59. Lisberger, SG, Miles, FA, and Optican, LM: Frequency-selective adaptation: Evidence for channels in the vestibulo-ocular reflex? J Neurosci 3:1234, 1983.

60. Lopez, I and Meza, G: Neurochemical evidence for afferent gabaergic and efferent cholinergic neurotransmission in the frog vestibule. Neuroscience 25:13, 1988.

61. Lorente De Nó, R: Anatomy of the eighth nerve. The central projection of the nerve endings of the internal ear. Laryngoscope. 43:1, 1933.

62. Lorente De Nó, R: Etudes Sur L'Anatomie et la Physiologie due Labyrinthe de L'Ovreille et due VIII Nerf. Madrid Univ Lab Recherches Biologiques Travaux 24:53, 1926.

63. Lowenstein, O and Roberts, TDM: Oscillographic analysis of the responses of the otolith organs of the thornback ray. J Physiol 110:392, 1949.

64. Lowenstein, O and Sand, A: The individual and integrated activity of the semicircular canals of the elasmobranch labyrinth. J Physiol 99:89, 1940.

65. Lowenstein, O and Wersäll, J: A functional interpretation of the electron-microscopic structure of the sensory hairs in the cristae of the elasmobranch raja clavata in terms of directional sensitivity. Nature 184:1807, 1959.

66. Lundquist, P-G: The endolymphatic duct and sac in the guinea pig. Acta Otolaryngol (Suppl) 201:1, 1965.

67. Mach, E: Grundlinien der Lehre von den Bewegungsempfindungen. Engelmann, Leipzig, 1875; Bonset, Amsterdam, 1967 (translation).

68. Mazzoni, A: Internal auditory artery supply to the petrous bone. Ann Otol Rhinol Laryngol 81:13, 1972.

69. Mazzoni, A: Internal auditory canal, arterial relations at the porus acusticus. Ann Otol Rhinol Laryngol 78:797, 1969.

70. McLaren, JW and Hillman, DE: Displacement of the semicircular canal cupula during sinusoidal rotation. Neuroscience 4:2001, 1979.

71. O'Leary, DP, Dunn, R, and Honrubia, V: Functional and anatomical correlation of afferent responses from the isolated semicircular canal. Nature 251:255, 1974.

72 Osborne, MP and Thornhill, R: The effect of monoamine depleting drugs upon the synaptic bars in the inner ear of the bullfrog (Rana catesbiana). Z Zellforsch mikrosk Anat 127:347, 1972.

73. Perlman, HB, Kimura, RS and Fernández, C: Experiments on temporary obstruction of the internal auditory artery. Laryngoscope 69:591, 1959.

74. Perlman, H and Lindsay, J: Relation of the internal ear spaces to the meninges. Arch Otolaryngol 29:12, 1939.

75. Precht, W, Illinás, R, and Clarke, M: Physiological responses of frog vestibular fibers to horizontal angular rotation. Exp Brain Res 13:378, 1971.

76. Ramprashad, F, Landolt, JP, Money, KE, and Laufer, J: Dimensional analysis and dynamic response characterization of mammalian peripheral vestibular structures. Am J Anat 169:295, 1984.

77. Rasmussen, A: Studies of the VIIIth cranial nerve of man. Laryngoscope 50:67, 1940.

78. Rosenhall, U: Mapping of the cristae ampullares in man. Ann Otol 81:882, 1972.

79. Rosenhall, U: Vestibular macular mapping in man. Ann Otol 81:339, 1972.

80. Ryals, BM and Rubel, EW: Hair cell regeneration after acoustic trauma in adult coturnix quail. Science 240:1774, 1988.

81. Salt, AN and Konishi, T: The cochlear fluids: Perilymph and endolymph. In Altschuler, RA, Hoffman, DW, Bobbin, RP (eds): Neurobiology of Hearing: The Cochlea. Raven Press, New York, 1986.

82. Sando, I, Black, FO, and Hemenway, WG: Spatial distribution of vestibular nerve in internal auditory canal. Ann Otol 81:305, 1972.

83. Schneider, LW and Anderson, DJ: Transfer char-

acteristics of first and second order lateral and vestibular neurons in gerbil. Brain Res 112:61, 1976.

84. Schuknecht, H and El Seifi, A: Experimental observations on the fluid physiology of the inner ear. Ann Otol Rhinol Laryngol 72:687, 1963.

85. Silverstein, H and Schuknecht, H: Biochemical studies of inner ear fluid in man. Arch Otolaryngol 84:395, 1966.

86. Silverstein, H: Biochemical studies of the inner ear fluids in the cat. Ann Otol Rhinol Laryngol 75:48, 1966.

87. Silverstein, H: Inner ear fluid proteins in acoustic neuroma. Meniere's disease and otosclerosis. Ann Otol Rhinol Laryngol 80:27, 1971.

88. Smith, CA, Lowry, OH, and Wu, ML: The electrolytes of the labyrinthine fluids. Laryngoscope 64:141, 1954.

89. Smith, CA: The capillaries of the vestibular membranous labyrinth in the guinea pig. Laryngoscope 63:87, 1953.

90. Steinhausen, W: Über Sichtbarmachung and Funktionsprufung der Cupula terminalis in den Bogengangs-ampullen der Labyrinths. Arch Ges Physiol 217:747, 1927.

91. Suh, KW, and Cody, DTR: Obliteration of vestibular and cochlear aqueducts in animals. Trans AAOOO 84:359, 1977.

92. Tomko, DL, Peterka, RJ, Schor, RH, and O'Leary, DP: Response dynamics of horizontal canal afferents in barbiturate-anesthetized cats. J Neurophysiol 45:376, 1981.

93. Valli, P, Costa, J, and Zucca, G: Local mechanisms in vestibular receptor control. Acta Otolar (Stockh) 97:611, 1984.

94. Valli, P, et al: The effect of glutamate on the frog semicircular canal. Brain Res 330:1, 1985.

95. Van Egmond, AAJ, Groen, JJ, and Jongkees, LBW: The mechanics of the semicircular canal. J Physiol 110:1, 1949.

96. Von Békésy, G and Rosenblith, W: The mechanical properties of the ear. In Stevens, SS (ed): Handbook of Experimental Psychology. John Wiley & Sons, New York, 1951.

97. Wersäll, J, Flock, A, and Lundquist, P-G: Structural basis for directional sensitivity in cochlear and vestibular sensory receptors. Cold Spring Harbor Symposia on Quantitiative Biology 30:115, 1965.

98. Wever, E and Lawrence, M: Physiological Acoustics. Princeton University Press, Princeton, 1954.

99. Wilson, VJ and Melvill Jones, G: Mammalian vestibular physiology. Plenum Press, New York, 1979.

Chapter 3

THE CENTRAL VESTIBULAR SYSTEM

VESTIBULAR NUCLEI

Anatomy

The axons of the primary vestibular neurons enter the brainstem at the inner aspect of the restiform body and divide into secondary ascending and descending branches, which form a clearly defined vestibular tract (Fig. 3–1).[35, 67, 90, 115, 143] The tract runs in the ventrolateral part of the superior and the descending vestibular nuclei. Branches from fibers in the ascending tract end either in the rostral end of the vestibular nuclei or in the cerebellum, and branches from the descending tract end in the caudal vestibular nuclei. The vestibular nuclei consist of a group of neurons located on the floor of the fourth ventricle bounded laterally by the restiform body, rostrally by the brachium conjunctivum, ventrally by the nucleus and spinal tract of the trigeminal nerve, and medially by the pontine reticular formation. Four distinct anatomic groups of neurons have traditionally been considered to constitute the vestibular nuclei, although not all of the neurons in these nuclei receive primary afferent vestibular nerve fibers. The largest contingent of afferent fibers to the vestibular nuclei originates in the cerebellum.[29] The main vestibular nuclei are the superior, also known as the angular, or Bechterew's nucleus; the lateral, or Deiters' nucleus; the medial, or triangular, nucleus of Schwalbe; and the descending, or inferior or spinal, vestibular nucleus. In addition, the vestibular nuclear complex includes several small groups of cells that are closely associated topographically with the main nuclei but have distinct morphologic characteristics and anatomic connections. In the chinchilla the vestibular nuclei contain approximately 4,500 neurons, 1,500 each in the lateral and descending nuclei and 1,500 in the remaining nuclei.[143]

How do the multiplicity of signals originating in different receptor organs distribute within the vestibular nuclei? Recent studies using intracellular labeling techniques are beginning to answer this important question.[75, 76, 84] Individual primary afferent neurons provide multiple branches (e.g., in the bullfrog an average of 82 branches per afferent fiber),[90] usually innervating secondary neurons in all four of the vestibular nuclei. At the same time, there are clear separations of afferent fibers such that specific areas in each nucleus preferentially receive afferents from specific receptors (as illustrated in Fig. 3–1). Many secondary vestibular neurons receive a converging input from different sensory organs (e.g., horizontal and vertical canal, canal and otolith) and from different size axons originating in the same end-organ. The emerging picture is a complex one of both separation (channeling) and convergence of afferent signals at the level of the vestibular nuclei (see below).

SUPERIOR VESTIBULAR NUCLEUS

The superior vestibular nucleus in the human being extends from the caudal pole of the trigeminal motor nucleus to approximately the level of the abducens nucleus.[175] It mainly contains medium-size neurons with some large multipolar cells at the cen-

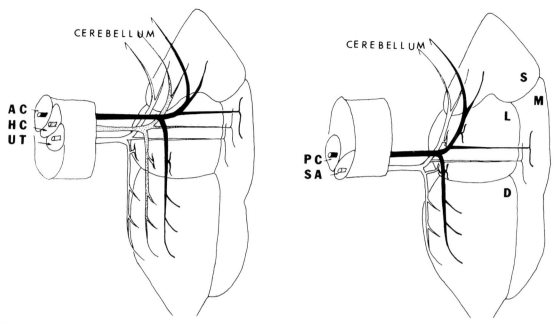

Figure 3–1. Distribution of primary vestibular afferent fibers within the vestibular nucleus of the chinchilla. Fibers were labeled by injecting individual receptors with horseradish peroxidase. *AC*, anterior canal; *HC*, horizontal canal; *PC*, posterior canal; *UT*, utriclus; *SA*, sacculus; *S*, superior nucleus; *L*, lateral nucleus; *M*, medial nucleus; *D*, descending nucleus. (Courtesy W. Lee, M.D., and A. Newman, M.D., Head and Neck Surgery, UCLA).

ter. The bulk of primary afferent projections to the superior vestibular nucleus originates in the cristae of the semicircular canals. Large fibers terminate preferentially on the larger neurons in the center of the nucleus.[29, 67] This area, however, also receives input from medium and small primary neurons.[106] Fibers from the anterior semicircular canal are found medially, those from the horizontal and posterior canals more laterally (see Fig. 3–1). Fibers from the utriculus and sacculus innervate only the periphery of the nucleus. Another major group of afferent fibers originate in the cerebellum. Those from the flocculus end in the central region; and those from the fastigial nucleus, nodulus, and uvula end in the peripheral region.[29, 109] A group of fibers from the contralateral medial and descending nucleus connect the two sides.

Axons from the neurons in the superior nucleus run in the ipsilateral and contralateral medial longitudinal fascicle (MLF) to innervate the motor nuclei of the extrinsic eye muscles; others project to the cerebellum and dorsal pontine reticular formation.[140, 141] The dendrites of neurons in

the periphery of the nucleus extend into the adjacent reticular formation and into the principal trigeminal nucleus. Because of the pattern of afferent and efferent connections, the superior vestibular nucleus is a major relay center for ocular reflexes mediated by the semicircular canals.

LATERAL VESTIBULAR NUCLEUS (DEITERS' NUCLEUS)

Beginning at the caudal end of the superior nucleus and ending below the level of the abducens nucleus, the lateral nucleus is transversed by the initial segments of the vestibular tract fibers corresponding to the root entry zone. The lateral nucleus is distinguished by the presence of giant cells (30 to 60μm) which are relatively more numerous in the dorsocaudal than in the rostroventral part.[29, 175] No sharp anatomic distinction divides these two parts of the nucleus; in cats, only the rostroventral part receives primary vestibular afferents (the majority originating from the utricular macula). The dorsocaudal part receives afferent fibers from the vermis and fastigial nucleus of the cerebellum (see Fig. 3–23). Afferent components from other sources (spinal and commissural fibers) are few in comparison with those from the cerebellum and vestibular nerve. The lateral nucleus sends most of its efferent fibers to the spinal cord as the ipsilateral vestibulospinal tract (see Fig. 3–22). This projection is somatotopically organized in that fibers to the cervicothoracic cord originate from the rostroventral part of the nucleus, whereas fibers to the lumbosacral cord originate from the dorsocaudal part.[157] The lateral nucleus also sends efferent fibers to the MLF bilaterally, which connect with the various oculomotor nuclei. Based on its fiber connections, the lateral vestibular nucleus is an important station for the control of vestibulospinal reflexes, particularly those involving the forelimbs.[34]

MEDIAL VESTIBULAR NUCLEUS

The medial vestibular nucleus is located beneath the floor of the fourth ventricle caudal to the superior, and medial to the descending nucleus. It consists of cells of many different sizes and shapes relatively close together, embedded in a fine meshwork of very thin fibers that course in almost all directions.[29, 175] It differs from the other nuclei in that it does not receive large-diameter fibers.[84] Anatomic separation from the superior nucleus is not well defined. Neurons in the upper part of the nucleus receive afferent fibers from the cristae of the semicircular canals as well as from the fastigial nucleus and flocculus of the cerebellum. Saccular and utricular afferents project to the middle section of the nucleus.[67] The caudal part receives its main afferents from the cerebellum (the ipsilateral and contralateral fastigial nucleus and the ipsilateral nodulus). Other afferent contributions include a large projection from the contralateral medial vestibular nucleus and a small projection from the reticular formation.

Efferent connections from the medial nuclei run in the descending MLF to the cervical and thoracic spinal levels by way of the vestibulospinal tract (see Fig. 3–22). From the rostral area (receiving afferent input from the cristae), efferent fibers pass to the ascending MLF bilaterally to reach the nuclei of the oculomotor nerves.[131] Other efferents are distributed to the vestibular cerebellum, the reticular formation, and the contralateral vestibular nuclei.[34] Because of its projections in the MLF to extraocular muscles and the cervical cord, the medial vestibular nucleus appears to be an important center for coordinating eye, head, and neck movements. The prominent commissural connections are probably important for the compensatory processes following peripheral vestibular lesions (see Mechanism of Compensation after Labyrinthectomy).

DESCENDING VESTIBULAR NUCLEUS

The descending or inferior vestibular nucleus is difficult to differentiate anatomically from the adjacent medial vestibular nucleus. It consists of small and medium-size cells with occasional giant cells.[29, 175] Projections from the cristae are to the center and those from the maculae to the periphery (utricular-ventral, saccular-dorsal). Cerebellar afferents from the flocculus, nodulus, and uvula are scattered throughout the nucleus, intermingling with the vestibular afferents. Projections from other sources, including spinal afferents, are minimal. Most of the efferent fibers from the descending nucleus pass to the cerebellum and to the reticular formation.[34] Numerous commissural fibers supply the contralateral superior, descending, medial, and lateral nuclei.[27] The descending nucleus apparently integrates vestibular signals from the two sides with signals from the cerebellum and reticular formation.

INTERSTITIAL NUCLEUS OF THE VESTIBULAR NERVE

Of the small groups of cells associated with the vestibular nuclei, the interstitial nucleus is most clearly defined.[29] It consists of small strands of elongated cells, some as large as the giant cells of the lateral nucleus, interspersed between the root fibers of the vestibular nerve near the brainstem entry zone. In the chinchilla, the interstitial nucleus receives numerous short afferent collaterals from the maculae of the utriculus (rostral) or sacculus (caudal), but only a few from the cristae of the semicircular canals. Efferent projections from the interstitial nucleus enter the ascending MLF and may be important in mediating vestibulo-ocular reflexes.

Physiology

INTRODUCTION

Vestibular signals originating in the two labyrinths first interact with signals from other sensory systems in the neurons of the vestibular nuclei. Only a fraction of the neurons receive direct vestibular connections and, with perhaps the exception of the interstitial nucleus of the vestibular nerve, the neurons that receive primary vestibular afferent fibers also may receive afferents from the cervical area, the cerebellum, the reticular formation, the spinal cord, and the contralateral vestibular nuclei.[163] Consequently, efferent signals from the vestibular nuclei reflect the interaction of these various afferent systems. For example, visual signals relayed through the cerebellar flocculus to neurons in the superior and medial nucleus modulate the activity of the vestibulo-ocular reflexes.[96] Inputs from the neck proprioceptors modulate the vestibulocollic reflexes.[85] The cerebellum influences the vestibulospinal reflexes by means of connections between the vermis and the lateral and descending vestibular nuclei.[158] Through connections with the reticular substance, vestibular neuron outflow interacts with descending corticobulboreticular and reticulospinal signals.[154]

TYPES OF SECONDARY VESTIBULAR NEURONS

Following stimulation of the vestibular nerve with a single brief electric pulse, two different groups of secondary vestibular neurons have been identified on the basis of their relationship to the field potential produced in areas of the brainstem receiving vestibular inputs[160, 163, 183] (Fig. 3–2). This field potential consists of three components: an initial positive-negative deflection from action currents in the primary vestibular fibers; a negative deflection wave (N_1) with a short latency less than 1.0 msec, generated by monosynaptically activated secondary vestibular neurons and fibers; and a delayed negative deflection (N_2) with a latency of about 2.5 msec, generated by multisynaptically activated neurons and fibers (Fig. 3–2A). By carefully placing microelectrodes in the vicinity of or inside secondary vestibular neurons and tailoring the electric stimuli, it has been demonstrated that some neurons produce action potentials at the time of the extracellular N_1 wave with latencies between 0.5 and 1.0 msec (Fig. 3–2B), suggesting that they receive monosynaptic input. Other neurons produce delayed action potentials (Fig. 3–2C), suggesting that they might be activated through multisynaptic connections. Only about 75 per-

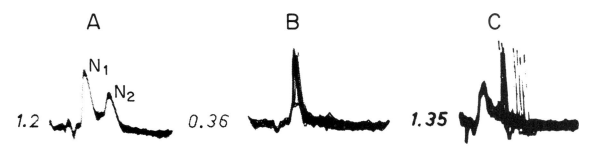

Figure 3–2. *(A)* Field potential recorded in the medial vestibular nucleus after electric stimulation of the ipsilateral vestibular nerve. N_1 is generated by monosynaptic activated secondary vestibular neurons and N_2 by multisynaptic activated neurons. *(B)* Response of a monosynaptic activated neuron. N_1 field potential is not seen because of superposition of spikes. *(C)* Response of a multisynaptic activated neuron demonstrating spikes timed with N_2 field potential. Each recording is composed of about 20 superimposed traces. (Adapted from Precht and Shimazu.[160])

cent of neurons are activated by nerve stimulation, and approximately half of these are monosynaptically activated.[160, 183] All monosynaptic connections are ipsilateral and excitatory. Among the monosynaptically activated neurons, about 37 percent respond to small electrical stimuli with very short latencies that activate only the thickest, most sensitive irregular primary afferents.[71] The rest of the neurons respond to larger electrical currents suggesting that they receive a predominant input from thinner, regular afferents. Goldberg and colleagues[71] emphasized, however, that it would be wrong to view secondary vestibular neurons as narrowly tuned channels, each receiving only a single kind of primary afferent input. Most vestibular nuclei neurons, even those predominantly related to regular and irregular afferents, receive a broad range of afferent inputs.

The simplest classification of secondary vestibular neurons derived from experiments in decerebrate cats consists of two major groups:[182] Type I neurons are excited, type II, inhibited, by ipsilateral rotation of the head (Fig. 3–3). The former are monosynaptically activated by ipsilateral primary afferents, whereas the latter receive their input via commissural connections either from neurons in the reticular substance or directly from contralateral type I neurons (see Fig. 3–3).[182] Contralateral labyrinth stimulation excites type II neurons, and they, in turn, inhibit ipsilateral type I neurons. It follows that during head rotation the activity of ipsilateral type I neurons is enhanced by excitation from the ipsilateral labyrinth and by decreased inhibition from neighboring type II neurons (whose input from the contralateral type I neurons has simultaneously decreased). Type I neurons are also affected by another crossed inhibitory pathway mediated by neurons within the reticular substance. (see Fig. 3–3). This inhibitory pathway is activated by electrical stimulation in the contralateral vestibular nuclei and is interrupted by shallow incisions of the midline of the floor of the fourth ventricle.[163, 182]

MECHANISM OF COMPENSATION AFTER LABYRINTHECTOMY

Knowledge of the different types of secondary vestibular neurons and their inter-

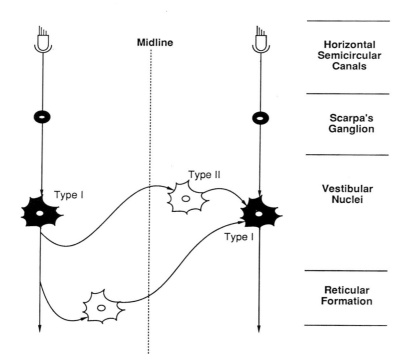

Figure 3–3. Interrelation of type I and type II secondary vestibular neurons. Dark neurons are excitatory and light neurons inhibitory. (Adapted from Precht and Shimazu.[160])

connecting pathways is important for understanding the sequence of recovery following a unilateral loss of labyrinthine function.[162] On the basis of connections depicted in Figure 3–3 it can be postulated that immediately after a labyrinthectomy the ipsilateral type I neurons lose their spontaneous activity and become unresponsive to ipsilateral angular rotation. At the same time, contralateral healthy type I neurons lose their inhibitory contralateral input, and their spontaneous activity increases in comparison to normal.[159] Contralateral type II neurons lose their inputs from excitatory type I neurons and cannot be identified electrophysiologically. An imbalance in the tone of body and eye musculature results and the clinical signs of labyrinthectomy are produced: nystagmus, past pointing, and imbalance. A few days after a labyrinthectomy, the previously silent type I neurons on the damaged side recover their spontaneous activity and begin to respond to physiologic stimulation of the contralateral labyrinth.[167, 185, 214] As a result of their connections with ipsilateral type II neurons, these reactivated type I units are inhibited when the type I neurons on the healthy side are excited and disinhibited when the contralateral type I neurons are inhibited. Although the responses of the type I neurons on the damaged side are not as intense as those on the normal side, they are qualitatively similar. The recovery of sensitivity in the ipsilateral type I neurons after a labyrinthectomy parallels the time course or improvement in clinical symptoms and signs.

The genesis of the renewed tonic input to ipsilateral type I neurons several days after a complete labyrinthectomy is not really known.[108] It doesn't come from the healthy side, because afferent activity on that side doesn't change.[162] It might result from the sprouting of axons from other sources (e.g., the commissural pathways) or from an increased efficacy of the remaining intact synapses.[66] In animal studies the course of compensation is affected by exercise,[95] visual experience[61] and drugs (as a rule, stimulants accelerate and sedatives slow compensation).[108] If a second labyrinthectomy is performed after compensation for the first occurs, the animal again develops signs of acute unilateral vestibular

loss with nystagmus directed toward the previously operated ear (Bechterew's compensatory nystagmus),[20] as if the first labyrinthectomy had not taken place. Compensation after the second labyrinthectomy is slightly faster than the first, but still requires several days.

VESTIBULO-OCULAR REFLEXES

Experimental Methods

Experiments employing a variety of research methods have documented that precisely organized projections connect the vestibular end-organs to motoneurons innervating the extrinsic eye muscles. The experimental data include (1) anatomic studies in normal animals using Golgi-stained preparations, cell and axon labeling techniques, and demonstration of wallerian and retrograde cellular changes following sectioning of nerve fibers; (2) electrophysiologic studies monitoring action potentials in eye muscles, oculomotor nerves and neurons, secondary vestibular neurons, and interconnecting pathways within the brainstem following stimulation of the vestibular end-organs and vestibular nerves; (3) precise recordings of eye movements induced by physiologic and electric stimulation of vestibular pathways (the individual peripheral receptors, afferent nerves, and the brainstem nuclei); and (4) more recently intracellular labeling of neurons that have been identified as part of the vestibulo-ocular reflex based on their location and their response to physiologic stimulation.

Organization of the Vestibulo-Ocular Reflex Arcs

The basic organization of the vestibulo-ocular reflexes is shown in Figure 3–4A. Type I secondary neurons make direct contact with oculomotor neurons and provide axon collaterals to chains of interneurons located on the same side of the brainstem and cerebellum.[117] These interneurons along with the commissural connections from the contralateral side provide positive

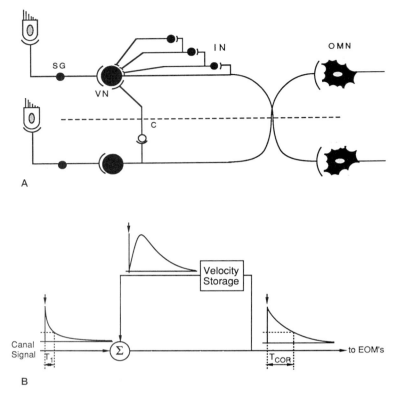

Figure 3–4. Schematic drawing of the anatomical organization of the vestibulo-ocular reflex. *(A) SG,* scarpas ganglion; *VN,* vestibular nucleus neuron; *IN,* ipsilateral interneurons; *c,* commissural interneuron; *OMN,* oculomotor neuron; *dark neurons,* excitatory; *light neurons,* inhibitory; *dashed line,* midline. Reciprocal pathways are omitted to simplify. *(B)* Prolongation of the dominant time constant of the canal ocular reflex (T_{COR}) by velocity storage within the positive feedback pathways shown in *A.* A step change in head angular velocity occurred at time *0* (*vertical arrows*). T_1 represents the long time constant of the cupula measured from the average response of primary afferent neurons.

feedback to the secondary vestibular neurons.[182] While the response of the contralateral neurons during physiologic stimulation is opposite in sign to that of the ipsilateral neurons, the inhibitory interneurons convert the commissural pathway to a positive feedback loop. The net effect is to provide a temporal integration of signals from different vestibular receptors and from other sensory systems while sustaining activity in the vestibular nuclei beyond that of the primary afferent signal, so-called velocity storage.[166]

The effect of velocity storage is graphically illustrated in Figure 3–4B. After an impulse of head acceleration, the time constant of the oculomotor response (T_{COR}) is prolonged beyond that of the primary afferent response (T_1) due to feedback onto the secondary vestibular neurons. The positive feedback loops perform the equivalent of a mathematical integration on the primary afferent signal.[172] The interneurons in these feedback pathways can be viewed as valves controlling the spontaneous ac-

tivity and dynamic properties of the secondary vestibular neurons.

Many of the direct connections from the vestibular nuclei to the oculomotor neurons are part of a large fiber bundle, the medial longitudinal fascicle (MLF), lying along the floor of the fourth ventricle. This fiber bundle extends from the cervical cord to the reticular substance of the midbrain and thalamus, providing an interconnecting pathway between the vestibular and the oculomotor complex in the rostral brainstem as well as connections to the abducens nuclei in the middle brainstem.[60] In addition to sending axons into the third and fourth nuclei, the MLF also sends collaterals into the reticular substance of the midbrain and thalamus.

SEMICIRCULAR CANAL–OCULAR REFLEXES

Detailed information about the connections that link vestibular receptors and different eye muscles was initially obtained by recording the eye muscle response following either physiologic or electric stimulation of each receptor.[45, 98, 116] By measuring the muscle tonus, the excitatory or inhibitory nature of each connection was established. Table 3–1 summarizes the primary excitatory and inhibitory connections of each semicircular canal with the muscles of both eyes.[98] Note that each semicircular canal is connected to the eye muscles in such a way that stimulation of the canal nerve results in eye movement approximately in the plane of that canal. For example, stimulation of the left posterior canal nerve causes excitation of the ipsilateral superior oblique and the contralateral inferior rectus muscles while inhibiting the ipsilateral inferior oblique and the contralateral superior rectus. An oblique downward movement in the plane of the left posterior canal is the end result. As suggested in Chapter 1 (see Classification of Vestibular Reflexes), tonic activity arriving at each eye muscle from all the labyrinthine organs provides an important background upon which these specific reflexes act.[116]

By systematically recording in different vestibular and oculomotor nuclei after selective stimulation of each semicircular canal, it has been possible to trace the main *disynaptic* excitatory and inhibitory pathways connecting the semicircular canals with the extraocular muscles (Fig. 3–5).[195, 196] As a general rule, excitatory connections run in the contralateral MLF and inhibitory connections in the ipsilateral MLF.[148] The connections illustrated in Figure 3–5 are only part of the picture, however. In as much as the planes of the semicircular canals are not exactly aligned with the planes of the three pairs of eye muscles, a spatial transformation from the canal to muscle coordinates must occur if eye movements are to compensate for head movements. In other words, it is not adequate to simply connect afferents from a single canal to a set of eye muscles (as shown in Fig. 3–5); other connections must also exist. Preliminary studies of labeled secondary vestibular neurons identified as part of the canal ocular reflex indicate that the spatial transformations occur through both a convergence of signals at the level of the vestibular nuclei and a divergence of signals at the level of the oculomotor nuclei.[152]

OTOLITH–OCULAR REFLEXES

The pathways from the maculae to the extraocular muscles are less clearly defined than are those from the semicircular canals. The latency of eye muscle activation after stimulation of the utricular and saccular nerves is similar to that recorded after semicircular canal nerve stimulation; disynaptic pathways also exist from the maculae to the extraocular muscles.[23, 58, 179] Because of the varied orientation of hair cells within the maculae, simultaneous stimulation of all the nerve fibers coming from a macula produces a nonphysiologic excitation, and the induced eye movements fail to represent the naturally occurring ones. Selective stimulation of different parts of the utriculus and sacculus results in mostly vertical and vertical-rotatory eye movements.[63, 189] As one would expect, stimulation on each side of the striola produces oppositely directed rotatory and vertical components. Each of the vertical eye muscles appears to be connected to specific areas of the maculae so that groups of hair cells whose kinocilia are oriented in opposite directions excite agonist and antagonist muscles.

SUMMARY

Several basic principles underlie the connections between the labyrinthine end-organs and eye muscles. First, a receptor organ is connected to a group of motoneu-

Table 3–1. CONNECTIONS OF THE SEMICIRCULAR CANALS WITH MUSCLES OF THE EYES

Semicircular Canal	Excitation	Inhibition
Horizontal	I — MR	C — MR
	C — LR	I — LR
Posterior	I — SO	I — IO
	C — IR	C — SR
Anterior	I — SR	I — IR
	C — IO	C — SO

I = Ipsilateral; C = contralateral; MR = medial rectus; LR = lateral rectus; SO = superior oblique; IO = inferior oblique; SR = superior rectus; IR = inferior rectus.

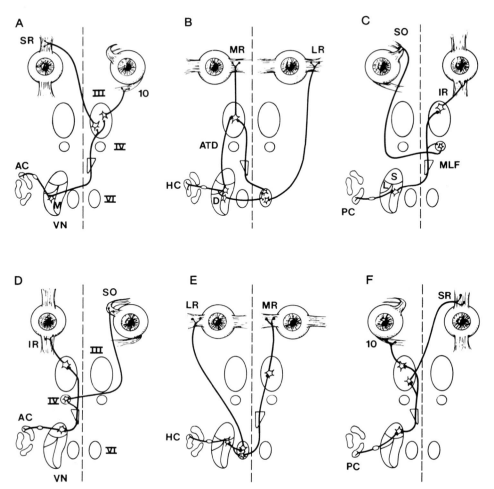

Figure 3–5. Excitatory *(a, b, c)* and inhibitory *(d, e, f)* pathways between the individual semicircular canals and eye muscles in the cat.[195, 196] *SR,* superior rectus; *IO,* inferior oblique; *MR,* medial rectus; *LR,* lateral rectus; *SO,* superior oblique; *IR,* inferior rectus; *AC,* anterior canal; *HC,* horizontal canal; *PC,* posterior canal; *VN,* vestibular nuclei; *S,* superior vestibular nucleus; *M,* medial vestibular nucleus; *L,* lateral vestibular nucleus; *D,* descending vestibular nucleus; *ATD,* ascending tract of Dieters; *VI,* abducens nucleus; *IV,* cochlear nucleus; *III,* oculomotor complex.

rons whose activity produces an eye muscle contraction that compensates for a specific head movement with the objective of maintaining gaze stability. Second, blind spots do not exist in the receptive field of the inner ear organs because the organs in each ear form a complementary set of acceleration sensors capable of reacting to the individual components of linear and angular acceleration associated with head movement in any direction in three-dimensional space. Third, each receptor organ simultaneously activates an excitatory and inhibitory pathway to agonist

and antagonist muscles resulting in a push-pull system of control (as illustrated in Fig. 1–7) Fourth, most natural head movements activate several receptors simultaneously, and inputs from multiple receptors converge on secondary neurons. Fifth, alternate pathways complement the elementary disynaptic connections. These pathways consist of interneurons that form reverberating circuits by means of which different reflexes interact and "fine-tune" the more specific end-organ reflexes. Finally, the strength and even the specificity of some connections can be modified by multisensory interactions, as will be discussed later (see Adaptive Modification of the Vestibulo-Ocular Reflex with Vision).

Characteristics of Eye Movements Induced by Stimulation of Semicircular Canals

COMPENSATORY EYE MOVEMENTS

The semicircular canal-ocular reflexes produce eye movements that compensate for head rotations. This is easily demonstrated in lower animals, such as the rabbit, who have few spontaneous eye movements. Angular head rotation of small amplitude within the frequency range of natural head movements (0.1 to 4.0 Hz) results in compensatory sinusoidal eye movements 180 degrees out of phase with the head (as illustrated in Figs. 1–3a, 3b) The various transformations involved in this process are illustrated in Figure 3–6. The natural stimulus for the semicircular canals is head angular acceleration as shown in Figure 3–6b. During sinusoidal rotation at the frequencies of natural head movements, the viscoelastic properties of the canal-cupula complex (as defined by the pendulum model, Chapter 2) produce the equivalent of one step of mathematical in-

tegration (a 90-degree phase shift), so that the vestibular nerve firing rate (e) is in phase with head velocity rather than head acceleration. The normal reflex response produces a compensatory eye movement equal and opposite to that of the head movement (compare a and g in Fig. 3–6). This eye movement results from activation of, among others, the abducens nerve to the left lateral rectus muscle (f) during ampullopetal stimulation of the right cupula-vestibular nerve (d and e). However, the recorded activity in the abducens nerve lags behind the activity in the vestibular nerve by an additional 90-degree delay. This raises a key question first asked by Skavinski and Robinson:[186] What produces the phase shift between the firing rates of the vestibular and abducens nerves [between e and f]? To answer the question, they introduced the concept of an oculomotor integrator, a hypothetical neural network that integrates, in a mathematical sense, velocity-coded signals (such as those originating in the vestibular end-organ) to position-coded signals required by the oculomotor neurons. Although the concept of neural integration is now generally accepted, the specifics are still debated. Some feel it is "localized" in a region of the brainstem[33, 37] or cerebellum,[36] but others consider it a "distributed property" of the multiple feedback pathways shown in Fig-

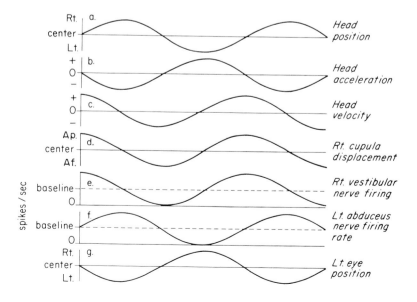

Figure 3–6. Mechanism by which sinusoidal changing head position (a) is converted to an equal and opposite eye position (g). Ap, ampullopetal; Af, ampullofugal. See text for details.

ure 3–4A. Galiana and Outerbridge[68] developed a mathematical model to show how these feedback pathways, particularly those via the commissural connections, could produce the necessary integration.

Although the VOR operates as an integrating angular accelerometer for frequencies greater than 0.1 Hz, at lower frequencies there is a progressive phase lead of eye velocity relative to head velocity reaching a maximum of 90 degrees at about 0.001 Hz (see Fig. 3, Appendix). Velocity storage within the central VOR feedback pathways (those illustrated in Fig. 3–4A) improves the low-frequency phase deficit of incoming primary afferent signals but does not correct it completely. As will be shown later, this low-frequency phase shift of the VOR is of little functional significance, inasmuch as natural head movements combine visual and vestibular stimulation and the visuovestibulo-ocular responses are perfectly compensatory even at the lowest frequencies. It does have important implications for clinical testing, however, because an increase in the low-frequency phase lead is a nonspecific sign of damage to the canal-ocular reflexes (see Chapter 7).

In summary, the vestibulo-ocular reflex involves the activity of many nuclei and a countless number of neurons, the group behavior of which may differ from that of the isolated units. This complexity must be kept in mind when attempting to evaluate the effects of lesions on vestibulo-ocular reflex activity. It is often impossible to interpret the results of vestibular tests in terms of deficits in a single neural pathway.

NYSTAGMUS

Description. If the stimulus to the semicircular canals is of large magnitude—one that cannot be compensated for by the motion of the eye in the orbit—the slow vestibular-induced eye deviation is interrupted with a quick movement in the opposite direction (Fig. 1–4c,d). This combination of rhythmic slow and fast movements in opposite directions is called nystagmus. Although the eye movement during the slow component takes place in different locations in the orbit, gaze stabi-

lization is still possible because the eye velocity during the slow component is approximately equal and opposite to that of the head. Because of the resetting fast components, the trajectory of the eye motion during the slow components effectively compensates for the head rotation, as if the eye had unlimited freedom of motion.

Neuronal Mechanisms for the Production of Nystagmus. The relationship between the firing rate of oculomotor neurons and the movements of the eyes during each phase of nystagmus has been studied extensively. Figure 3–7 shows the membrane potential changes of an abducens motoneuron associated with nystagmus in both directions. During the production of an agonist slow component (Fig. 3–7b), the membrane potential is slowly depolarized by excitatory postsynaptic potentials arriving via the vestibulo-ocular pathways discussed in the previous sections.[7, 121] Toward the end of the slow component, the membrane potential rapidly becomes hyperpolarized, and the motoneuron abruptly terminates its discharge. This hyperpolarization is produced by inhibitory burst neurons located in the pontomedullary reticular formation just caudal to the contralateral abducens nucleus.[86] The firing rate of the abducens nerves shown in the middle and lower traces of Figure 3–7 reflect the build-up of excitatory and inhibitory activity recorded intracellularly in the motoneuron. The opposite membrane potential changes and abducens nerve firing rate occur when the neuron is participating antagonistically in the production of the slow component of nystagmus (Fig. 3–7d).

Figure 3–8 illustrates the firing rate of a single right abducens nerve fiber during sinusoidal angular rotation at three different magnitudes.[93] The concurrent nystagmus of the left eye is shown above each firing record. With slow components to the right, the right abducens nerve is innervating an agonist muscle, and a steady increase in nerve firing occurs that is roughly proportional to the eye displacement. Just before initiation of the fast component in the opposite direction (to the left), the firing of the right abducens nerve suddenly decreases and, in many in-

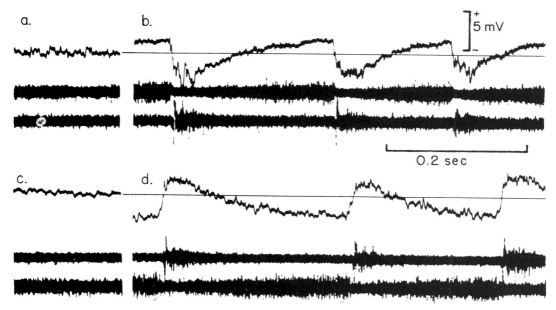

Figure 3–7. Intracellular recording of membrane potential changes in a left abducens motoneuron *(upper traces)* and firing rate of the left *(middle traces)* and right *(lower traces)* abducens nerve before *(a and c)* and during nystagmus induced by stimulation of the right *(b)* and left *(d)* vestibular nerve. Horizontal lines indicate the membrane potential levels (– 41 mv in *b* and – 43 mv in *d*). (From Maeda et al.,[121] with permission.)

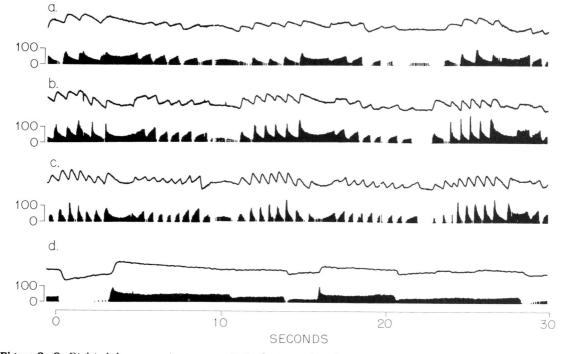

Figure 3–8. Right abducens motoneuron activity during induced nystagmus in the cat. In each pair of traces, the *top trace* represents the EOG recording of eye movement and the *bottom trace* the motoneuron firing frequency. In *a*, *b*, and *c*, the animal was rotated at the frequency of 0.1 Hz at peak velocities of 30, 60, and 120 deg/sec, respectively. Spontaneous eye movements (saccades) are shown in *d*.

stances, stops completely. During the subsequent slow component, the nerve fiber remains silent until the eye reaches a position in the orbit that is above threshold for this particular abducens neuron. With slow components to the left, an abrupt increase in firing rate occurs just before the onset of the fast component, followed by a slow decrease during the slow components. Although the change in nerve firing rate during the slow component bears a close relationship to the change in eye position, during the fast component a much larger increase in action potentials occurs per unit of time.

Measurement of the relationship between motoneuron firing rates and eye movement induced by vestibular or visual stimuli has shown that the motoneurons behave the same, regardless of the nature of the stimulus.[171] Almost all oculomotor neurons exhibit a threshold above which they increase their firing rate roughly in proportion to the change in eye position in the orbit. A small percentage of the change in firing rate (approximately 20 percent) is proportional to the velocity of the eye movement. It is as though the firing rate of the oculomotor neurons were designed to overcome the elastic and viscous forces (roughly in a ratio of 5 to 1) restraining the eye in the orbit. This relationship can best be appreciated by examining the rate of firing of an oculomotor neuron associated with a visually induced refixation saccade (Fig. 3–8d), in which the goal is to move the eyes as rapidly as possible from one position in the orbit to another and to maintain the new position once it is reached. During the high-velocity saccade, the oculomotor neuron increases its firing rate to a high level to compensate for the viscous drag of the eye ligaments.[161] Once the new position is reached, a much lower rate of discharge produces compensation for the elastic restraining force and maintains the new position. Although the reflex pathways for vestibular and visually induced eye movements involve different neuronal circuits, the motoneuorns governing the extrinsic eye muscles fire in the same manner regardless of the original sensory input.

Fast Component Generation. Groups of neurons in the paramedian pontine reticular formation (PPRF) fire in short bursts of activity just before the onset of horizontal fast components and voluntary saccades.[41, 102, 187] Apparently, fast eye movements, whether voluntary or involuntary, are generated by a common neuronal mechanism.[41] The PPRF is not a discrete anatomic structure but rather a region that has been designated because of its apparent functional specificity. Stimulation in the PPRF produces ipsilateral slow and rapid eye movements depending on the stimulus variables.[102] The latency of induced eye movements suggests that one or two synapses lie between the pontine neurons and the oculomotor neurons. Anatomic pathways between this area of the reticular formation and the eye muscle motor nuclei were first reported by Lorente de Nó[117] and subsequently confirmed by other investigators.[81] Numerous documented anatomic pathways also interconnect the vestibular nuclei with the PPRF.[81] Apparently, neurons in the PPRF monitor vestibulo-ocular signals and intermittently discharge to produce corrective fast components based on certain features of the vestibulo-ocular signal (see below).

Pattern of Eye Motion. Intuitively one might assume that the slow phases of nystagmus deviate the eyes toward the periphery of the orbit, and the fast components reset them back to the center. Indeed, this pattern occurs in the rabbit (see Fig. 1–3). In animals with more developed visual oculomotor function, however, the fast components act as anticipatory movements taking the eyes toward the periphery.[135] The fast components of the initial beats of nystagmus are larger than the preceding slow components, and the eyes deviate in the direction of the fast component (see Fig. 7–6). In the human being, the exact threshold position varies with the velocity of the slow component of nystagmus, but it is usually near the midposition.[92] The apparent advantage of this strategy is that the eyes are ready to focus on newly arriving targets in the field of rotation, and fixation can be maintained during the subsequent slow component.

Effect of Experimental Lesions

Spontaneous Nystagmus. Spontaneous vestibular nystagmus is produced in animals by lesions of the labyrinth, the vestibular nerve, and the vestibular nuclei.[45] A key ingredient for the production of spontaneous nystagmus is an imbalance in the vestibulo-ocular pathways. Damage to one labyrinth results in spontaneous nystagmus, the slow component of which is directed toward the lesion side; the tonic input from the intact side is no longer balanced by input from the damaged side. This spontaneous nystagmus is indistinguishable from nystagmus produced by stimulation of the normal labyrinth. If a process simultaneously removes both labyrinths, spontaneous nystagmus does not result, demonstrating that, for production of nystagmus, the relative balance of input is more important than the absolute magnitude of input.

Spontaneous nystagmus produced by sectioning of the vestibular nerve duplicates that resulting from labyrinthectomy. The slow component is directed toward the side of the lesion. The direction of spontaneous nystagmus associated with lesions of the vestibular nuclei, however, is less predictable and depends on the location and extent of the lesion. Uemura and Cohen[197] produced spontaneous nystagmus in monkeys with small focal lesions in the vestibular nuclei. They found that the slow phase of nystagmus developed contralateral to lesions in the superior and rostral medial nuclei and ipsilateral to lesions in the lateral and caudal medial nuclei. The imbalance between inhibitory and excitatory secondary vestibular neurons undoubtedly determined the direction of spontaneous nystagmus.

Induced Nystagmus. Lesions involving the vestibulo-ocular pathways in animals may affect either the slow or the fast component and occasionally both phases of induced nystagmus. Interruption of the connections linking the semicircular canals to the oculomotor neurons decreases the velocity of the slow components of induced nystagmus. Lesions involving the peripheral vestibular structures (end-organ and nerve) affect the nystagmus in both eyes equally, because the central pathways are symmetrically connected. A single remaining labyrinth senses angular rotation in both directions and produces conjugate nystagmus in both directions. The maximum slow component velocity of induced nystagmus may be asymmetric, however, because of the asymmetry in afferent nerve firing rate produced by ampullopetal and ampullofugal endolymph flow (see Characteristics of Primary Afferent Neurons, Chapter 2). Central lesions lying anywhere from the vestibular nuclei to the oculomotor neurons often produce disconjugate nystagmus, because the pathways to the eye muscles diverge beginning at the vestibular nuclei. A lesion of the MLF, for example, impairs slow and fast components made by the ipsilateral medial rectus muscle but leaves normal slow and fast components at the contralateral lateral rectus (see Fig. 7–6).

The proposed role of the PPRF in the production of rapid horizontal eye movements is largely based on the results of experimental lesions in several species of animals. Animals with unilateral lesions of the PPRF lose all types of rapid ipsilateral eye movement, and the eyes move in the contralateral hemifield.[43, 82] Ipsilateral voluntary saccades and quick phases of vestibular and optokinetic nystagmus are affected equally. Stimuli that normally would produce nystagmus with ipsilateral fast components simply cause a strong tonic contralateral deviation of the eyes (see Fig. 7–6). On the other hand, vestibular stimuli that produce contralateral fast components result in normal nystagmus (i.e., ipsilateral slow phases are normal). Lesions in the pretectal region have a similar effect on vertical rapid eye movements without affecting horizontal eye movements[21, 83]— an effect consistent with the separate neural organization of horizontal and vertical saccades.[81]

Level of Arousal and Habituation. Since the turn of the century, numerous investigators have noted a relationship between the magnitude of induced nystagmus and the state of arousal of the animals or human subjects receiving vestibular stimulation.[48] In animal studies amphetamines are routinely used to maintain alertness. Collins[49] first began a systemic evaluation of the instructions given to human subjects aimed at controlling alertness during rotational and caloric testing and found that the velocity of the slow components of induced nystagmus depended on the type of mental activity. If the subject was instructed to relax and daydream, the velocity was less than when the subject was instructed to perform continuous mental arithmetic (successive division). Although other techniques of mental alerting, such as having the subject report on the turning sensation or estimate the time of auditory stimuli, were also effective, mental arithmetic tasks were most effective in maintaining mental alertness. The mental task had to achieve a certain degree of complexity, inasmuch as simple forward-counting was not effective in maintaining the nystagmus response.[48]

If a normal subject is continuously rotated at low sinusoidal frequencies in the dark, there is a gradual decrease in gain and an increase in the phase lead of eye velocity relative to head velocity (so-called habituation).[9, 99] The effect peaks in about an hour and can persist for days. Presumably, with habituation, there is a gradual decrease in velocity storage within the multineural pathways illustrated in Figure 3–4, shifting the low-frequency response of the canal-ocular reflex toward that of primary afferent signal (i.e., the VOR time constant decreases towards that of the cupula—see Appendix). Because a caloric stimulus is equivalent to a low-frequency rotational stimulus, habituation with repeated caloric testing is explained on a similar basis. Alerting techniques (including stimulant drugs) probably work by activating the multineural feedback pathways and thereby improving the low-frequency response of the canal ocular reflex.

Characteristics of Eye Movements Induced by Otolith Stimulation

GENERAL PROPERTIES

Because the sensory cells of each macula are oriented in multiple directions, the firing rate of the macular afferent nerve reflects a complex pattern of excitation and inhibition of different units within the macula. By comparison, all the sensory cells of a semicircular canal crista are aligned in the same direction and are ei-

ther excited or inhibited by a stimulus acting in the plane of the canal. The organization of the otolith-ocular reflexes is, therefore, more complex than that of canal-ocular reflexes. To simplify the discussion of otolith-ocular reflexes, it has been traditional to consider the otolith organs (utriculus and sacculus combined) as a unitary sensor capable of resolving all of the linear forces acting on the head into a single resultant vector force. This "unitary" three-dimensional otolith receptor is positioned at the center of the head with the x and y axes orthogonal to, and the z axis parallel to, the earth's vertical axis. The receptor computes the angle (θ) between the resultant vector force and the earth's vertical axis and sends this information to the central nervous system (CNS), where a compensatory eye deviation is generated with the goal of maintaining the eyes normal to the earth's vertical axis. The perfect macular reflex would be one that rotates the eyes at an angle equal and opposite to θ. In the case of head tilt in the sagittal plane, as illustrated in Figure 3–9, the efficiency or gain of the reflex can be represented by the relation of the angle of the eye deviation α to the angle of head tilt θ (gain equals α/θ). With these concepts in mind, it is interesting to compare the eye movements produced by head tilt (Fig. 3–9b) with those produced by linear acceleration of the head (Figure 3–9c).

EYE MOVEMENTS PRODUCED BY HEAD TILT

Compensatory eye movements produced by static head tilt in different animals are either rotational or torsional, depending on the direction of tilt and the position of the orbits in the skull. In rabbits and fish, lateral tilt causes a vertically directed rotational movement, and forward-backward tilt causes a torsional eye movement. In humans, compensatory torsional movements are produced by lateral tilt (ocular counterrolling), and vertical rotation results from forward-backward tilt (see Fig. 3–9). Eye movements associated with static tilt have been studied most extensively in the rabbit. Head tilt in the dark within a range of ±45 degrees about the

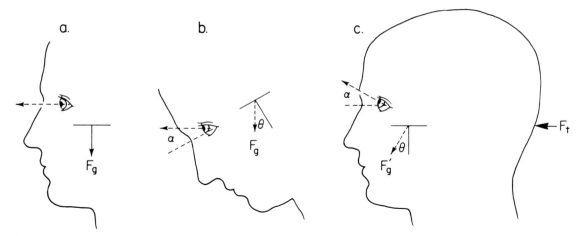

Figure 3–9. Compensatory eye movement induced by static head tilt *(b)* and by linear acceleration tangential to the "unitary" otolith receptor *(c)*. α equals the angle of eye rotation and θ equals the angle between the resultant force of gravity and a line orthogonal to the receptor.

normal position causes a compensatory eye deviation with a gain of approximately 0.6[3] That is, the angle of eye rotation (α) is approximately 60 percent of the angle of tilt (θ). In human subjects, the ocular response to tilt is much less efficient. The maximum ocular torsion for a lateral tilt of 50 degrees is only 5 to 6 degrees (a gain of approximately 0.1).[139]

EYE MOVEMENTS PRODUCED BY LINEAR ACCELERATION OF THE HEAD

Linear Track Acceleration. Continuous linear acceleration in a vehicle along a straight track theoretically constitutes an ideal stimulus to test the function of the otolith-ocular reflex arc. The direction of the linear acceleration vector lies perpendicular to the earth-vertical, and the effective stimulus is the result of interaction of the force due to the vehicle acceleration with that of gravity (e.g., see Figs. 1–1C and 3–9c). Unfortunately, from a clinical point of view, the length of track required to produce measurable otolith-ocular reflexes is much greater than is feasible.

Niven and coworkers[144] used a linear track to produce periodic linear accelerations in human subjects at different frequencies and in different head orientations. Linear acceleration along the

interaural axis induced compensatory horizontal eye movements (including nystagmus), but acceleration in the head-foot axis (lying) or occipitonasal axis (sitting) did not induce vertical eye movements. The horizontal eye movements induced by linear acceleration in the interaural axis were about the same whether the subjects were lying or sitting. The magnitude and phase of the horizontal nystagmus induced by linear acceleration (so-called L-nystagmus) were different from those associated with periodic angular acceleration of the canals in a comparable frequency range, so it is unlikely that they resulted from unanticipated stimulation of the horizontal canals. Buizza and associates[22] also produced horizontal L-nystagmus in seated normal subjects during horizontal acceleration along the interaural axis in the dark.

Parallel Swing. The parallel swing consists of a platform suspended from the ceiling by four stiff bars about 2 to 3 meters in length. The moving parts are connected by ball bearings so that the platform can be displaced in only one direction. The natural period (T) in seconds of the swing is dependent on the length of arms (λ) in meters by $T = 2\pi\sqrt{\lambda/g}$. The oscillation amplitude and hence the acceleration depend on the initial deviation of the platform, which, once released, exhibits a damped oscillation with a frequency of 1/T. The parallel swing has a vertical as well as a horizontal displacement, although the former is small if the amplitude is small.

Eye movements induced in a normal subject sitting on a parallel swing in the dark are shown in Figure 3–10.[8] Displacement along the interaural axis (upper three traces) produced sinusoidal horizontal eye movements with occasional corrective fast components. Vertical eye movements were approximately sinusoidal with a frequency twice that of the swing frequency. When subjects sat facing forward so that the linear acceleration occurred in the occipitonasal axis, almost identical vertical but no consistent horizontal eye movements were induced (lower three traces). Frequency analysis of similar data from 10 normal subjects revealed a mean gain (peak eye velocity/peak swing velocity) of 3.8 to 4.7 deg/m and a mean phase shift (eye velocity re swing velocity) of − 152 to − 160 degrees for horizontal and vertical displacements over a range of swing amplitudes. The values for horizontal eye movements are comparable to those obtained with a linear sled by Niven and colleagues[144] and Buizza and associates[22] (see Table 3–6, Reference 8).

FUNCTIONAL IMPLICATIONS

Following the simple model of otolith function illustrated in Figure 3–9 one would predict that linear acceleration along the occipitonasal axis (y axis) would result in vertical eye movements and linear acceleration along the interaural axis (x axis), torsional eye movements (just as lateral tilt produces ocular counter rolling). As noted above, however, linear acceleration in the occipitonasal axis produces minimal vertical eye movements and acceleration along the interaural axis induces predominantly horizontal eye movements. The brain must be able to distinguish between gravity and other linear acceleration components (transient or oscillating) of the otolith signal. This is reasonable from a functional point of view, since the logical function of the reflex is to augment visual pursuit during linear displacement of the head (analogous to the role of the canal-ocular reflex during angular displacement of the head). Lateral head movements require horizontal, not torsional, eye movements to maintain fixation on an earth-fixed target. Similarly, with fore-aft movements, vertical eye movements would impair rather than improve fixation on an

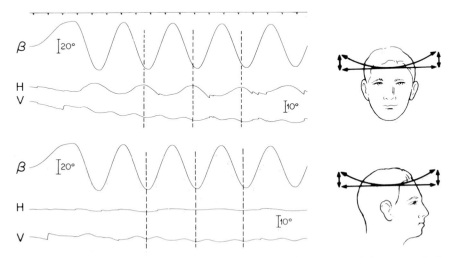

Figure 3–10. Horizontal *(H)* and vertical *(V)* eye movements induced on the parallel swing with the subject sitting with eyes open in the dark *(mental alerting)*. In the *upper three traces* horizontal linear acceleration occurred along the interaural axis; in the *lower three traces*, along the occipitonasal axis. *Vertical dashed lines* demonstrate the phase shift between zero eye velocity and zero swing velocity. Interval between tick marks: 1 second. The *horizontal* and *vertical lines* and *arrows (right side)* indicate direction and relative magnitude of the horizontal and vertical components of swing displacement; *curved lines* indicate actual swing trajectory. (From Baloh et al.,[8] with permission.)

earth-fixed target in the axis of movement. How this distinction is achieved at the cellular level is yet to be determined.

Interaction of Semicircular Canal and Otolith-Induced Eye Movements

Most natural head movements are composed of a combination of linear and angular displacements so that the canal and otolith-ocular reflexes must work together to assure steady fixation. There is an important difference, however, between the geometry of target displacement with angular and linear accelerations. With the latter the angle of the required compensatory eye movement increases as the target moves closer to the subject. Buizza and colleagues[30] proposed a model of canal-otolith-ocular reflex interaction that assumes that the gain of the canal-ocular reflex is fixed while the otolith-ocular reflex gain increases with decreasing target distance. Their simple model ignores interocular spacing and the separation of the vestibular organs from the eyes (i.e., it assumes a central cyclopean eye), but this is not a major problem as long as the target distance is greater than a meter. With this model, if the head rotates with angular velocity A and translates with linear velocity T, then the eye angular velocity $\omega = -A - KT$, where K inversely depends on target distance. Virre and associates[200] recently showed that the magnitude of induced eye movements measured in monkeys during combined linear and angular accelerations (by varying the radius of head rotation) was dependent on target location. Furthermore, they observed that the adjustments occurred too fast (within 10 ms) to be visually guided. They proposed that the oculomotor system makes use of a rapid, nonvisual estimate of current target location relative to the head by combining available visual, auditory, and proprioceptive information.

A series of recent studies in animals indicate that the velocity storage feedback pathways within the central VOR provide a key mechanism for otolith-canal interaction.[40, 165] This can best be illustrated by the response of a monkey to off-vertical axis rotation (OVAR) (Fig. 3–11). If the animal is rotated at a constant velocity about a tilted vertical axis, the slow phase velocity of induced nystagmus does not decay to zero (as when the monkey is vertical) but rather persists at a steady state level. If the animal is suddenly stopped, the postrotatory nystagmus after OVAR is much less than that when the animal is stopped in the upright position (in Fig. 3–11, compare B and C with A). Blocking the semicir-

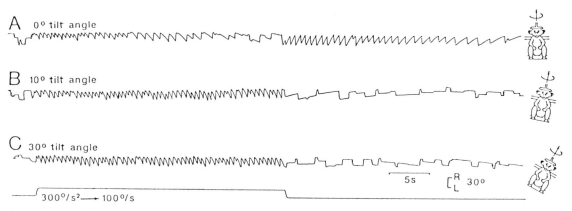

Figure 3–11. Off-axis vertical rotation (OVAR) in monkey. In *A* the animal is rotated about the earth-vertical axis; after the step change in angular velocity (0–100 deg/sec, acceleration 300 deg/sec²), the nystagmus slow phase velocity slowly declines with the time constant of the canal ocular reflex; deceleration induces similar nystagmus in the opposite direction. In *B* and *C*, with varying off-vertical angles, nystagmus persists during rotation at a constant velocity, and there is little nystagmus after the deceleration. (Adapted from Waespe, W and Henn, V: Gaze stabilization in the primate. The interaction of the vestibulo-ocular reflex, optokinetic nystagmus, and smooth pursuit. Rev Physiol Biochem Pharmacol 1987, 106:37.)

cular canals does not alter the steady state response during OVAR, indicating that the otoliths generate the signals necessary for the continuous nystagmus. It has been postulated that sequential excitation and inhibition of the otolith hair cells by the rotating gravity vector produces a traveling wave the velocity of which is estimated centrally and then passed on to the velocity storage integrator which produces the continuous horizontal nystagmus.[165] Raphan and Cohen[164] demonstrated that the velocity storage system can be activated by many types of stimuli (canal, otolith, vision), and through a three-dimensional gravity-dependent structure the system is capable of storing information to produce eye movements in all planes.

VESTIBULO-OCULAR REFLEX INTERACTION WITH OTHER SYSTEMS

Neck-Vestibular Interaction

INTRODUCTION

Ocular stability during most natural head movements results from a coordinated interaction of signals originating in vestibular, visual, and neck receptors. The compensatory nature of neck-induced eye movements has been documented in animals. In 1924, De Kleyn[53] showed that if one holds an animal's head stationary and displaces the body, a compensatory eye deviation occurs, which tends to preserve the relationship between gaze and the body axis. Nonfoveated animals, such as the rabbit, exhibit clear compensatory eye deviations because they possess almost no spontaneous eye movements.[78] Cervicoocular and vestibulo-ocular reflex interaction is more difficult to study in humans because of the dominance of voluntary and visually controlled eye movements. Very few investigators have quantitatively assessed eye, head, and neck movement coordination in humans, and the clinical significance of lesions involving the cervicoocular reflex pathways is uncertain (see Cervical Dizziness and Vertigo, Chapter 17).

ANATOMIC AND PHYSIOLOGIC BASIS

Animal studies have shown that the cervico-ocular reflex originates from nerve endings in the ligaments and capsules of the upper cervical articulations.[85, 130] The reflex can be induced by electrically stimulating the capsules of the upper cervical joints, the C_1 to C_3 dorsal roots, and the high cervical spinal cord. The reflex is not induced by stimulating the superficial muscles or skin of the neck. Bilateral sectioning of the high cervicodorsal roots or the application of local anesthetic around the cervical articulations abolishes the cervico-ocular reflexes. Unilateral interruption of the neck-ocular reflex pathways produces nystagmus in rabbits, cats, and monkeys when fixation is inhibited, although no consistent relationship exists between the side of dorsal root involvement and the direction of nystagmus.[52, 94] As with the vestibulo-ocular reflexes, the eye muscles are either excited or inhibited by neck stimulation, depending on whether the muscle is agonistic or antagonistic for the required compensatory movement.

Electrophysiologic experiments suggest that the cervico-ocular reflexes are mediated via the vestibular nuclei (primarily in the medial and descending nuclei).[85, 174] The precise projections of the neck afferents to each vestibular nucleus are only partially known, but it can be anticipated that inasmuch as the neck-induced eye movements compensate for displacement in the precise plane of body motion, the vestibular nuclei must contain a discrete topographic representation of cervical afferents in a manner similar to that of the vestibular afferents.

Electric stimulation of the high cervicodorsal roots in the cat produces evoked potentials in the contralateral vestibular nuclei[85] followed by excitation of the abducens nucleus ipsilateral to the neck stimulation and inhibition of the contralateral abducens nucleus. In addition, stimulation of the cervicodorsal roots enhances the amplitude of action potentials in the ipsilateral abducens nerve induced by contralateral vestibular nerve stimulation and inhibits action potentials in the contralateral abducens nerve induced by ipsilateral vestibular nerve stimulation. Vestibulo-ocular and cervico-ocular reflex interaction, therefore, results from a convergence of neck and semicircular canal afferents on secondary vestibular neurons.

CHARACTERISTICS OF NECK-INDUCED EYE MOVEMENTS

Figure 3–12 illustrates the synergistic interaction of neck and vestibulo-ocular reflexes. When the rabbit's head is turned to the right (clockwise about the cephalocaudal axis) the eyes turn counterclockwise in the orbit because the movement stimulates the horizontal semicircular canals and neck reflexes. (see Fig. 3–12b). The direction of the eye movement is the same as if the whole animal had been rotated, stimulating only the semicircular canals (see Fig. 3–12c). The characteristics of the neck-ocular reflex alone are evaluated by rotating the body while the head is stationary (see Fig. 3–12a). The same relationship between head and torso is produced as in Figure 3–12b, and the eyes deviate in the same direction. In both instances the normal relationship between eyes and torso is maintained.

Since the time of Bárány, rotating the body with the head stationary and measuring the eye movements has been considered a potential functional test of the human neck-ocular reflex pathways.[15, 17, 133, 190] Several methodologic problems have been encountered, however. It is difficult to induce body motion and concurrently maintain the head completely stationary so as to avoid vestibular stimulation. As with vestibular-induced eye movements, care must be taken to inhibit fixation while monitoring the neck-induced eye movement. Even if these problems are overcome, a body torsion of 50 to 60 degrees results in a compensatory eye deviation of only 4 to 5 degrees.[133] The magnitude of the reflex response varies with the frequency of sinusoidal body rotation, being optimal 0.1 and 1.0 Hz (when eye and body motion are in phase).[190] Compensatory sinusoidal eye movements induced by sinusoidal body rotation take on the appearance of nystagmus if the stimulus is large enough. The direction of the slow phase of nystagmus is such that the eye is driven in phase with the motion of the trunk.

The neck-ocular reflexes exert influence on both vestibular- and optokinetic-induced nystagmus. Tonic neck deviation in the rabbit produces an imbalance in the otherwise symmetrical nystagmus that results from rotating the animal sinusoidally

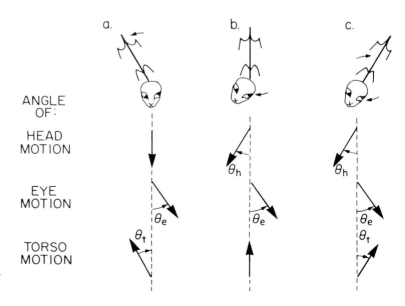

Figure 3–12. Synergistic interaction of cervico-ocular and vestibulo-ocular reflexes. See text for details.

ANGLE OF:

HEAD MOTION

EYE MOTION

TORSO MOTION

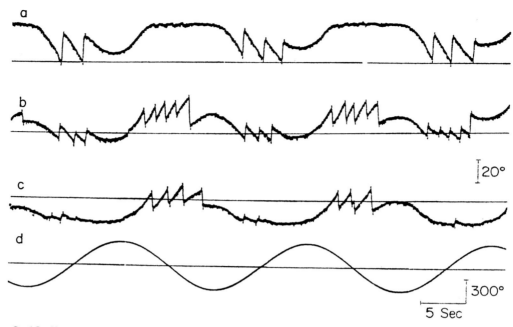

Figure 3–13. Nystagmus induced in a rabbit by sinusoidal angular rotation *(d)* with the head maintained at three orientations with respect to the torso. In *a*, *b*, and *c* the head is to the left, straight ahead, and to the right, respectively. In *a*, the mean eye position is displaced to the right, and left beating nystagmus is inhibited. The reverse occurs in *c*.

with the head and body normally aligned. When the slow components of nystagmus are in the direction of the neck-induced tonic ocular deviation, the amplitude of the fast components and the velocity of the slow components are smaller than those of the nystagmus in the opposite direction. Figure 3–13 illustrates cervicovestibuloocular reflex interaction when a rabbit is sinusoidally rotated with the head maintained at three different positions with respect to the body. When the head is turned to the left (see Fig. 3–13*a*), the mean eye position and slow components are displaced to the right and fast components to the left are inhibited. The reverse occurs when the head is tonically deviated to the right (see Fig. 3–13*c*).

Visual-Vestibular Interaction

INTRODUCTION

The relationship between the head and an object in the environment may change in several ways. The object may move relative to the head, the head may move relative to the object, or the head and object may move simultaneously. The visual and vestibular signals interact synergistically to stabilize gaze during most natural head movements. As discussed in the previous section, if the neck is also turned, the neck-ocular reflex participates in the compensatory movement. The effect is better ocular stability than would be possible if each system worked alone. Occasionally vestibular and visual signals conflict and one signal must override the other in order to maintain gaze stability. In these instances the visually mediated ocular reflexes override the vestibulo-ocular reflex. For example, when the head and visual target are moving at the same velocity, the vestibulo-ocular reflex is supressed and gaze is maintained on the target (see Fig. 1–9).

Three visually controlled ocular stabilizing systems produce versional eye movements: the saccadic, the smooth pursuit, and optokinetic systems.[55, 170, 202, 209, 210] In everyday life these three systems interact for the maintenance of gaze as subjects attempt to identify moving objects in space and maintain stability in gaze.[170, 202] The optokinetic is the phylogenetically older system; the other two are related to the anatomic development of the fovea. The saccade system responds to an error in the direction of gaze with respect to the position of an object of interest by initiating a rapid eye movement (a saccade) to correct the "retinal position error," bringing the object to the fovea in the shortest possible time. The anatomy and physiology of saccades was briefly discussed earlier (see Fast Component Generation). The smooth pursuit system is responsible for maintaining gaze on a moving target; that is, it keeps the target within the foveal visual field. It compares the eye velocity with that of the target velocity and produces a continuous match of the eye and target velocity. The optokinetic system is generally considered to be a primitive form of smooth pursuit involving the whole retina instead of the fovea alone. The eye tracking motion is periodically interrupted by corrective saccades in the opposite direction to relocate the gaze on new targets coming into the visual field.

OPTOKINETIC NYSTAGMUS (OKN)

In afoveate animals, such as the rabbit, monocular stimulation results in a prominent asymmetry in response; temporonasal target motion induces much greater slow-phase velocity than nasotemporal motion.[4, 47] Also, there is a gradual build-up in slow phase velocity after the step onset of an optokinetic stimulus (over 20 to 30 seconds). In afoveate animals the peak OKN slow phase velocity rarely exceeds 30 deg/sec, whereas in foveate animals—including the human, OKN slow phase velocity may exceed 100 deg/sec.[170]

Although OKN can be elicited in primates with parafoveal stimulation, the strongest responses are induced when the fovea is included in the field of stimulation.[57, 198] Monocular asymmetry as seen in afoveate animals is not observed in adult monkeys or humans, but human infants exhibit a temporonasal preponderance during monocular stimulation in the first few months of life while the fovea is immature.[142] Also, monocular asymmetry has been observed in patients with maldeveloped foveas[11] and with congenital or early acquired amblyopia.[2]

In monkeys the OKN response to a step change in stimulus velocity has two dynamic components (Fig. 3–14B), a rapid initial jump in slow phase velocity (a) followed by a gradual rise to a steady state level (b).[44] If the lights are turned off after the steady state is achieved, the eye velocity immediately drops to a value near that achieved after the initial rapid rise (c) from which it slowly decays as optokinetic after nystagmus (OKAN) (d). The eye velocity reached after the initial fast jump varies from 40 to 80% of the stimulus velocity; the steady state values are almost equal to stimulus velocities up to 60 deg/sec but progressively decrease for higher stimulus velocities.[44] Also, OKN is more irregular at high stimulus velocities (see Fig. 3–14A), so that average gain values are less than peak values. The maximum initial velocity of OKAN varies with stimulus velocity but can exceed 70 deg/sec.[44] With sinusoidal optokinetic stimulation in monkeys, the gain of OKN is near 1 at low frequencies (<0.1 Hz) but progressively decreases at higher frequencies. (e.g., 0.3 to 0.5 at 2 to 4 Hz).[24, 150]

A slow build-up in OKN slow phase velocity is not observed in normal humans,[198] but it has been seen in patients with lesions of the retina,[2, 11] parietal lobe[12] and cerebellum.[10] If a normal subject is instructed to follow the stripes on an optokinetic drum, he or she produces a large-amplitude, low-frequency nystagmus ("look" OKN), and if he or she is instructed to stare straight ahead at the drum surface, the subject produces a small-amplitude high-frequency nystagmus ("stare" OKN). In normal human subjects the slow phase velocity of "look" OKN can exceed 100 deg/sec, but that of "stare" OKN rarely exceeds 60 deg/sec.[91] OKAN responses in humans are much less consistent than those in monkeys; the maximum initial slow phase velocity does not exceed 20 deg/sec.[103, 180]

SMOOTH PURSUIT

In foveate animals the smooth pursuit system functions to stabilize a moving target on the fovea. The system operates opti-

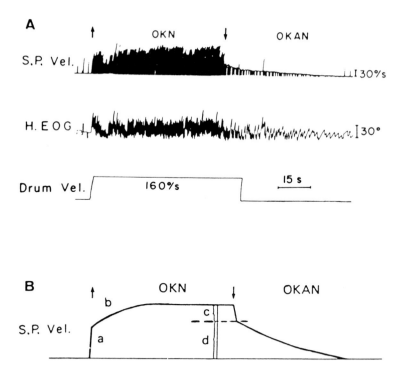

Figure 3–14. *(A)* Optokinetic nystagmus (OKN) and optokinetic after nystagmus (OKAN) in response to a velocity step of the optokinetic drum. *First trace,* velocity of horizontal eye movements, fast phases clipped; *second trace,* horizontal eye position; *third trace,* velocity profile of the optokinetic drum. *Upward arrow,* lights on; *downward arrow,* lights out. *(B)* Velocity envelope of the slow phases of OKN and OKAN redrawn schematically from the first trace in *A.* (From Waespe, W and Henn, V: Gaze stabilization in the primate. The interaction of the vestibulo-ocular reflex, optokinetic nystagmus and smooth pursuit. Rev Physiol Biochem Pharmacol 106:37, 1987, with permission.)

mally for low velocities and low frequencies of target motion.[18, 137] As the velocity and frequency increase (e.g., above 60 deg/sec or 1 Hz in humans), the eyes continually fall behind, and frequent corrective saccades are required to bring the target to the fovea. The gain of smooth pursuit is a function not only of target velocity but also of target acceleration.[111] Subjects pursue a target with constantly changing velocity better if the pattern of movement is predictable (as with a sinusoidal pattern).[18] Steinbach[188] suggested that the stimulus for smooth pursuit may be perceived target motion rather than actual target motion because subjects can pursue apparent target motion in the absence of a target moving across the retina. Also, subjects can pursue a stabilized retinal image eccentric to the fovea.[105, 156] Probably retinal velocity error is the main driving force for smooth pursuit eye movements with a lesser contribution from retinal position error and perceived target motion.

PURSUIT-OPTOKINETIC INTERACTION

When a subject tracks a moving target across a structured background an optoki-

netic stimulus is generated in the opposite direction yet pursuit remains smooth. Collewijn and colleagues[46] reported that the velocity of smooth pursuit in the human decreased by 20 to 30% in the presence of a stationary background (compared to pursuit in the dark). We and others[215] observed a small but predictable affect of a moving background on attempted smooth pursuit in the human; pursuit velocity increased with background movement in the same direction as the target and decreased with background movement in the opposite direction. In a later study of stationary and moving backgrounds, Kowler and coworkers[107] concluded that any observed effects on pursuit could be attributed to the subjects' effort or attention rather than to an involuntary integration of velocity information from the peripheral retina. Cerebral cortical pathways (see below) undoubtedly determine which targets are to be followed and which are to be neglected.

ORGANIZATION OF VISUALLY GUIDED TRACKING EYE MOVEMENTS

A simple scheme of visually guided tracking eye movements based on the concepts of Cohen and colleagues[42] is shown in Fig. 3–15. Visual motion information reaches the oculomotor neurons via two pathways: a direct pathway with fast dynamics and an indirect pathway with slower dynamics. A key feature of the indirect pathway is the velocity storage element shared with the vestibulo-ocular reflex. Optokinetic stimulation activates both pathways, whereas pursuit (according to Robinson[172]) activates only the direct pathway. The velocity storage element accounts for the slow build-up in optokinetic nystagmus and for OKAN. The direct pathway accounts for the initial rapid rise in OKN and the rapid drop after turning off the lights.

In 1936 Ter Braak[193] performed a series of experiments in which he confirmed the presence of cortical and subcortical optokinetic pathways in several animal species. Cortical OKN was elicited by movement of a series of relatively small objects that attracted the animal's attention (so-called active nystagmus), and subcortical OKN was produced by movement of the whole optical environment (passive nystagmus). Presumably, the cortical pathway corresponds to the direct (pursuit) pathway, and the subcortical pathway, to the indirect (velocity storage) pathway. In animals without a fovea, such as the rabbit, only passive OKN can be induced, and bilateral occipital lobectomy produces a minimal effect on induced OKN.[87] In cats and dogs, passive and active OKN can be induced, but only the latter is abolished by bilateral occipital lobectomy.[193] In monkeys, bilateral occipital lobectomy abolishes smooth pursuit and the initial rapid rise in OKN (leaving the slow build-up and OKAN intact), but after a few months the animals regain some smooth pursuit and part of the rapid phase of OKN.[216]

Inasmuch as human subjects have poor OKAN and do not exhibit a build-up in OKN slow phase velocity, the subcortical (indirect) pathway must be less prominent in humans than in other animals. It has been a general clinical dictum that patients with cortical blindness do not produce OKN. Ter Braak and associates,[192] however, reported a patient with cortical blindness due to infarction of the occipital lobes and lateral geniculate nuclei who exhibited a slow build-up of OKN in one direction only. This interesting patient denied seeing any movement despite the presence of OKN. As noted earlier, patients with lesions of the parietal lobe and midline cerebellum also exhibit a slow build-up in OKN; the indirect pathway is uncovered after loss of the direct pathway.

COMPARISON OF VESTIBULAR AND VISUAL INDUCED EYE MOVEMENTS

The schematic diagrams of the visuo-ocular (pursuit and optokinetic) and the vestibulo-ocular reflexes in Figure 3–16 il-

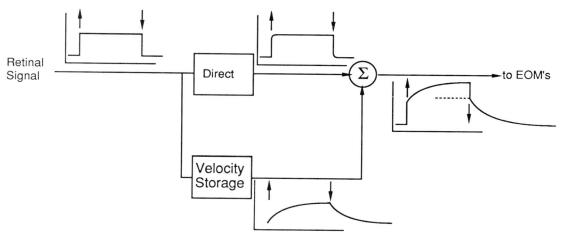

Figure 3–15. Schematic drawing of the direct and indirect (velocity storage) visuomotor pathways. A constant velocity optokinetic stimulus begins at the first arrow and the lights are turned off at the second arrow. The signals from the two pathways are added together to produce the characteristic slow phase velocity envelope of OKN and OKAN *(far right)*.

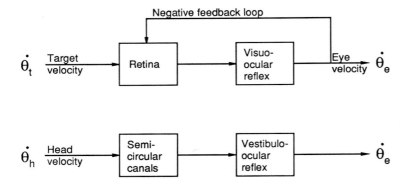

Figure 3–16. Schematic diagrams of the visuo-ocular reflex and the vestibulo-ocular reflex. The former is a closed-loop negative feedback system, and the latter is an open-loop system.

lustrate important similarities and differences between the two types of reflexes. In both instances the objective of the reflex eye movement $\dot{\Theta}_e$ is to match the stimulus velocity if the system is functioning perfectly. In the case of the visuomotor system, the stimulus is the target velocity $\dot{\Theta}_t$ (or optokinetic drum velocity), whereas for the vestibular system it is the head velocity $\dot{\Theta}_h$. The eye movement takes the form of either smooth pursuit or nystagmus. In the latter case, the $\dot{\Theta}_e$ response is that of the slow component of the nystagmus. The target velocity and head velocity must have opposite signs in order to produce ($\dot{\Theta}_e$) with the same sign. The visuomotor system functions as a closed-loop system with negative feedback to compare eye and target velocity, whereas the vestibulo-ocular reflex is an open-loop system.

For both systems, the gain of induced eye movements is dependent on the velocity and frequency of the stimulus. The visuomotor system is most efficient at low target velocities and frequencies. Normal human subjects can track a target moving sinusoidally at 0.1 Hz, peak velocity 30 deg/sec, with a gain near 1.[13, 111] The gain rapidly falls off for target velocities greater than 100 deg/sec and frequencies greater than 1 Hz. By contrast the gain of the vestibulo-ocular reflex is about 0.6 when a normal human subject is sinusoidally rotated in the dark at 0.1 Hz and a maximum velocity of 30 deg/sec. Unlike the visuomotor system, however, the vestibulo-ocular reflex responds with a gain near 1 for frequencies from 1 to 4 Hz and velocities greater than 100 deg/sec.[18, 42] The reader can test the increased efficiency of the ves-

tibular system over the visuomotor system at high input velocities and frequencies by a simple maneuver: rapidly move your hand back and forth with increasing velocity with your head stationary until your hand appears blurred. Then hold your hand stationary and move your head back and forth at the same high speed. Despite the rapid head movement the smallest detail of the palm remains clear.[134]

ANATOMY AND PHYSIOLOGY OF VISUAL-VESTIBULAR INTERACTION

The existence of neurons in the vestibular nuclei whose responses reflect visual inputs represented a new concept in the organization of the vestibular reflexes. Shortly after it was demonstrated by Dichgans and coworkers[54] that neurons in the vestibular nuclei of goldfish responded to visual inputs, similar observations were made by other investigators in a variety of animals under a variety of experimental conditions. Waespe and Henn [201–205] found that every neuron in the vestibular nucleus of alert monkeys that responded to horizontal rotation of the animal in the dark also responded to horizontal rotation of the visual surround. During combined visual-vestibular stimulation neurons were maximally excited (or inhibited) when the vestibular and optokinetic nystagmus were in the same direction (i.e., the background moved in the opposite direction of the monkey). If the optokinetic drum was mechanically coupled to the turntable so that both rotated together, nystagmus was reduced and neuronal activity was attenuated, compared with pure vestibular stimulation in the dark (Fig. 3–17).[201] The need for a site for interaction of vestibular and visual inputs had been recognized, but the realization that the interaction took place within the vestibular nuclei represented a departure from the rules of sensory specificity for the vestibular system.

Afoveate Animals. In afoveate animals the subcortical, accessory optic system is the predominant pathway for visual-vestibular interaction.[47, 161, 184] This system includes a group of nuclei at the mesodiencephalic border, which, like the lateral geniculate nucleus, receives direct retinal

projections but, unlike the lateral geniculate, projects directly to the brainstem and cerebellum. The most prominent cell group of the accessory optic system, the nucleus of the basal optic root, is identifiable in all classes of vertebrates. Lázár[110] found that optokinetic responses are abolished in frogs after destruction of the basal optic root nuclei, whereas ablation of the lateral geniculate nuclei and superior colliculi did not affect optokinetic responses. As in the rabbit, only subcortical passive OKN can be elicited in the frog.

Electrophysiologic studies in rabbits have demonstrated projections from the retina to the flocculonodular lobe of the cerebellum via the accessory optic system.[70, 122, 124] Microelectrode recordings in the accessory optic nucleus of the rabbit and the cat reveal units that show a strong response to a slow full-field retinal stimulation.[47, 88] Temporonasal movements of large patterns (rich in texture) evoke the strongest response. Neuroanatomic studies using horseradish peroxidase to map the connections between the accessory optic system and the flocculus reveal two separate pathways: one direct and the other an indirect pathway synapsing in the inferior olive.[25, 213]

The principal anatomic pathways for visual-vestibular interaction in the rabbit as proposed by Ito[98] are shown in Figure 3–18. Retinal sensory information reaches the inferior olives by way of the accessory optic tract and the central tegmental tract. Neurons in the inferior olives activate Purkinje cells in the flocculus, nodulus, and adjacent parts of the cerebellum. These areas of the cerebellum also receive primary vestibular afferent fibers and secondary vestibular fibers originating mostly in the medial and descending vestibular nuclei (not shown). Outflow from the cerebellar Purkinje cells terminates at secondary vestibular neurons and neurons in the adjacent reticular substance. Although Purkinje cell outflow to the vestibular nuclei is inhibitory (as with all Purkinje cell output), because it ends on both excitatory and inhibitory vestibular neurons it can enhance or inhibit the vestibulo-ocular reflex. Several types of experimental data confirm the floccular role in mediating visual-vestibular interaction in the rabbit.

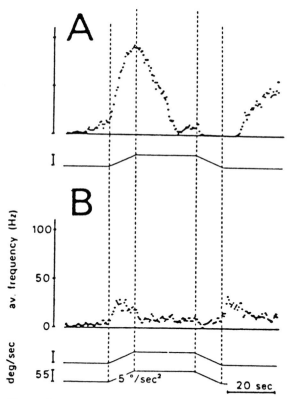

Figure 3–17. Type I neuron during vestibular (A, rotation of the monkey in the dark) and during conflicting visual-vestibular stimulation (B, turntable and optokinetic drum rotating together in the same direction). Neuronal frequency averaged over 1 second and displayed every 0.5 second. Below stimulus profile with acceleration of 5 deg/sec[2] and constant velocity of 55 deg/sec. During the conflict stimulation in B the response is strongly attenuated. (From Waespe, W and Henn, V: Motion information in the vestibular nuclei of alert monkeys: Visual and vestibular input vs. optomotor output. Prog Brain Res 50:683, 1979, with permission.)

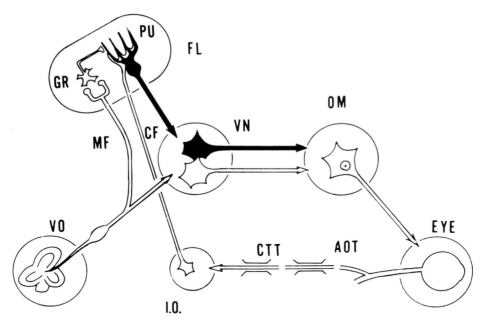

Figure 3–18. Anatomic pathways of visual-vestibular interaction in the rabbit. *AOT*, accessory optic tract; *CTT*, central tegmental tract; *IO*, inferior olive; *VO*, vestibular end organ; *MF*, mossy fiber; *CF*, climbing fiber; *GR*, granule cell; *PU*, Purkinje cell; *FL*, flocculus; *VN*, vestibular nucleus; *OM*, ocular motoneuron. Inhibitory neurons are filled in black. (From Ito,[98] with permission.)

Electric stimulation of the flocculus inhibits nystagmus induced by physiologic and electric stimulation of the vestibular nerve.[96] The reflex contraction produced in agonist extraocular muscles by electric stimulation of an isolated canal nerve is inhibited by prior stimulation of the flocculus, the accessory optic tract, or the optic chiasm.[123] Finally, in animals with lesions of the flocculus or inferior olives, the vestibulo-ocular reflex cannot be modulated by visual stimulation.[96]

Foveate Animals. With the development of the fovea, cortical pathways become progressively more important in visual-vestibular interaction. Recent anatomic and physiologic studies in primates indicate that visual signals reach the brainstem for interaction with vestibular signals via a complex cascade of interconnecting pathways (Fig. 3–19). In contrast to the rabbit and cat, neurons in the pretectal complex of the monkey receive predominant input from the visual cortex and respond equally well to small spots or large random dot patterns moving through their receptive field.[89] Furthermore, they respond the same to monocular or binocular stimulation, that is, they do not exhibit the temporal-nasal preponderance seen in afoveate animals. Electrical stimulation of the nucleus of the optic tract (NOT) in alert monkeys evokes horizontal nystagmus with a slow build-up in slow phase velocity followed by after-nystagmus in the same direction.[177] The rising time course in slow phase velocity is similar to the slow build-up in OKN and the falling time course of the after-nystagmus parallels that of OKAN. The striate cortex,[56] the superior temporal sulcus (particularly areas MT and MST)[1, 127, 191, 218] and the posterior parietal cortex[173, 176] are the key cortical areas in the monkey for processing retinal motion information. These cortical centers project heavily to the dorsolateral pontine nucleus (DLPN) which is a primary source of afferents to the flocculus and vermal areas VI and VII, two cerebellar areas involved in the regulation of eye movements.[128, 129] Neurons in DLPN exhibit a directionally selective response to movement of discrete spots and large backgrounds, and microstimulation in the region of the DLPN

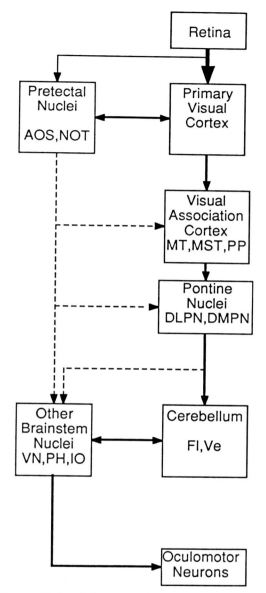

Figure 3–19. Schematic drawing of visual-vestibular pathways in the primate (see text for details). *AOS,* accessory optic system; *NOT,* nucleus of the optic tract; *MT,* middle temporal area; *MST,* medial superior temporal area; *PP,* posterior parietal cortex (area 7a); *DLPN,* dorsal lateral pontine nuclei; *DMPN,* dorsal medial pontine nuclei; *VN,* vestibular nucleus; *PH,* prepositus hypoglossi nucleus; *IO,* inferior olive; *Fl,* flocculus; *Ve,* vermis. *Dashed lines* indicate probable pathways.

causes a short-latency modification of the velocity of an ongoing pursuit eye movement.[129]

In the monkey, lesions of the parieto-

temporal region,[119] DLPN,[129] and the flocculus[217] result in an impairment of (1) smooth pursuit, (2) the initial rapid rise in OKN slow phase velocity, and (3) visual vestibular interaction requiring the "direct" visuomotor pathway (e.g., fixation suppression of vestibular nystagmus with a foveal target). By contrast, lesions of the pretectal nuclei (nucleus of the optic tract) impair OKN but not pursuit.[101] Taken together, these data suggest that the cortical and subcortical pathways illustrated in Figure 3–19 roughly correspond to the direct and indirect visuomotor pathways of the model shown in Figure 3–15.

MODEL OF VISUAL-VESTIBULAR INTERACTION

Figure 3–20 gives a simple linear interaction model for the visual and vestibular oculomotor systems.[165] The two independent block diagrams in Figure 3–16 have been interrelated to produce a single output eye velocity ($\dot{\Theta}_e$). When the target (foveal or full field) is stationary, movement of the head results in an equivalent movement of the target in the opposite direction relative to the head. When both the target and the head move, the driving stimulus to the visuomotor system is the angular velocity of the target relative to the head; that is, the difference between the target velocity relative to space ($\dot{\Theta}_t$) and the head angular velocity relative to space ($\dot{\Theta}_h$). In the absence of head movement ($\dot{\Theta}_h = 0$), the eye movement response is under the control of the closed-loop visuomotor system; whereas if the head is rotated in the dark, the visual system is inoperative and the eye movement response is under the control of the vestibular system.

A quantitative assessment of this model is presented in the Appendix, but a few general features deserve emphasis because of their relevance to clinical testing. A full-field target activates both the direct (pursuit) and indirect (velocity storage) pathways, the latter shared with the vestibular system. Optokinetic after nystagmus (OKAN) provides the only independent measure of the indirect pathway. A foveal target, on the other hand, activates predominantly the direct pathway (pursuit after responses are minimal).[111] Therefore, pursuit testing is almost exclusively a mea-

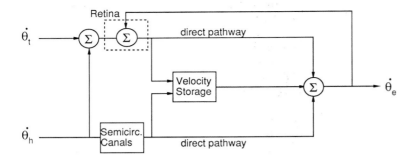

Figure 3–20. Model of visual-vestibular interaction after Cohen et al.[126] $\dot{\Theta}_t$, target (foveal or full field) velocity; $\dot{\Theta}_h$, head velocity; $\dot{\Theta}_e$, eye velocity. See text for details.

sure of the direct visuomotor pathway. At low-input frequencies and velocities (head or target), the gain of the direct visuomotor pathway is an order of magnitude higher than that of the other pathways (see Appendix). This explains why normal subjects can completely inhibit the VOR when rotated with a fixation target at the low frequencies commonly used for clinical testing (i.e., ≤ 0.1 Hz) (see Fig. 1–9).

ADAPTIVE MODIFICATION OF THE VESTIBULO-OCULAR REFLEX WITH VISION

Although clinicians have long been aware of the adaptive changes that occur within the VOR after lesions, quantitative assessment of these capabilities in normal subjects has only recently been undertaken. Based on the psychophysical studies of Kohler,[104] Gonshor and Melvill Jones[72–74] began a series of experimental studies in the early 1970s designed to investigate the potential for adaptive plasticity within the VOR. Probably the most dramatic example of this plasticity was the complete reversal of the VOR that occurred in normal subjects after wearing optically reversing prisms.[74] After about two weeks of wearing goggles that produced continuous left-right reversal of the visual environment, the VOR measured in the dark adaptively changed such that the direction of the slow and quick phases of induced nystagmus was the reverse of normal. The process occurred gradually over days, initially with a drop in gain followed by a pro-

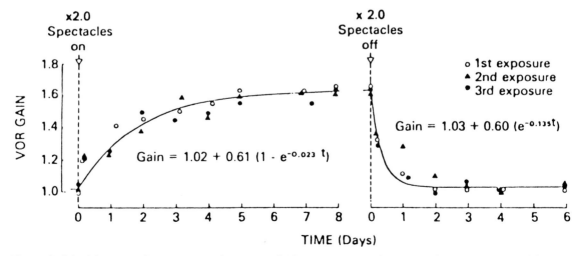

Figure 3–21. Adaptive enhancement and recovery of VOR gain in a monkey exposed to continuous ×2 binocular vision. The different symbols represent data from the same animal obtained on different occasions. The similarity of the curves they depict emphasizes the "machinelike" characteristics of the adaptive process. (From Miles, FA and Eighmy, BB: Long-term adaptive changes in primate vestibulo-ocular reflex: I. Behavioral observations. J. Neurophysiol, 43:1406, 1980, with permission.)

gressive change in phase (although never quite reaching the desired 180-degree phase shift). After the goggles were removed, the VOR gradually returned to normal somewhat faster than the original adaptation. Subsequent studies using magnifying and minifying lenses in normal humans[134] and a variety of animals[126, 138, 169, 206] showed that the dark-measured VOR gain could be increased and decreased, respectively, almost with a "machine-like precision" (Fig. 3–21). Furthermore, these adaptive changes were not restricted to a single plane.[155] For example, if an animal was sinusoidally rotated in one plane (the horizontal) while the visual surround was simultaneously rotated in another plane (the vertical), the VOR measured with horizontal rotation in the dark developed a vertical component.[178] Although the site of these induced plastic changes in the VOR remain uncertain, the cerebellum appears to play a key role. Lesions of the cerebellum in a variety of animals block adaptive plasticity of the VOR.[97, 138, 169] Recent work of Lisberger and colleagues[112] indicates that although the cerebellum provides a critical signal needed for the adaptive process, the modifiable synapse is on neurons within the vestibular nucleus.

VESTIBULOSPINAL REFLEXES

Comparison of Ocular and Spinal Vestibular Reflexes

It is helpful to consider the similarities and differences between the ocular and spinal vestibular reflexes as an introduction to the organization of vestibulospinal reflexes. If a rabbit is rotated at a constant speed on a turntable and suddenly stopped (producing an impulse of acceleration to the horizontal semicircular canals), a burst of ocular nystagmus results with the slow phase in the direction of the rotation prior to the deceleration (in the direction of endolymph flow). In addition, if the head is mobile it deviates slowly in the same direction as the slow phase eye deviation. In some animals, if the stimulus is large enough, quick return movements regularly interrupt the slow head deviation, resulting in head oscillation ("head nystag-

mus"). The relationship between the magnitude of reflex head movement and nystagmus changes along the phylogenetic scale. For example, in pigeons the head movement predominates, in rabbits head movement and nystagmus are equally prominent, and in primates nystagmus predominates. When present, head movement occurs in the plane of the stimulated canal; one can infer a highly organized pattern of connections between the individual semicircular canals and neck muscles similar to the connections between the individual canals and the eye muscles.[6, 211]

If unrestrained and standing on four legs, the rabbit on the turntable tends to fall in the direction of the slow phase of eye and head deviation when the table is suddenly stopped. This falling tendency is counteracted by reflex activation of the antigravity muscles of the limbs on the side toward which the rabbit is falling, producing an increased extensor thrust in those limbs. At the same time the extensor tone of the contralateral limbs is diminished and the rabbit maintains his balance. These extremity muscle reflexes are mediated via the semicircular canals and are always appropriate to prevent falling regardless of the direction of the acceleration force.[168]

The effector organs of the vestibulo-ocular reflexes are the extraocular muscles, and those of the vestibulospinal reflexes are the "antigravity" muscles—the extensors of the neck, trunk, and extremities. Figure 3–22 illustrates the organization of the vestibulospinal reflexes. Note the similarities between this figure and Figure 1–7, which illustrates the organization of the horizontal semicircular canal-ocular reflex. The same push-pull mechanism exists for controlling the balance between the extensor and flexor skeletal muscles as for the lateral and medial recti. A major difference between the organization of ocular and spinal reflexes is the increased complexity of the spinal muscle response, compared with the eye movement produced by an agonist and antagonist muscle acting in the horizontal plane. Even a simple movement about an extremity joint in a two-dimensional plane requires a complex pattern of contraction and relaxation in numerous muscles. Multiple agonist and antagonist muscles on both sides must

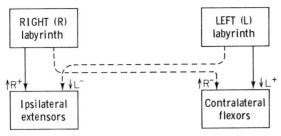

Figure 3—22. Organization of vestibulospinal reflexes. See text for details.

receive appropriate signals to ensure a smooth coordinated movement. Unfortunately, a simple recording technique does not exist for quantifying this complex skeletal muscle response. These factors have hindered the mapping of connections between the labyrinthine receptors and the individual skeletal muscles.

Vestibulospinal Pathways

Secondary vestibular neurons influence spinal anterior horn cell activity by means of three major pathways: (1) the lateral vestibulospinal tract, (2) the medial vestibulospinal tract, and (3) the reticulospinal tract. The first two arise directly from neurons in the vestibular nuclei, but the third arises from neurons in the reticular formation, which are influenced by vestibular stimulation (as well as several other kinds of input). The cerebellum is highly interrelated with each of these pathways.

LATERAL VESTIBULOSPINAL TRACT

It is generally agreed that the vast majority of fibers in the lateral vestibulospinal tract originate from neurons in the lateral vestibular nucleus (Fig. 3–23).[29] A somatotropic pattern of projections originates in the lateral vestibular nucleus such that neurons in the rostroventral region supply the cervical cord, whereas neurons in the dorsocaudal region innervate the lumbosacral cord. Neurons in the intermediate region supply the thoracic cord.

In the spinal cord the fibers run ipsilaterally in the ventral half of the lateral funicle and the lateral part of the ventral funi-

cle. (see Fig. 3–23). The tract terminates throughout the length of the cord in the eighth lamina and the medial part of the seventh lamina, either directly on dendrites of anterior horn cells or on interneurons that project to anterior horn cells of the axial and proximal limb musculature.[146] Some of the cells of the eighth lamina send their axons to the contralateral cord, probably accounting for the bilateral effects that have been observed after stimulation in the lateral vestibular nucleus. Activation of vestibulospinal fibers by electric stimulation in the lateral nucleus produces monosynaptic excitation of extensor motoneurons and disynaptic inhibition of flexor motoneurons.[59, 118] Both alpha and gamma motoneurons of extensor muscles receive monosynaptic excitatory postsynaptic potentials. Gamma motoneurons fire at lower magnitudes of stimulation, however, so that muscle spindles are activated before stronger stimulation evokes alpha discharge and muscle contraction.[69] The gamma system appears to function as a sensitizing device, ensuring smooth, continuous control; whereas the alpha system provides a rapid forceful contraction. Consistent with this interpretation is the fact that interrupting the gamma loop by cutting the dorsal roots only slightly reduces the tension that vestibular stimulation produces in the gastrocnemius muscle.[69]

MEDIAL VESTIBULOSPINAL TRACT

The fibers of the medial vestibulospinal tract originate from neurons in the medial vestibular nucleus and enter the spinal cord in the descending MLF (see Fig. 3–23).[29] The fibers travel in the ventral funicle as far as the midthoracic level. The majority end on interneurons in the seventh and eighth lamina of the cervical cord.[145] No monosynaptic connections appear to exist between the medial vestibulospinal tract and cervical anterior horn cells.[69, 212]

Functionally the medial vestibulospinal tract plays an important part in interaction of neck-vestibular-ocular reflexes. It has far fewer fibers than either the lateral vestibulospinal or reticulospinal tracts. Long latency excitatory and inhibitory postsynaptic potentials have been recorded intracellularly from both flexor and

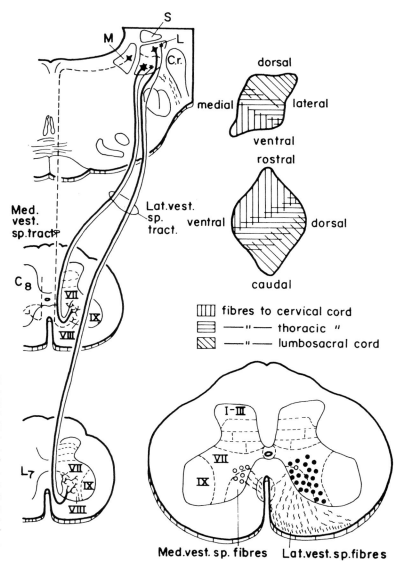

Figure 3–23. Lateral and medial vestibulospinal tracts. Topographical organization within the lateral vestibular nucleus *(upper right)* and endings within the spinal cord *(lower right)*. M, medial vestibular nucleus; L, lateral vestibular nucleus; S, superior vestibular nucleus. (From Brodal, A: Anatomical organization of cerebello-vestibulo-spinal pathways. In De Renck, AVS and Knight, J (eds): CIBA Foundation Symposium: Myotatic, kinesthetic and vestibular mechanisms. Churchill, London, 1967, with permission.)

extensor cervical motoneurons after stimulation of the descending MLF.[69, 212]

RETICULOSPINAL TRACT

The reticulospinal tract originates from neurons in the bulbar reticular formation.[154] The nuclei reticularis gigantocellularis and pontis caudalis provide most of the long fibers passing into the spinal cord, although the majority of neurons in the caudal reticular formation also contribute fibers. Both crossed and uncrossed fibers transverse the length of the spinal cord, terminating in the seventh and eighth laminae of the gray matter.[147]

Stimulation of the pontomedullary reticular formation in the regions where the long descending spinal projections originate results in inhibition of both extensor and flexor motoneurons throughout the spinal cord.[113, 114] If localized electric stimulation is applied to the more rostral or lateral regions of the reticular formation, facilitation is produced rather than inhibition.[194] This facilitatory influence must involve multisynaptic connections, because the neurons in these regions have short axons and do not send fibers into the spinal cord. The inhibitory and facilitatory reticulospinal fibers do not form well-defined tracts within the spinal cord, although some separation of the inhibitory and facilitatory fibers occurs in the lateral funicle. As in the case of the lateral vestibulospinal tract, both alpha and gamma motoneurons are influenced by excitatory and inhibitory input from the reticulospinal tract.

The vestibular nuclei are one of many structures that send fibers to the reticular formation. Axonal branches and collaterals of cells in all four main vestibular nuclei are distributed to the pontomedullary reticular formation. Only a small number of primary vestibular fibers end in the reticular formation, so that the main vestibular influence on reticulospinal outflow is mediated by way of the secondary vestibular neurons. A pattern exists within the vestibuloreticular projections such that each nucleus projects to different areas of the

reticular formation, but no detailed somatotropic organization has been identified.[29]

Cerebellar-Vestibular Interaction

The "spinal" cerebellum provides a major source of input to neurons whose axons form the lateral vestibulospinal and reticulospinal tracts. A somatotopic organization of projections to the lateral nucleus occurs in both the vermian cortex and fastigial nuclei (Fig. 3–24).[28, 158, 168] Direct projections connect the vermian cortex to the lateral vestibular nucleus, and indirect projections pass through the fastigial nuclei. The caudal part of the fastigial nucleus gives rise to a bundle of fibers that cross the midline (Russell's hook bundle), curving around the brachium conjunctivum before running to the contralateral lateral vestibular nucleus and dorsolateral

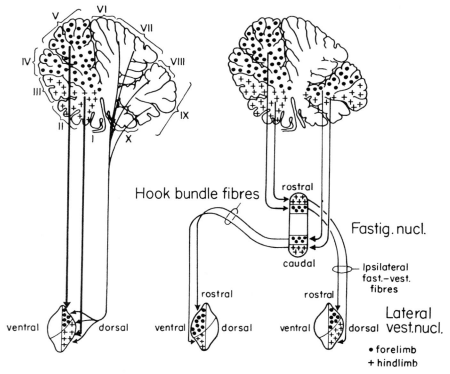

Figure 3–24. Topographical organization of cerebellar vermian, fastigial nucleus and lateral vestibular nucleus connections. (From Brodal, A: Anatomy of the vestibular nuclei and their connections. In Kornhuber, HH (ed): Handbook of Sensory Physiology, Vol VI, Part I. Springer-Verlag, New York, 1974, with permission.)

reticular formation. In addition, direct ipsilateral outflow passes from the fastigial nucleus to areas of the reticular formation that send long fibers to the spinal cord in the reticulospinal tract. The cerebellar-reticular pathways do not exhibit somatotopic organization.[158]

The cerebellar vermis and fastigial nuclei receive input from secondary vestibular neurons, the spinal cord, and the pontomedullary reticular formation. The result is a close-knit vestibular-reticular-cerebellar functional unit for the maintenance of equilibrium and locomotion.

Vestibular Influence in the Control of Posture and Equilibrium

The elementary unit for the control of tone in the trunk and extremity skeletal muscles is the myotatic reflex (the deep tendon reflex). The myotatic reflexes of the antigravity muscles are under the combined excitatory and inhibitory influence of multiple supraspinal neural centers (Fig. 3–25).[14] At least in the cat one finds two main facilitatory centers (the lateral vestibular nucleus and rostral reticular formation) and four inhibitory centers (the

pericruciate cortex, basal ganglia, cerebellum, and caudal reticular formation). The balance of input from these different centers determines the degree of tone in the antigravity muscles. If one removes the inhibitory influence of the frontal cortex and basal ganglia by sectioning the animal's midbrain, a characteristic state of contraction in the antigravity muscles results—so-called decerebrate rigidity. The extensor muscles increase their resistance to lengthening, and the deep tendon reflexes become hyperactive. One may conclude that the vestibular system contributes largely to this increased extensor tone after witnessing the marked decrease upon bilateral destruction of the labyrinths.[5] Unilateral destruction of the labyrinth or the lateral vestibular nucleus results in an ipsilateral decrease in tone, indicating that the main excitatory input to the anterior horn cells arrives from the ipsilateral lateral vestibulo-spinal tract.[65]

In a decerebrate animal with normal labyrinths the intensity of the extensor tone can be modulated in a specific way by changing the position of the head in space.[125, 181] The tone is maximal when the animal is in the supine position with the angle of the mouth 45 degrees above horizontal and minimal when the animal is

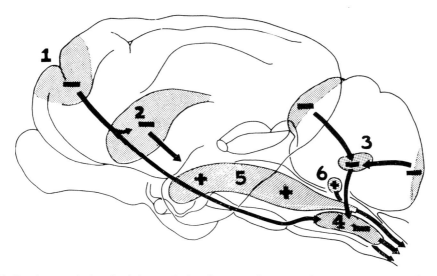

Figure 3–25. Facilitatory (+) and inhibitory (−) pathways influencing the myotatic spinal reflex in the cat. Inhibitory pathways are (1) corticobulboreticular, (2) caudatospinal, (3) cerebelloreticular, and (4) reticulospinal. Facilitatory pathways are (5) reticulospinal and (6) vestibulospinal. (From Lindsley, DB, Schreiner, LH, and Magoun, HW: An electromyographic study of spasticity. J Neurophysiol 12:197, 1949, with permission.)

prone with the angle of the mouth 45 degrees below the horizontal. Intermediate positions of rotation of the animal's body about the transverse or longitudinal axis result in intermediate degrees of extensor tone. If the head of the upright animal is tilted upward (without neck extension), extensor tone in the forelegs increases; downward tilting of the head causes decreased extensor tone and flexion of the forelegs. Lateral tilt produces extension of the extremities on the opposite side.

These tonic labyrinthine reflexes, mediated by way of the otoliths, seldom occur in intact animals or human subjects because of the inhibitory influence of the higher cortical and subcortical centers. They can be demonstrated in premature infants, however, and in adults with lesions releasing the brainstem from the higher neural centers.[132]

SUBJECTIVE VESTIBULAR SENSATION

INTRODUCTION

Unlike those sensory organs that respond to energy sources external to the body, the labyrinths respond to self-generated forces. During natural head movements these forces are not under voluntary control, and therefore the vestibular responses are more automatic than those of the other sensory modalities. For example, one can remove vision simply by closing one's eyes, whereas one cannot suppress vestibular stimuli during head movement.

The existence of a separate sense organ for the perception of motion was first appreciated over a hundred years ago through the imaginative experiments of Mach.[120] A sensory illusion experienced while traveling on a railroad train aroused Mach's interest in the study of vestibular sensation. He wrote:

On the railroad, when riding a great curve, the horses and the trees often seem to deviate considerably from the vertical. . . . This could be explained if one assumes that the direction of the vertical is perceived, and that the direction of the mass acceleration resulting from the interaction of the force of gravity and the centrifugal force, is always considered to be in the vertical direction.

Through a series of experiments Mach became aware that it was the acceleration (or change in velocity of movement) that was perceived. When rotating a subject inside a box about an earth vertical axis he found that

every rotatory movement will be recognized immediately according to direction and approximate amount. But if the rotation is maintained uniformly for several seconds, the sensation of rotation will gradually cease entirely. . . . As soon as the apparatus is stopped, one has the impression that one is executing, together with the box, a contrary rotation. If the rotating box is opened quickly, the entire visible space and its contents will rotate.

He made a similiar observation regarding linear acceleration by producing vertical oscillations in a subject seated on a seesaw platform. The subject

always stated that he is sinking shortly before arriving at the highest point of the oscillation. . . . Likewise the rise was always noticed shortly before, or at the lowest point (of displacement) itself, of course always with the eyes closed. Hence, one is very sensitive to oscillations of the amount of the gravity acceleration, and one does not perceive the position or the velocity in the vertical movements, but rather the accelerations.

Mach observed that the perception of motion in his different experiments could be altered by changing the position of the head in relation to the body, which suggested to him that the sensory organs were located in the head. His findings, along with the physiologic and histologic work of contemporaries such as Flourens,[62] Crum-Brown,[51] and Breuer,[26] led him to the conclusion that the semicircular canals and the otoliths were responsible for the perception of angular and linear acceleration, respectively.

Several important clinical observations support the existence of a specific vestibular sensation. Probably the most convincing is that patients without vestibular function (either on an acquired or congenital basis) do not experience a turning sensation when rotated in the dark if visual and tactile cues are eliminated.[79] Patients with complete spinal transections in the cervical region, on the other hand, perceive acceleration normally.[207] The sensation of movement is not dependent on vision or associated nystagmus, inasmuch as blind subjects and patients with complete oculomotor paralysis experience a spinning sensation comparable to that of normal subjects when their vestibular endorgans are stimulated. Focal cortical lesions in the nondominant parietal lobe interfere with spatial orientation and the performance of three-dimensional construction tasks, and epileptic discharges from many different areas of the cortex can be associated with a subjective illusion of movement (usually spinning).[16, 50, 151] These observations imply a cerebrocortical representation for vestibular sensation.

Anatomy and Physiology of Vestibular Sensation

The first electrophysiologic identification of vestibulocortical projections was made in the cat by Watzl and Mountcastle.[208] Following electric stimulation of the contralateral vestibular nerve, they recorded short-latency monophasic potentials in the suprasylvian gyrus just anterior to the auditory area. The ascending vestibulocortical system includes at least three synaptic stations: the vestibular nuclei, the thalamus, and the cerebral cortex (Fig. 3–26).[32, 136] Vestibulothalamic projections originate from neurons in the superior and lateral vestibular nuclei. At least two thalamic regions receive projections from these secondary vestibular neurons.[80] A large anterior vestibulothalamic projection runs ventrally in the brainstem, passing lateral to the red nucleus and dorsal to the subthalamic nucleus, to terminate in the main sensory nucleus of the thalamus (nucleus ventralis posterior lateralis pars oralis). A smaller posterior vestibulothalamic projection runs in the lateral lemniscus along with the auditory projections and ends predominantly near the medial geniculate. The vast majority of vestibulothalamic projections run outside

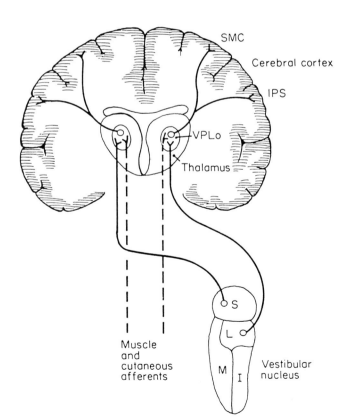

Figure 3–26. Vestibulothalamocortical projections. *S*, superior nucleus; *L*, lateral nucleus; *M*, medial nucleus; *I*, inferior nucleus; *VPLo*, nucleus ventralis posterior lateralis pars oralis; *IPS*, intraparietal sulcus; *SMC*, sensorimotor cortex.

the MLF. Two separate thalamocortical projection areas have been identified in the monkey: one near the central sulcus close to the motor cortex, and the other at the lower end of the intraparietal sulcus next to the face area of the post central gyrus.[31, 64] In humans, electrical stimulation of the superior sylvian gyrus and the region of the inferior intraparietal sulcus produces a subjective sensation of rotation or body displacement.[151]

The vestibulocortical pathway via the thalamus is concerned with the control of body position and orientation in space. Thalamic and cortical units that receive vestibular signals are also activated by proprioception and visual stimuli (as shown in Fig. 3–26). Most units respond in a similiar way to rotation in the dark, or to moving visual fields, indicating that they play a role in relaying information about self-motion. From a functional point of view the vestibulothalamocortical projections appear to integrate vestibular, proprioceptive, and visual signals to provide one with a "conscious awareness" of body orientation. Beginning at the vestibular nuclei, a stepwise integration of body-orienting signals occurs, reaching its maximum at the level of the cortex.

Psychophysical Studies

SEMICIRCULAR CANALS

As Mach[120] described, a subject rotated about an earth vertical axis on a rotatory platform will perceive turning that is dependent on the magnitude of angular acceleration. The perceived "speed of turning" progressively increases with prolonged constant acceleration, although the turning sensation increases at a lesser rate than the platform velocity. Below a minimum or threshold angular acceleration the subject does not perceive turning. Although considerable difference exists in reported values, the threshold to constant angular acceleration is in the range of 0.1 to 0.5 deg/sec^2.[39, 79] This is approximately an order of magnitude lower than the constant angular acceleration necessary to produce nystagmus.[100]

Attempts to correlate the threshold and magnitude of subjective sensation with the magnitude of angular acceleration represent the earliest tests of vestibular function. Cupulometry developed by van Egmond and associates[199] is still occasionally used for assessing vestibular function on the basis of subjective sensation. With this test the subject is maintained at a constant velocity of angular rotation and then suddenly stopped. The durations of "after-turning" sensation are measured for impulses of different amplitude (usually 15 to 60 deg/sec) and plotted versus the log of impulse magnitude (in the so-called cupulogram). The intercept of the line with the abscissa corresponds to a subjective sensation threshold; and the slope, a time constant of after-turning sensation. Normative data for the subjective threshold vary from 1 to 4 deg/sec, and the time constant of after turning sensation from 2 to 14 seconds.[100]

OTOLITH ORGANS

A subject undergoing horizontal linear oscillation (e.g., on a parallel swing) reports experiencing two separate types of motion. One is a sensation of linear movement in the horizontal plane and the other is a sensation of tilt. Both sensations vary with the changing velocity (acceleration) of the platform.[100] Beginning with low amplitudes of oscillation the subject initially perceives motion without a specific direction. This is followed by perception of the direction of linear movement and finally at higher intensities of stimulation by a perception of tilting. Using dynamic stimuli, estimates of the minimal horizontal linear acceleration that normal subjects can perceive range from 5 to 15 cm/sec^2.[79] Interestingly, these threshold values are similar to the values obtained by Mach for the perception of vertical linear acceleration (10 to 12 cm/sec^2).

The most complete data on threshold and accuracy of estimation of tilt have been obtained with static tilt experiments.[38, 77] The subject is strapped to a tilt platform in darkness and asked either to estimate the deviation of his head from the earth vertical or to adjust a luminous line on a dark field to a vertical position. Normal subjects respond with an accuracy of 2 to 4 degrees for tilt angles up to 40 degrees (accuracy falls off progressively for larger angles of tilt).[19, 77] The subjective estimate of tilt obviously depends on the gravitational force (F_g).[149] If the subject is asked to estimate the angle of tilt under different gravitational forces, the estimate will vary with F_g. For g values less than 1 the angle of tilt is underestimated, whereas for g values greater than 1 the angle of tilt is overestimated. In experiments carried out at "zero g" in parabolic aircraft flights and in orbiting spacecraft, the subjects are unable to perceive tilt.

REFERENCES

1. Albright, TD: Direction and orientation selectivity of neurons in visual area MT of the macaque. J Neurophysiol 52:1106, 1984.
2. Atkinson, J: Development of optokinetic nystagmus in the human infant and monkey infant: An analogue to development in kittens. In Freeman, RD (ed): Developmental Neurobiology of Vision. NATO Advanced Study Institute Series: Series A, Life Sciences. Plenum Press, New York, 1979, pp 277–287.
3. Baarsma, EA and Collewijn, H: Eye movements due to linear accelerations in the rabbit. J Physiol 245:227, 1975.
4. Baarsma, EA and Collewijn, H: Vestibulo-ocular and optokinetic reactions to rotation and their interaction in the rabbit. J Physiol 238:603, 1974.
5. Bach, LMN and Magoun, HW: The vestibular nuclei as an excitatory mechanism for the cord. J Neurophysiol 10:331, 1947.
6. Baker, J, Goldberg, JM, and Peterson, B: Spatial and temporal response properties of the vestibulocollic reflex in decerebrate cats. J Neurophysiol 54:735, 1985.
7. Baker, R and Berthoz, A: Organization of vestibular nystagmus in oblique oculomotor system. J Neurophysiol 37:195, 1974.
8. Baloh, RW, Beykirch, K, Honrubia, V, and Yee, RD: Eye movements induced by linear acceleration on a parallel swing. J Neurophysiol 60:200, 1988.
9. Baloh, RW, Henn, V, and Jäger, J: Habituation of the human vestibulo-ocular reflex by low frequency harmonic acceleration. Am J Otolaryngol 3:235, 1982.
10. Baloh, RW, Yee, RD, and Honrubia, V: Late cortical cerebellar atrophy: Clinical and oculographic features. Brain 109:159, 1986.
11. Baloh, RW, Yee, RD, and Honrubia, V: Optokinetic asymmetry in patients with maldeveloped foveas. Brain Res 186:211, 1980.
12. Baloh, RW, Yee, RD, and Honrubia, V: Optokinetic nystagmus and parietal lobe lesions. Ann Neurol 7:269, 1980.
13. Baloh, RW, Yee, RD, Honrubia, V, Jacobson, K: A comparison of the dynamics of horizontal and vertical smooth pursuit in normal human subjects. Aviat Space Environ Med 59:121, 1988.
14. Bard, P: Postural coordination and locomotion and their central control. In Bard, P (ed): Medical Physiology, ed 11. CV Mosby, St Louis, 1961.
15. Barlow, D and Freeman, W: Cervico-ocular reflex in the normal adult. Acta-Otolaryngol 89:487, 1980.
16. Barlow, JS: Vestibular and non-dominant parietal lobe disorders. Dis Nerv Syst 31:624, 1970.
17. Barnes, GR and Forbat, LN: Cervical and vestibular afferent control of oculomotor response in man. Acta-Otolaryngol 88:79, 1979.
18. Barnes, GR, Benson, AJ, and Prior, ARJ: Visual-vestibular interaction in the control of eye movement. Aviat Space Environ Med 49:557, 1978.
19. Bauermeister, M: Effect of body tilt on apparent verticality, apparent body position, and their relation. J Exp Psychol 67:142, 1964.
20. Bechterew, W: Ergebnisse der Durchschneidung des N. acusticus, nebst Erörterung der Bedeutung der semicirculären Canäle für das Körpergleichgewicht. Pfuegers Arch Ges Physiol 30:312, 1883.
21. Bender, MB: Brain control of conjugate horizontal and vertical eye movements. A survey of the structural and functional correlates. Brain 103:23, 1980.
22. Buizza, A, Leger, A, Droulez, J, et al: Influence of otolithic stimulation by horizontal linear acceleration on optokinetic nystagmus and visual motion perception. Exp Brain Res 39:165, 1980.
23. Blanks, RHI, Anderson, JH, and Precht, W: Response characteristics of semicircular canal and otolith systems in cat. II. Responses of trochlear motoneurons. Exp Brain Res 32:509, 1978.
24. Boyle, R, Büttner, U, and Markert, G: Vestibular nuclei activity and eye movements in the alert monkey during sinusoidal optokinetic stimulation. Exp Brain Res 57:362, 1985.
25. Branth, SE and Karten, HJ: Direct accessory optic projections to the vestibulocerebellum: A possible channel for oculomotor control systems. Exp Brain Res 28:73, 1977.
26. Breuer, J: Über die Funktion der Bogengänge des Ohrlabyrinthes. Wein Med Jahrb 4:72, 1874.
27. Brodal, A: Organization of the commissural connections: Anatomy. Progress in Brain Research 37:167, 1972.
28. Brodal, A: Anatomical organization of cerebello-vestibulo-spinal pathways. In De Renck, AVS and Knight, J (eds): CIBA Foundation Symposium: Myotatic, kinesthetic and vestibular mechanisms. Churchill, London, 1967.
29. Brodal, A: Anatomy of the vestibular nuclei and their connections. In Kornhuber, HH (ed): Handbook of Sensory Physiology, The Ves-

tibular System, Vol. VI, Part 1. Springer-Verlag, New York, 1974.

30. Buizza, A, Avanzini, P, and Schmid, R: Visual-vestibular interaction during angular and linear body acceleration: modelling and simulation. In Fedina, L, Kanyar, B, Kocsis, B, and Kollai, M (eds): Mathematical and Computational Methods in Physiology. Pergamon, Oxford, UK, 1981, pp 13–19.

31. Büttner, U and Lang, W: The vestibulocortical pathway: Neurophysiological and anatomical studies in the monkey. Progr Brain Res 50:581, 1979.

32. Büttner-Ennever, JA: Vestibular oculomotor organization. In Fuchs, AF and Becker, W (eds): The Neural Control of Eye Movements. Elsevier, Amsterdam, 1981.

33. Cannon, SC and Robinson, DA: Neural integrator failure from brain stem lesions in monkey. Investigative Ophthalmology and Visual Science (suppl 3) 26:47, 1985.

34. Carleton, SC and Carpenter, MB: Afferent and efferent connections of the medial, inferior and lateral vestibular nuclei in the cat and monkey. Brain Res 278:29, 1983.

35. Carleton, SC and Carpenter, MB: Distribution of primary vestibular fibers in the brainstem and cerebellum of the monkey. Brain Res 294:281, 1984.

36. Carpenter, RHS: Cerebellectomy and the transfer function of the vestibulo-ocular reflex in the decerebrate cat. Proc Roy Soc B 181:353, 1972.

37. Cheron, G and Godaux, E: Disabling of the oculomotor neural integrator by kainic acid injections in the prepositus-vestibular complex of the cat. J Physiol 394:267, 1987.

38. Clark, B: The vestibular system. Ann Rev Psychol 21:273, 1970.

39. Clark, B: Thresholds for the perception of angular acceleration in man. Aerospace Med 38:443, 1967.

40. Cohen, B, Susuki, JI, and Raphan, T: Role of the otolith organs in generation of horizontal nystagmus: Effects of selective labyrinthe lesions. Brain Res 276:159, 1983.

41. Cohen, B and Henn, V: The origin of quick phases of nystagmus in the horizontal plane. Bibl Ophthalmol 82:36, 1972.

42. Cohen, B, Henn V, Raphan, T, and Dennett, D: Velocity storage, nystagmus, and visual-vestibular interactions in humans. Ann NY Acad Sci 374:421, 1981.

43. Cohen, B, Komatsuzaki, A, and Bender, MB: Electro-oculographic syndrome in monkeys after pontine reticular formation lesions. Arch Neurol 18:78, 1968.

44. Cohen, B, Matsuo, V, and Raphan, TH: Quantitative analysis of the velocity characteristics of optokinetic nystagmus and optokinetic after-nystagmus. J Physiol 270:321, 1977.

45. Cohen, B: The vestibulo-ocular reflex arc. In Kornhuber, HH (ed): Handbook of Sensory Physiology, The Vestibular System, Vol VI, Part 1. Springer-Verlag, New York, 1974.

46. Collewijn, H, et al: Control of gaze in man: Synthesis of pursuit, optokinetic and vestibulo-ocular systems. In Roucouz, A and Crommelink, M (eds): Physiological and Pathological Aspects of Eye Movements. W Junk, The Hague, 1982, pp 3–22.

47. Collewijn, H: Direction-selective units in the rabbit's nucleus of the optic tract. Brain Res 100:489, 1975.

48. Collins, WE: Arousal and vestibular habituation. In Kornhuber, HH (ed): Handbook of Sensory Physiology, The Vestibular System, Vol VI, Part 2. Springer-Verlag, New York, 1974.

49. Collins, WE: Manipulation of arousal and its effects upon human vestibular nystagmus induced by caloric irrigation and angular accelerations. Aerospace Med 34:124, 1963.

50. Critchley, M: The Parietal Lobes. Arnold, London, 1953.

51. Crum-Brown, A: On the sense of rotation and the anatomy and physiology of the semicircular canals of the internal ear. J Anat Physiol 8:327, 1874.

52. De Jong, PTVM, et al: Ataxia and nystagmus induced by injection of local anesthetics in the neck. Ann Neurol 1:240, 1977.

53. De Kleyn, A: Recherches quantitatives sur les positions compensatories l'oeil chez de lapin. Arch Neerl Physiol 7:138, 1922.

54. Dichgans, J, Schmidt, CL and Graf, W: Visual input improves the speedometer function of the vestibular nuclei in the goldfish. Exp Brain Res 18:319, 1973.

55. Dodge, R: Five types of eye movements in the horizontal meridian plane of the field of regard. Am J Physiol 8:307, 1903.

56. Dow, B: Functional classes of cells and their laminar distribution in monkey visual cortex. J Neurophysiol 37:927, 1974.

57. Dubois, MFW and Collewijn, H: Optokinetic reactions in man elicited by localized retinal motion stimuli. Vision Research 19:1105, 1979.

58. Eckmiller, R: Concerning the linear acceleration input to the neural oculomotor control system in primates. In Roucoux, A and Crommelinck, M (eds): Physiological and Pathological Aspects of Eye Movements. W Junk, The Hague, 1982, pp 131–138.

59. Erulkar, SD, et al: Organization of the vestibular projection to the spinal cord of the cat. J Neurophysiol 29:626, 1966.

60. Evinger, LC, Fuchs, AF, and Baker, R: Bilateral lesions of the medial longitudinal fasciculus in monkeys: Effects on the horizontal and vertical components of voluntary and vestibular induced eye movements. Exp Brain Res 28:1, 1977.

61. Fetter, M, Zee, DS, and Proctor, LR: Effect of lack of vision and of occipital lobectomy upon recovery from unilateral labyrinthectomy in rhesus monkey. J Neurophysiol 59:394, 1988.

62. Flourens, P: Recherches Expérimentals sur les Propriétés et les Fonctions due Systéme Nerveaux dans les Animaux Vertébrés. Crevot, Paris, 1842.

63. Fluur, E and Mellström, A: The otolith organs

and their influence on oculomotor movements. Exp Neurol 30:139, 1971.

64. Fredrickson, JM, Kornhuber, HH, and Schwarz, JM: Cortical projections of the vestibular nerve. In Kornhuber, HH (ed): Handbook of Sensory Physiology, The Vestibular System, Vol VI, Part 2. Springer-Verlag, New York, 1974.

65. Fulton, JF, Liddell, EGT, and Rioch, DM: The influence of unilateral destruction of the vestibular nuclei upon posture and the knee jerk. Brain 53:327, 1930.

66. Gacek, RR, Lyon, MJ, and Schoonmaker, J: Ultrastructural changes in vestibulo-ocular neurons following vestibular neurectomy in the cat. Ann Otol Rhinol Laryngol 97:42, 1988.

67. Gacek, R: The course and central termination of first order neurons supplying vestibular endorgans in the cat. Acta Otolaryngol (Suppl) 254, 1969.

68. Galiana, HL and Outerbridge, JS: A bilateral model for central neural pathways in vestibulo-ocular reflex. J Neurophysiol 51:210, 1984.

69. Gernandt, BF: Vestibulo-spinal mechanisms. In Kornhuber, HH (ed): Handbook of Sensory Physiology: The Vestibular System, Vol VI, Part 2. Springer-Verlag, New York, 1974.

70. Ghelarducci, B, Ito, M, and Yagi, N: Impulse discharges from flocculus Purkinje cells of alert rabbits during visual stimulation combined with horizontal head rotation in the rabbit. Brain Res 87:66, 1975.

71. Goldberg, JM, Highstein, SM, Moschovakis, AK, and Fernández, C: Inputs from regularly and irregularly discharging vestibular nerve afferents to secondary neurons in the vestibular nuclei of the squirrel monkey. I. An electrophysiological analysis. J Neurophysiol 58:700, 1987.

72. Gonshor, A and Melvill Jones, G: Plasticity in the adult human vestibulo-ocular reflex arc. Proc Can Fed Biol Soc 14:11, 1971.

73. Gonshor, A and Melvill Jones, G: Short-term adaptive changes in the human vestibulo-ocular reflex arc. J Physiol 256:361, 1976.

74. Gonshor, A and Melvill Jones, G: Extreme vestibulo-ocular adaptation induced by prolonged optical reversal of vision. J Physiol 256:381, 1976.

75. Graf, W and Ezure, K: Morphology of vertical canal related second order vestibular neurons in the cat. Exp Brain Res 63:35, 1986.

76. Graf, W, Baker, JF, Peterson, BW, and Wickland, CR: Differential canal-canal convergence on second-order vestibulo-oculomotor neurons in the cat. Soc Neurosci Abstr 12:774, 1986.

77. Graybiel, A: Measurement of otolith function in man. In Kornhuber, HH (ed): Handbook of Sensory Physiology: The Vestibular System, Vol VI, Part 2. Springer-Verlag, New York, 1974.

78. Gresty, MA: A reexamination of "neck reflex" eye movements in the rabbit. Acta Otolaryngol 81:386, 1976.

79. Guedry, FE: Psychophysics of vestibular sensation. In Kornhuber, HH (ed): Handbook of Sensory Physiology: The Vestibular System, Vol. VI, Part 2. Springer-Verlag, New York, 1974.

80. Hawrylshyn, PA, et al: Vestibulothalamic projections in man, a sixth primary sensory pathway. J Neurophysiol 41:394, 1978.

81. Henn, V, Hepp, K, and Büttner-Ennever, JA: The primate oculomotor system. II. Premotor system. Human Neurobiol 1:87, 1982.

82. Henn, V, Lang, W, Hepp, K, and Reisine, H: Experimental gaze palsies in monkeys and their relation to human pathology. Brain 107:619, 1984.

83. Henn, V, Schnyder, H, Happ, K, and Reisine, H: Loss of vertical rapid eye movements after Kainic acid lesions in the restrol mesencephalon in the rhesus monkey. Soc Neurosci Abst 9:749, 1983.

84. Highstein, SM, Goldberg, JM, Moschovakis, AK, and Fernandez, C: Inputs from regularly and irregularly discharging vestibular-nerve afferents to secondary neurons in the vestibular nuclei of the squirrel monkey. II. Correlation with output pathways of secondary neurons. J Neurophysiol 58:719, 1987.

85. Hikosaka, O and Maeda, M: Cervical effects on abducens motoneurons and their interaction with vestibulo-ocular reflex. Exp Brain Res. 18:512, 1973.

86. Hikosaka, O, Igusa, Y, Nakao, S, and Shimazu, H: Direct inhibitory synaptic linkage of pontomedullary reticular burst neurons with abducens motoneurons in the cat. Exp Brain Res 33:337, 1978.

87. Hobbelen, JF and Collewijn, H: Effect of cerebro/cortical and collicular ablations upon the optokinetic reactions in the rabbit. Doc Ophthalmol 30:227, 1971.

88. Hoffman, KP and Schoppman, A: Retinal input to direction selective cells in the nucleus tractus opticus of the cat. Brain Res 99:359, 1975.

89. Hoffman, KP, Distler, C, Erickson, RG, and Mader, W: Physiological and anatomical identification of the nucleus of the optic tract and dorsal terminal nucleus of the accessory optic tract in monkeys. Exp Brain Res 69:635, 1988.

90. Honrubia, V et al: Central projections of primary vestibular fibers in the bullfrog. III. The anterior semicircular canal afferents. Laryngoscope 95:1526, 1985.

91. Honrubia, V et al: Experimental studies on optokinetic nystagmus. II. Normal humans. Acta Otolaryngol 65:441, 1968.

92. Honrubia, V et al: The patterns of eye movements during physiologic vestibular nystagmus in man. Trans Am Acad Ophthalmol Otolaryngol 84:339, 1977.

93. Honrubia, V, Reingold, DB, Lau, CGY, and Ward, PH: Neural correlates of nystagmus in abducens nerve. J Neurophysiol 42:1282, 1979.

94. Igarashi, M et al: Nystagmus after experimental

cervical lesions. Laryngoscope 82:1609, 1972.

95. Igarashi, M, Levy, JK, O-Uchi, T, and Reschke, MF: Further study of physical exercise and locomotor balance compensation after unilateral labyrinthectomy in squirrel monkeys. Acta Otolaryngol 92:101, 1981.

96. Ito, M et al: Visual influence on rabbit horizontal vestibulo-ocular reflex presumably effected via the cerebellar flocculus. Brain Res 65:170, 1974.

97. Ito, M, et al: The cerebellar modification of rabbit's horizontal vestibulo-ocular reflex induced by sustained head rotation combined with visual stimulation. Proc Jpn Acad 50:85, 1974.

98. Ito, M: The vestibulo-cerebellar relationships: Vestibulo-ocular reflex arc and flocculus. In Naunton, RF (ed): The Vestibular System. Academic Press, New York, 1975.

99. Jäger, J and Henn, V: Habituation of the vestibulo-ocular reflex (VOR) in the monkey during sinusoidal rotation in the dark. Exp Brain Res 41:108, 1981.

100. Jongkees, LBW and Groen, JJ: The nature of the vestibular stimulus. J Laryngol 61:529, 1946.

101. Kato, I, et al: Role of the nucleus of the optic tract in monkeys in relation to optokinetic nystagmus. Brain Res 364:12, 1986.

102. Keller, EL: Participation of medial pontine reticular formation in eye movement generation in monkey. J Neurophysiol 37:316, 1974.

103. Koenig, E and Dichgans, J: Aftereffects of vestibular and optokinetic stimulation and their interaction. In Cohen B (ed): Vestibular and oculomotor physiology. Ann NY Acad Sci 374:434, 1981.

104. Kohler, I: Experiments with goggles. Sci Am 206:62, 1962.

105. Kommerell, G and Täumer, R: Investigations of the eye tracking system through stabilized retinal images. Bibl Ophthalmol 82:288, 1972.

106. Korte, GE and Friedrich, VL, Jr: The fine structure of the feline superior vestibular nucleus: Identification and synaptology of the primary vestibular afferents. Brain Res 176:3, 1979.

107. Kowler, E, Van den Steen, J, Tamminga, EP, and Collewijn, H: Voluntary selection of the target for smooth eye movements in the presence of superimposed, full-field stationary, and moving stimuli. Vision Res 24:1789, 1984.

108. Lacom, M and Xerri, C: Vestibular compensation: New perspectives. In Flohr, H, Precht, W (eds): Lesion-induced Neuronal Plasticity in Sensorimotor Systems. Springer-Verlag, Berlin, 1984, pp 240–253.

109. Langer, T, et al: Floccular efferents in the rhesus macaque as revealed by autoradiography and horseradish peroxidase. J Comp Neurol 235:26, 1985.

110. Lázár, G: Role of the accessory optic system in the optokinetic nystagmus of the frog. Brain Behav Evol 5:443, 1973.

111. Lisberger, SG, et al: Relationship between eye acceleration and retinal image velocity during foveal smooth pursuit in man and monkey. J Neurophysiol 46:229, 1981.

112. Lisberger, SG: The neural basis for learning of simple motor skills. Science 242:728, 1988.

113. Llinás, R and Terzuolo, CA: Mechanisms of supraspinal actions upon spinal cord activities. Reticular inhibitory mechanisms on alpha-extensor motoneurons. J Neurophysiol 27:579, 1964.

114. Llinás, R and Terzuolo, CA: Mechanisms of supraspinal actions upon spinal cord activities. Recticular inhibitory mechanisms upon flexor motoneurons. J Neurophysiol 28:413, 1965.

115. Lorente De Nó, R: Anatomy of the eighth nerve: The central projection of the nerve endings of the internal ear. Laryngoscope 43:1, 1933.

116. Lorente De Nó, R: The regulation of eye positions and movements induced by the labyrinth. Laryngoscope 42:233, 1932.

117. Lorente De Nó, R: Vestibulo-ocular reflex arc. Arch Neurol Psychiatr 30:245, 1933.

118. Lund, S and Pompeiano, O: Descending pathways with monosynaptic action on motoneurones. Experientia 21:602, 1965.

119. Lynch, JC and McLaren, JW: The contribution of parieto-occipital association cortex to the control of slow eye movements. In Lennerstrand, G, Zee, DS, and Keller, EL (eds): Functional Basis of Ocular Motility Disorders. Pergamon, Oxford, UK, 1982, pp 501–510.

120. Mach, E: Grundlinien der Lehre von den Bewegungsempfindungen. Engelmann, Leipzig, 1875; Bonset, Amsterdam (translation), 1967.

121. Maeda, M, Shimazu, H, and Shinoda, Y: Nature of synaptic events in cat abducens motoneurons at slow and quick phase of vestibular nystagmus. J Neurophysiol 35:279, 1972.

122. Maekawa, K and Takeda, T: Electrophysiological identification of the climbing and mossy fiber pathways from the rabbit's retina to the contralateral cerebellar flocculus. Brain Res 109:169, 1976.

123. Maekawa, K and Simpson, JI: Climbing fiber activation of Purkinje cells in the flocculus by impulses transferred through the visual pathway. Brain Res 39:245, 1972.

124. Maekawa, K and Takeda, T: Mossy fiber responses evoked in the cerebellar flocculus of rabbits by stimulation of the optic pathway. Brain Res 98:590, 1975.

125. Magnus, R: Körperstellung. Springer-Verlag, Berlin, 1924.

126. Mandl, G, Melvill Jones, G, and Cynader, M: Adaptability of the vestibulo-ocular reflex to vision reversal in strobe reared cats. Brain Res 209:35, 1981.

127. Maunsell, JHR and Van Essen, DC: Functional properties of neurons in middle temporal visual area of the macaque monkey. I. Selectivity for stimulus direction, speed and orientation. J Neurophysiol 49:1127, 1983.

128. May, JG and Anderson, RA: Different patterns

of cortico-pontine projections from separate cortical fields within the inferior parietal lobule and dorsal prelunate gyrus of the macaque. Exp Brain Res 63:265, 1986.

129. May, JG, Keller, EL, and Suzuki, DA: Smooth pursuit eye movement deficits with chemical lesions in the dorsolateral pontine nucleus of the monkey. J Neurophysiol 59: 952, 1988.

130. McCouch, GP, Deering, ID, and Ling, TH: Location of receptors for tonic neck reflexes. J Neurophysiol 14:191, 1951.

131. McCrea, RA, Strassman, A, May, E, and Highstein, SM: Anatomical and physiological characteristics of vestibular neurons mediating the horizontal vestibulo-ocular reflex of the squirrel monkey. J Comp Neurol 264:547, 1987.

132. McNally, WJ and Stuart, EA: Physiology of the Labryinth. A manual prepared for graduates in medicine. Am Acad Ophthalmol Otolaryngol McGill University and Royal Victoria Hospital, Montreal, 1967.

133. Meiry, JL: Vestibular and proprioceptive stabilization of eye movements. In Bach-Y-Rita, P, Collins, CC, and Hyde, JE (eds): The Control of Eye Movements. Academic Press, New York, 1971.

134. Melvill Jones, G: Adaptive modulation of VOR parameters by vision. In Berthoz, A, Melvill Jones, G (eds): Adaptive Mechanisms in Gaze Control: Reviews in Oculomotor Research. Elsevier, Amsterdam, 1985, pp 21–50.

135. Melvill Jones, G: Predominance of anti-compensatory oculomotor responses during rapid head rotation. Aerospace Med 35:965, 1964.

136. Mergner, T, Deeke, L, and Wagner, HJ: Vestibulo-thalamic projection to the anterior suprasylvian cortex of the cat. Exp Brain Res 44:455, 1981.

137. Meyer, CH, Lasker, AG, and Robinson, DA: The upper limit of human smooth pursuit velocity. Vision Res 25:561, 1985.

138. Miles, FA, Braitman, DJ, and Dow, BM: Long term adaptive changes in primate vestibulo-ocular reflexes: IV. Electrophysiological observations in flocculus of adapted monkeys. J Neurophysiol 43:1477, 1980.

139. Miller, EF II: Counterrolling of the human eye produced by head tilt with respect to gravity. Acta Otolaryngol 54:479, 1962.

140. Mitsacos, A, Reisine, H, and Highstein, SM: The superior vestibular nucleus: An intracellular HRP study in the cat. II. Non-vestibulo-ocular neurons. J Comp Neurol 215:92, 1983.

141. Mitsacos, A, Reisine, H, and Highstein, SM: The superior vestibular nucleus: An intracellular HRP study in the cat. I. Vestibulo-ocular neurons. J Comp Neurol 215:78, 1983.

142. Naegele, JR, and Held, R: The postnatal development of monocular optokinetic nystagmus in infants. Vision Res 22:391, 1982.

143. Newman, A, Suarez, C, and Lee, W: The histo-morphology and innervation of the vestibular nuclei of the chinchilla. Abstracts of the Association for Research in Otolaryngology 1989, p 329.

144. Niven, JI, Hixson, WC, and Correia, MJ: Elicitation of horizontal nystagmus by periodic linear acceleration. Acta Otolaryngol 62: 429, 1965.

145. Nyberg-Hansen, R: Origin and termination of fibers from the vestibular nuclei descending in the medial longitudinal fasciculus. An experimental study with silver impregnation methods in the cat. J Comp Neurol 122:355, 1964.

146. Nyberg-Hansen, R: Sites and mode of termination of fibers of the vestibulo-spinal tract in the cat. An experimental study with silver impregnation methods. J Comp Neurol 122:369, 1964.

147. Nyberg-Hansen, R: Sites and mode of termination of reticulospinal fibers in the cat. An experimental study with silver impregnation methods. J Comp Neurol 124:71, 1965.

148. Ohgaki, T, Curthoys, IS, and Markham, CH: Morphology of physiologically identified second order vestibular neurons in cat, using intracellularly injected HRP. J Comp Neurol 276:387, 1988.

149. Ormsby, CC and Young, LR: Perception of static orientation in a constant gravitoinertial environment. Aviat Space Environ Med 47: 159, 1976.

150. Paige, GD: Vestibulo-ocular reflex and its interactions with visual following mechanisms in the squirrel monkey. I. Response characteristics in normal animals. J Neurophysiol 49:134, 1983.

151. Penfield, W: Vestibular-sensation and the cerebral cortex. Ann Otol 66:691, 1957.

152. Perlmutter, ST, Fukushima, K, Peterson, BW, and Baker, JF: Spatial properties of second order vestibulo-ocular reflex neurons in the alert cat. Soc Neurosci Abstr 14:137.9, 1988.

153. Peterson, BW, Graf, W, and Baker, JF: Spatial properties of signals carried by second order vestibulo-ocular relay neurons in the cat. Soc Neurosci Abstr 13:1093, 1987.

154. Peterson, BW: The reticulospinal system and its role in the control of movement. In Barnes, CD (ed): Brainstem Control of Spinal Cord Function. Academic Press, New York, 1984, pp 27–86.

155. Peterson, BW, Baker, J, and Wickland, C: Plastic changes in the cervicoocular and vestibuloocular reflexes elicited by labyrinthine lesions or altered visual feedback. In Keller, E and Zee, D (eds): Adaptive Processes in Visual and Oculomotor Systems. Pergamon Press, New York, 1986, pp 399–408.

156. Pola, J and Wyatt, HJ: Target position and velocity: The stimuli for smooth pursuit eye movements. Vision Res 20:523, 1980.

157. Pompeiano, O and Brodal, A: Spino-vestibular fibers in the cat. An experimental study. J Comp Neurol 108:353, 1957.

158. Pompeiano, O: Cerebello-vestibular interrelations. In Kornhuber, HH (ed): Handbook of Sensory Physiology. The Vestibular System,

Vol VI, Part 1. Springer-Verlag, New York, 1974.

159. Precht, W and Dieringer, N: Neuronal events paralleling functional recovery (compensation) following peripheral vestibular lesions. In Berthoz, A, Melvill Jones, G (eds): Adaptive Mechanisms in Gaze Control: Facts and Theories. Elsevier, Amsterdam, 1985, p 25.

160. Precht, W and Shimazu, H: Functional connections of tonic and kinetic vestibular neurons with primary vestibular afferents. J Neurophysiol 28:1014, 1965.

161. Precht, W and Strata, P: On the pathway mediating optokinetic responses in the vestibular nuclear neurons. Neuroscience 5:777, 1980.

162. Precht, W, Shimazu, H, and Markham, CH: A mechanism of central compensation of vestibular function following hemilabyrinthectomy. J Neurophysiol 29:996, 1966.

163. Precht, W: Vestibular mechanisms. Ann Rev Neurosci 2:265, 1979.

164. Raphan, T and Cohen, B: Multidimensional modelling of the vestibulo-ocular reflex. In Keller, E and Zee, D (eds): Adaptive Processes in Visual and Oculomotor Systems. Pergamon Press, New York, 1986.

165. Raphan, T and Cohen, B: Velocity storage and the ocular response to multidimensional vestibular stimuli. In Berthoz, A, Melville Jones, G (eds): Adaptive Mechanisms in Gaze Control. Elsevier, Amsterdam, 1985, pp 123–143.

166. Raphan, T, Matsuo, V, and Cohen, B: Velocity storage in the vestibulo-ocular reflex arc (VOR). Exp Brain Res 35:229, 1979.

167. Ried, S, Maioli, C, and Precht, W: Vestibular nuclear neuron activity in chronically hemilabyrinthectomized cats. Acta Otolaryngol 98:1, 1984.

168. Roberts, TDM: Neurophysiology of Postural Mechanisms. Plenum Press, New York, 1967.

169. Robinson, DA: Adaptive gain control of vestibulo-ocular reflex by the cerebellum. J Neurophysiol 39:954, 1976.

170. Robinson, DA: Control of eye movements. In Brooks, VB (ed): Handbook of Physiology. The nervous system II. American Physiological Society, Washington, DC, 1981, pp 1275–1313.

171. Robinson, DA: Oculomotor unit behavior in the monkey. J Neurophysiol 33:393, 1970.

172. Robinson, DA: The use of control systems analysis in the neurophysiology of eye movements. Ann Rev Neurosci 4:463, 1981.

173. Robinson, DL, Goldberg, ME, and Stanton, GB: Parietal association cortex in the primate: Sensory mechanisms and behavioral modulation. J Neurophysiol 41:910, 1978.

174. Rubin, AM, et al: Vestibular-neck integration in the vestibular nuclei. Brain Res 96:99, 1975.

175. Sadiadpour, K and Brodal, A: The vestibular nuclei in man. A morphological study in the light of experimental findings in the cat. J Hirnforsch 10:299, 1968.

176. Sakata, H, Sibutani, H, and Kawano, K: Functional properties of visual tracking neurons in posterior parietal association cortex of the monkey. J Neurophysiol 49:1364, 1983.

177. Schiff, D, Cohen, B, and Raphan, T: Nystagmus induced by stimulation of the nucleus of the optic tract in the monkey. Exp Brain Res 70:1, 1988.

178. Schultheis, LW and Robinson, DA: Directional plasticity of the vestibulo-ocular reflex in the cat. Ann NY Acad Sci 374:504, 1981.

179. Schwindt, PC, Richter, A, and Precht, W: Short latency utricular and canal input to ipsilateral abducens motoneurons. Brain Res 60:259, 1973.

180. Segal, BN and Liben, S: Modulation of human velocity storage sampled during intermittently-illuminated optokinetic stimulation. Exp Brain Res 59:515, 1985.

181. Sherrington, CS: The Integrative Action of the Nervous System. Yale University Press, New Haven, 1906.

182. Shimazu, H and Precht, W: Inhibition of central vestibular neurons from the contralateral labyrinth and its mediating pathway. J Neurophysiol 29:467, 1966.

183. Shimazu, H and Precht, W: Tonic and kinetic responses of cat's vestibular neurons to horizontal angular acceleration. J Neurophysiol 28:991, 1965.

184. Simpson, JT: The accessory optic system. Ann Rev Neurosci 7:13, 1984.

185. Sirkin, DW, Precht, W, and Courjon, JH: Initial, rapid phase of recovery from unilateral vestibular nerve lesion not dependent on survival of central portion of vestibular nerve. Brain Res 302:245, 1984.

186. Skavenski, AA, and Robinson, DA: Role of abducens neurons in vestibulo-ocular reflex. J Neurophysiol 36:724. 1973.

187. Sparks, DL and Travis, Jr., RP: Firing patterns of reticular formation neurons during horizontal eye movements. Brain Res 33:477, 1971.

188. Steinbach, MJ: Pursuing the perceptual rather than the retinal stimulus. Vision Res 16:1371, 1976.

189. Suzuki, J-I, Tokumasu, K, and Goto, K: Eye movements from single utricular nerve stimulation in the cat. Acta Otolaryngol 68:350, 1969.

190. Takemori, S and Suzuki, J-I: Eye deviations from neck torsion in humans. Ann Otol 80:439, 1971.

191. Tanaka, K, et al: Analysis of local and wide-field movements in the superior temporal visual areas of the macaque monkey. J Neurosci 6:134, 1986.

192. Ter Braak, JWG, Schenk, VWD, and Van Vliet, AGM: Visual reactions in a case of long-lasting cortical blindness. J Neurol Neurosurg Psychiatr 34:140, 1971.

193. Ter Braak, JWG: Untersuchungen über optokinetischen Nystagmus. Arch Neerl Physiol 21:309, 1936. (Translated "Investigations of optokinetic nystagmus" in Collewijn, H (ed): The Oculomotor System of the Rabbit and its Plasticity. Studies of Brain Func-

tion, Vol 5. Springer-Verlag, Berlin, 1981.)

194. Terzuolo, CA, Llínas, R, and Green, KT: Mechanisms of supraspinal sections upon spinal cord activities; Distribution of reticular and segmental inputs in cat's alpha-motoneurons. Arch Ital Biol 103:635, 1965.

195. Uchino, Y and Suzuki, S: Axon collaterals to the extraocular motoneuron pools of inhibitory vestibulo-ocular neurons activated from the anterior, posterior and horizontal semicircular canals in the cat. Neuroscience Letters 37:129, 1983.

196. Uchino, Y, Hirai, N, and Suzuki, S: Branching pattern and properties of vertical- and horizontal-related excitatory vestibuloocular neurons in the cat. J Neurophysiol 48:891, 1982.

197. Uemura, T and Cohen, B: Effects of vestibular nuclei lesions on vestibulo-ocular reflexes and posture in monkeys. Acta Otolaryngol (Suppl.) 315, 1973.

198. Van Die, G and Collewijn, H: Optokinetic nystagmus in man. Hum Neurobiol 1:111, 1982.

199. Van Egmond, AAJ, Groen, JJ, and Jongkees, LBW: The turning test with small regulable stimuli. J Laryngol Otol 62:63, 1948.

200. Virre, E, Tweed, D, Milner, K, and Vilis, T: A re-examination of the gain of the vestibuloocular reflex. J Neurophysiol 56:439, 1986.

201. Waespe, W and Henn, V: Conflicting visual-vestibular stimulation and vestibular nucleus activity in alert monkeys. Exp Brain Res 33:203, 1978.

202. Waespe, W and Henn, V: Gaze stabilization in the primate: The interaction of the vestibulo-ocular reflex, optokinetic nystagmus, and smooth pursuit. Rev Physiol Biochem Pharmacol 106:38, 1987.

203. Waespe, W and Henn, V: Motion information in the vestibular nuclei of alert monkeys: Visual and vestibular input vs. optomotor output. In Granit, R and Pampeiano, O (eds): Reflex Control of Posture and Movement. Progress in Brain Research 50:693, 1979.

204. Waespe, W and Henn, V: Neuronal activity in the vestibular nuclei of the alert monkey during vestibular and optokinetic stimulation. Exp Brain Res 27:523, 1977.

205. Waespe, W and Henn, V: Vestibular nuclei activity during optokinetic after-nystagmus (OKAN) in the alert monkey. Exp Brain Res 30:323, 1977.

206. Wallman, J, et al: Avian vestibulo-ocular reflex: Adaptive plasticity and developmental changes. J Neurophysiol 48:952, 1982.

207. Walsh, EG: Role of the vestibular apparatus in the perception of motion on a parallel swing. J Physiol 155:506, 1961.

208. Watzl, E and Mountcastle, V: Projection of vestibular nerve to cerebral cortex of the cat. Am J Physiol 159:594, 1949.

209. Westheimer, G: Eye movement responses to a horizontally moving visual stimulus. Arch Ophthalmol 52:932, 1954.

210. Westheimer, G: Mechanism of saccadic eye movements. Arch Ophthalmol 52:710, 1954.

211. Wilson, VJ and Maeda, M: Connections between semicircular canals and neck motoneurons in the cat. J Neurophysiol 37:346, 1974.

212. Wilson, VJ, Wylie, RM, and Marco, LA: Organization of the medial vestibular nucleus. J Neurophysiol 31:166, 1968.

213. Winfield, JA, Hendrickson, A, and Kimm, J: Anatomical evidence that the medial terminal nucleus of the accessory optic tract in mammals provides a visual mossy fiber input to the flocculus. Brain Res 151:175, 1978.

214. Yagi, T and Markham, CH: Neural correlates of compensation after hemilabyrinthectomy. Exp Neurol 84:98, 1984.

215. Yee, RD, et al: Effects of an optokinetic background on pursuit eye movements. Invest Ophthalmol Vis Sci 24:115, 1983.

216. Zee, DS, et al: Effects of occipital lobectomy upon eye movements in primate. J Neurophysiol 58:883, 1987.

217. Zee, DS, et al: Effects of ablation of flocculus and paraflocculus on eye movements in primate. J Neurophysiol 46:878, 1981.

218. Zeki, SM: The responses of cells in the anterior bank of the superior temporal sulcus in macaque monkeys. J Physiol Lond 308:85P, 1980.

Part II

EVALUATION OF THE DIZZY PATIENT

Chapter 4

THE HISTORY IN THE DIZZY PATIENT

TYPES OF DIZZINESS

Dizziness is a nonspecific term that describes a sensation of altered orientation in space. Because visual, proprioceptive, and vestibular signals provide the main source of information about the position of the head and body in space, damage to any of these afferent systems can lead to a complaint of dizziness. Changes in the brain centers that integrate these orienting signals can also result in the sensation of dizziness. The initial task of the clinician is to obtain a description of what the patient means by dizziness. The patient should be encouraged to use his own words to describe the sensation and how the sensation interferes with his or her daily activities. In our experience less than half of patients complaining of dizziness actually have vertigo. Because the diagnostic evaluation and management differ markedly depending on the category of dizziness, it is critical that the examining physician determine the type of dizziness (Table 4–1) before proceeding with exhaustive diagnostic studies.

Vertigo

DEFINITION

Vertigo is an illusion of movement, usually that of rotation, although patients occasionally describe a sensation of linear displacement or tilt. The afferent nerves from the otoliths and semicircular canals of each labyrinth maintain a balanced tonic rate of firing into the vestibular nuclei. Asymmetric involvement of this baseline activity anywhere in the peripheral and central vestibular pathways leads to an illusion of movement. For example, damage to a semicircular canal or its afferent nerve produces a sensation of angular rotation in the plane of that canal similar to the sensation experienced during physiologic stimulation. More typically, lesions involve all the canals and otoliths of one labyrinth, producing a sensation of rotation in a plane determined by the balance of afferent signals from the contralateral labyrinth (usually near the horizontal plane, inasmuch as the vertical canal and otolith signals partially cancel out). If a patient with a unilateral vestibular lesion attempts to fixate on an object, it will appear blurred and seem to be moving in the direction opposite to that of the slow phase of the patient's spontaneous nystagmus (i.e., away from the side of the lesion). This illusion of movement occurs because the brain lacks eye proprioceptive information and interprets the target displacement on

Table 4–1. THE MECHANISM OF COMMON TYPES OF DIZZINESS

Type	Mechanism
Vertigo	Imbalance of tonic vestibular signals
Presyncopal light-headedness	Diffuse cerebral ischemia
Psychophysiologic dizziness	Impaired central integration of sensory signals
Dysequilibrium	Loss of vestibulospinal, proprioceptive, cerebellar, or motor function
Ocular dizziness	Visual-vestibular mismatch due to impaired vision
Multisensory dizziness	Partial loss of multiple sensory system function
Physiologic dizziness	Sensory conflict due to unusual combination of sensory signals

Table 4–2. DIFFERENTIATION BETWEEN PERIPHERAL (END-ORGAN AND NERVE) AND CENTRAL CAUSES OF VERTIGO

	Nausea and Vomiting	Imbalance	Hearing Loss	Oscillopsia	Neurologic Symptoms	Compensation
Peripheral	Severe	Mild	Common	Mild	Rare	Rapid
Central	Moderate	Severe	Rare	Severe	Common	Slow

the retina as object movement rather than eye movement. An illusion of linear movement or tilting suggests isolated involvement of an otolith or its central connections.

CENTRAL VERSUS PERIPHERAL CAUSES

Vertigo defined as an illusion of movement always indicates an imbalance within the vestibular system, although the symptom per se does not indicate where in the system the imbalance originates. The same sensation can result from lesions in such diverse locations as the inner ear, the deep paravertebral stretch receptors of the neck, the visual-vestibular interaction centers in the brainstem and cerebellum, or in the subjective sensation pathways of the thalamus or cortex. Distinction between peripheral and central causes of vertigo can usually be made, however, based on other features in the history (Table 4–2).

Well-documented lesions within the vestibular pathways sometimes produce only a nonspecific sensation of disorientation without a clearly defined illusion of movement. Normal subjects undergoing caloric stimulation (i.e., a physiologic imbalance in the vestibular system) occasionally describe the experience with terms such as floating or even giddiness. For these reasons one must not to be too restrictive in classifying dizziness based on the subjective description alone.

TIME COURSE

Vertigo invariably occurs in episodes, usually abrupt in onset followed by decreasing intensity as the inciting factor dissipates or as compensation occurs. Continuous dizziness without fluctuation

for long periods of time is not typical of vestibular disorders. Durations associated with several of the more common causes of vertigo are outlined in Table 4–3. Episodes lasting seconds suggest the diagnosis of benign positional vertigo.[6] During the acute phase such patients may report a nonspecific feeling of disorientation and imbalance along with nausea and vomiting that lasts for hours to days, but on careful questioning one can identify recurrent brief attacks of positional vertigo interspersed with a more persistent nonspecific dizziness. An episode of vertigo lasting minutes suggests a transient vascular ischemic attack.[24, 27] This is the typical duration of vertigo with transient ischemia within the basilar vertebral circulation and for migraine attacks (with or without headache). With a typical bout of Meniere's syndrome the vertigo reaches a peak within minutes, remains severe for an hour or two, and then gradually resolves over the next few hours.[3] Vertigo gradually resolving over several days occurs with viral vestibular neuritis, labyrinthine trauma, infarction of the labyrinth or any lesion that produces permanent damage to the inner ear or vestibular nerve.[27, 58] Even with a complete unilateral loss of vestibular function the vertigo will gradually resolve as central compensation occurs. The onset is abrupt with trauma and vascular occlusion, whereas it is more gradual in onset (over hours to days) with viral vestibular neuritis.

Table 4–3. DURATION OF COMMON CAUSES OF VERTIGO

Seconds	Benign positional vertigo
Minutes	Vertebrobasilar insufficiency, migraine
Hours	Meniere's syndrome
Days	Vestibular neuritis, infarction of labyrinth

PRECIPITATING FACTORS

The events just prior to an episode of vertigo are important in determining the cause. Rapid head movements commonly induce vertigo because they accentuate any imbalance within the vestibular pathways. Even after compensation has occurred, head movements or change in position can lead to a brief sensation of vertigo and disorientation. Positional vertigo is commonly induced by turning over in bed, sitting up from a lying position, extending the neck to look up, or bending over and straightening up. Patients with a perilymph fistula develop brief episodes of vertigo precipitated by changes in middle ear pressure (coughing, sneezing).[25] The pressure change in the middle ear is transferred directly to the inner ear (usually the horizontal semicircular canal) through the fistula. Occasionally loud noises induce transient vertigo in patients with inner ear lesions (Tulio phenomenon). For example, as the labyrinthine membranes dilate with Meniere's syndrome, adhesions may develop between the stapedius footplate and the membranous labyrinth, resulting in traction on the labyrinth with sudden movement of the stapes.[46]

ASSOCIATED SYMPTOMS

Autonomic symptoms such as sweating, pallor, nausea, and vomiting commonly accompany dizziness caused by vestibular lesions, but such symptoms are uncommon with other types of dizziness. Typically, the autonomic symptoms are more pronounced when the vertigo has a peripheral origin, although there are frequent exceptions to the rule. Occasionally, vegetative symptoms are the only manifestation of a vestibular lesion. Numerous interconnecting pathways between brainstem vestibular and autonomic centers account for this close association of vestibular and autonomic symptoms.

The site of the lesion determines the symptoms that accompany vertigo (Table 4–4). In addition to vertigo, lesions of the labyrinth or VIII nerve commonly produce auditory symptoms such as hearing loss, tinnitus, a sensation of pressure or fullness in the ear, or pain in the ear. Lesions

Table 4–4. SYMPTOMS ASSOCIATED WITH VERTIGO DUE TO LESIONS AT DIFFERENT ANATOMICAL LOCATIONS

Inner ear	Brainstem
Hearing loss	Diplopia
Tinnitus	Dysarthria
Pressure	Perioral numbness
Pain	Extremity weakness
	and numbness
Internal auditory canal	Drop attacks
Hearing loss	
Tinnitus	Cerebellum
Facial weakness	Imbalance
	Incoordination
Cerebellopontine angle	
Hearing loss	Temporal lobe
Tinnitus	Absence spells
Facial weakness and	Visual (formed), ol-
numbness	factory or gusta-
Extremity incoordination	tory hallucinations
	Occipital lobe
	Visual field loss
	Visual hallucinations
	(unformed)

of the internal auditory canal also produce hearing loss and tinnitus and may be associated with ipsilateral facial weakness, whereas those in the cerebellar pontine angle may be associated with ipsilateral facial numbness and weakness and ipsilateral extremity ataxia. As with vertigo the time course of an associated hearing loss can help determine the cause. Fluctuating hearing loss and tinnitus are characteristic of Meniere's syndrome. Patients with this disorder usually notice a build-up of pressure in the ear just prior to the onset of hearing loss, tinnitus, and vertigo. Abrupt complete unilateral deafness and vertigo occur with viral involvement of the labyrinth and/or VIII nerve and with vascular occlusion to the inner ear. A slow progressive unilateral hearing loss suggests the existence of an acoustic neuroma or other cerebellopontine angle tumor.

Because of the proximity of other neuronal centers and fiber tracts in the brainstem and cerebellum it is unusual to find lesions in these areas that produce isolated vestibular symptoms.[5] Lesions of the brainstem invariably are associated with other cranial nerve and long-tract symptoms. For example, vertigo caused by transient vertebrobasilar insufficiency is associated with other brainstem and occipital lobe symptoms such as diplopia, hemianoptic field defects, drop attacks, weakness, numbness, dysarthria, and ataxia.[61] Lesions of the cerebellum (e.g., infarction or hemorrhage) may be relatively silent but are always associated with extremity and truncal ataxia in addition to vertigo. Of note, hearing loss for pure tones is unusual with central lesions even in the late stages.

Vertigo can occur as part of an aura of temporal lobe seizures.[52] The cortical projections of the vestibular system are activated by a focal discharge within the temporal lobe. Such vertigo is nearly always associated with other typical aura symptoms such as an abnormal taste or smell and distortion of the visual world (hallucinations and illusions). Rarely, however, vertigo can be the only manifestation of an aura. In such cases, the association with typical absence spells should lead one to the correct diagnosis.

COMPENSATION

The severity of symptoms following a vestibular lesion depends on (1) the extent of the lesion, (2) whether the lesion is unilateral or bilateral, and (3) the rapidity with which the functional loss occurs. Patients who slowly lose vestibular function bilaterally (e.g., secondary to ototoxic drugs) often do not complain of vertigo but will report oscillopsia with head movements and instability when walking (due to loss of vestibulo-ocular and vestibulospinal reflexes, respectively). If a patient slowly loses vestibular function on one side over a period of months to years (e.g., with an acoustic neuroma), symptoms and signs may be absent. On the other hand, a sudden unilateral loss of vestibular function is a dramatic event. The patient complains of severe vertigo and nausea, is pale and perspiring, and usually vomits repeatedly. He prefers to lie quietly in a dark room but can walk if forced to (falling toward the side of the lesion). A brisk spontaneous nystagmus interferes with vision. These symptoms and signs are transient, however, and the process of compensation begins almost immediately. Within one week of the lesion a young patient can walk without difficulty and with fixation can inhibit the spontaneous nystagmus. Within one month most patients return to work with little if any residual symptoms. By contrast, patients with central vestibular lesions, (e.g., Wallenberg's syndrome or cerebellar infarction) often show only minimal compensation for the vestibular imbalance even after months or years. Presumably, the central pathways necessary for vestibular compensation are damaged with these central lesions.

PREDISPOSING FACTORS

The patient's general state of health just prior to the onset of dizziness should be carefully investigated. Most severe systemic disorders are associated with dizziness either due to partial involvement of all the body-orienting systems or due to a decreased capacity of the central nervous system (CNS) to deal with information from these systems (a type of multisensory dizziness). Some systemic disorders such as vasculitis, bacterial endocarditis, and septicemia selectively damage the vestibular system by interfering with its blood supply. Such patients may develop severe vertigo and vomiting typical of an acute peripheral vestibular loss. Patients with viral vestibular neurolabyrinthitis frequently report an upper respiratory tract illness either within 2 or 3 weeks before or at the time of onset of vertigo. Chronic middle ear infections may lead to bacterial labyrinthitis or serous labyrinthopathy, and patients with bacterial meningitis may develop bacterial labyrinthitis through the direct cerebrospinal fluid–perilymph connections.[17, 47] Patients with Meniere's syndrome may have an attack of vertigo precipitated by foods high in salt content.

Head injury commonly damages the delicate labyrinthine membranes with or without associated bone fracture.[37] Labyrinthine trauma may result in a single prolonged episode of vertigo or, more commonly, recurrent episodes of positional vertigo. The more common nonspecific lightheaded dizziness following head trauma is probably not related to vestibular damage, inasmuch as common associated symptoms and signs are absent. Surgery in or about the ear is a major cause of trauma to the labyrinthine membranes.

Vertigo not infrequently follows surgery confined to the middle ear. Past medical history should focus on past or chronic medical illnesses that might predispose the patient to vestibular system damage such as diabetes mellitus, atherosclerotic vascular disease, syphilis (congenital or acquired), and major allergies. Viral illnesses that damage the inner ear in utero or in infancy (e.g., rubella, mumps, rubeola) may be followed years later by recurrent episodes of vertigo.[45] This so-called delayed endolymphatic hydrops may not be associated with auditory symptoms such as hearing loss, tinnitus, or ear pressure because the patient may be deaf in the damaged ear.

A careful drug history is crucial in evaluating any patient with dizziness (Table 4–5). Ototoxic drugs such as the aminoglycosides and salicylates occasionally cause vertigo but more often produce gait unsteadiness and imbalance and oscillopsia from bilateral symmetrical vestibular endorgan damage. Antihypertensive medications produce a lightheaded dizziness secondary to postural hypotension. Anticoagulants can be associated with an acute inner ear hemorrhage causing a dramatic onset of severe vertigo and nausea. Alcohol and phenytoin produce acute reversible dysequilibrium and chronic irreversible dysequilibrium from cerebellar dysfunction. Positional vertigo and nystagmus commonly occur with acute alcohol intoxication. Sedative drugs (e.g., barbiturates, antihistamines, benzodiazepines) cause a nonspecific dizziness typically described as a fogginess, cloudiness, or giddiness that is presumably due to a diffuse depression of the central sensory integrating centers.

FAMILY HISTORY

Common vestibular disorders with a genetic predisposition include migraine, Meniere's syndrome, otosclerosis, neurofibromatosis, and spinocerebellar degeneration. Migraine can present as isolated episodes of vertigo (a migraine equivalent) in some members of a family, whereas other members have classic migraine headaches. Some varieties of Meniere's syndrome may be due to a congenitally narrow endolymphatic duct. Patients with otosclerosis usually present with a conductive hearing loss, although sensorineural hearing loss and vertigo may result from involvement of the otic capsule. Neurofibromatosis is inherited as an autosomal dominant trait and is manifested by the combination of pigmented skin lesions, multiple tumors of the spinal and cranial nerves, tumors of the skin, and intracranial gliomas and meningiomas. Acoustic neuromas and meningiomas in the CP angle are common; a central variant is manifested by bilateral acoustic neuromas without the typical peripheral manifestations. Central varieties of positional vertigo are commonly seen in patients with the inherited ataxia syndromes (particularly common with the late-onset cortical cerebellar atrophy syndromes). Positional vertigo and ataxia are also commonly seen with Hippel-Lindau disease. This autosomal dominant disorder is characterized by hemangioblastomas of the cerebellar hemispheres, angiomas of the retina, and cystic changes in the kidney and pancreas. The diagnosis should be considered in any patient with a cerebellar tumor or hemorrhage who manifests an elevated hematocrit.

Table 4–5. DRUGS COMMONLY ASSOCIATED WITH DIZZINESS

Class of Drug	Type of Dizziness	Mechanism
Alcohol	Positional vertigo, drunkenness	Changes cupula specific gravity, cerebellar dysfunction
Tranquilizers	Nonspecific disorientation	Depression of central integrative centers
Antihypertensives	Presyncopal lightheadedness	Orthostatic hypotension
Anticonvulsants	Drunkenness, dysequilibrium	Cerebellar dysfunction
Aminoglycoside antibiotics	Dysequilibrium, oscillopsia, occasional vertigo	Damage to labyrinthine hair cells

Congenital deformities of the inner ear may result from abnormal genes or from abnormal development *in utero*. Most of the inherited disorders of the inner ear are associated with multiple malformations in other organs producing a characteristic clinical profile (e.g., Alport's and Waardenburg's syndromes). Progressive atrophy of the cochlear and vestibular nerves may be seen as part of a more diffuse degenerative disorder (e.g., with Friedreich's ataxia or olivopontocerebellar atrophy) or may occur as an isolated phenomenon (both autosomal dominant and recessive inheritance). Although uncommon, the syndrome of familial periodic ataxia and vertigo is important to recognize because it has been shown to respond dramatically to acetazolamide. With this dominantly inherited disorder, episodes of vertigo and ataxia recur throughout the patient's life often without objective findings between episodes.

DIAGNOSIS AND MANAGEMENT

The reader is referred to Chapters 9–17 for discussion in detail of the diagnosis and management of common causes of vertigo.

Presyncopal Lightheadedness

Presyncopal lightheadedness can best be described as the sensation of an impending faint. It is often associated with a feeling of unsteadiness or even of falling. Presyncopal lightheadedness results from pancerebral ischemia. Common causes are summarized in Table 4–6. We emphasize

Table 4–6. COMMON CAUSES OF PRESYNCOPAL LIGHTHEADEDNESS

Cause	Precipitating Factors
Orthostatic hypotension	Reduced blood volume, hypotensive drugs, autonomic dysfunction
Vasovagal attack	Prolonged standing in hot sun, fear, severe pain, acute vertigo
Hyperventilation	Anxiety, stress, panic attacks
Decreased cardiac output	Arrhythmia, valvular disease, heart failure

that presyncopal lightheadedness is not a symptom of focal occlusive cerebrovascular disease (i.e., not a symptom of impending stroke).

ORTHOSTATIC HYPOTENSION

All of us have experienced lightheadedness after rapidly assuming the standing position from the supine or sitting position. This symptom is transient and of little consequence. Also, not uncommonly, susceptible subjects may develop presyncopal lightheadedness and may even faint after standing for a prolonged period in the hot sun. Recurrent symptoms of postural hypotension, however, can usually be traced to either reduced blood volume, the chronic use of hypotensive drugs, or autonomic dysfunction. Nearly all of the antihypertensive drugs and a large number of antidepressants and major tranquilizers will predispose a patient to orthostatic hypotension, as will long-term bedrest.[28]

Diagnosis and Management. Presyncopal lightheadedness with orthostatic hypotension can develop immediately on standing or insidiously after several minutes of standing. The diagnosis is made by documenting an acute or progressive decline in mean blood pressure of more than 10 to 15 torr while the patient is in the erect position. In patients with autonomic insufficiency the pulse rate will remain unchanged despite the hypotension. Autonomic impairment can be documented at the bedside by taking the pulse while the supine patient performs a vigorous Valsalva maneuver. Normally the pulse slows and the mean blood pressure increases by 10 to 30 torr in the immediate post-Valsalva period. Orthostatic hypotension can often be eliminated by removing offending drugs or by correcting the causes of blood-volume depletion. In patients with autonomic insufficiency, increased salt intake can increase blood volume, and elastic stockings can prevent pooling of blood in the lower extremities.[49] In severe cases the salt-retaining steroid fludrocortisone can aid in expanding blood volume.

VASOVAGAL ATTACKS

Prior to a common faint one experiences sensations of lightheadedness, giddiness, nausea, and an abdominal sinking sensation. Typically the subject is pale and there are associated signs of parasympathetic hyperactivity, including piloerection and sweating. These symptoms are induced when emotions such as fear and anxiety, initiated in the forebrain limbic system, activate the medullary vasodepressor centers.[53] The consequences are a fall in heart rate and blood pressure and a decline in cardiac output, leading to a decrease in cerebral blood flow. Parasympathetic hyperactivity accounts for the slowing of heart rate, and diminished sympathetic tone leads to vasodilation. Normal cardiovascular reflexes are reinstated if the subject lies supine or if there is loss of consciousness with a common faint.

Vasodepressor lightheadedness commonly occurs when a subject has fasted for a long period of time, is exposed to hot moist weather, and/or has stood for a prolonged period of time. Some individuals are clearly more susceptible to presyncopal lightheadedness and the common faint than others, and occasionally one can find a family history with members in several generations who are susceptible. Vasodepressor episodes can also be precipitated by acute visceral pain or by a sudden severe attack of vertigo. This explains the occasional patient with an acute peripheral vestibular lesion who will present with a history of syncope. In this case, it is important to obtain a history of severe vertigo and autonomic symptoms preceding the loss of consciousness.

Diagnosis and Management. Diagnosis of vasodepressor lightheadedness and syncope is based on finding the characteristic history in a patient without neurologic or cardiovascular disease and with a normal examination.[50] Routine laboratory studies, including electrocardiogram (ECG), are normal. Treatment is directed at increasing circulation to the brain by lowering the head and elevating the lower extremities to reverse the distal pooling of blood. Rarely, severe cardiac arrhythmia or asystole requires cardiopulmonary resuscitation.[22]

IMPAIRED CARDIAC OUTPUT

In older patients, episodes of presyncopal lightheadedness can often be traced to impaired cardiac output due to arrhythmia.[34] Vagal-mediated bradycardia (vagovagal attacks) can be induced by sudden emotional stimuli or by acute noxious or abnormal visceral sensations. Usually these attacks are accompanied by relatively minor vasodepressor changes in the peripheral vasculature, suggesting that the sympathetic nervous system plays a relatively minor role. It is obviously important to identify patients with cardiac-related presyncope or syncope because many of these patients have serious underlying cardiac disease and are at risk for sudden death if not appropriately treated. Common associated heart conditions include severe hypertension, recurrent myocardial infarction, congestive heart failure, and severe valvular disease (especially aortic stenosis).

Diagnosis and Management. Although physical examination and routine ECG will identify most of the serious heart diseases listed above, intermittent arrhythmias are not identified. Any patient with episodic presyncopal lightheadedness and/or syncope should undergo electrocardiographic monitoring to search for episodes of sinus pauses, sinus bradycardia, atrial fibrillation with slow ventricular rate, and sustained supraventricular tachycardia. Management of the arrhythmia obviously depends on the nature of the underlying heart disease, but many patients can be helped with the insertion of a pacemaker, even if the heart disease cannot be treated.[18]

HYPERVENTILATION

Chronic anxiety with associated hyperventilation is the most common cause of persistent presyncopal lightheadedness in a young patient.[40] From a series of 125 patients presenting to a university outpatient clinic with the complaint of dizziness, Drachman and Hart[21] found that hyperventilation was the single most common cause of dizziness (accounting for 23 percent of patients). Patients typically describe sensations of lightheadedness, faintness, and giddiness along with other sensations that will be described below under the category of psychophysiologic dizziness. Associated symptoms typically include frequent sighing, air hunger, perioral numbness, paresthesias of the extremities, lump in the throat, and tightness in the chest. Patients often report being unable to obtain the satisfaction of a full deep breath and they will sigh frequently as though they were trying to catch their breath. Hyperventilation causes presyncopal lightheadedness by lowering the carbon dioxide content of the blood, thus producing constriction of the cerebrovasculature.[26] In most subjects only a moderate increase in respiratory rate can drop the $Paco_2$ levels to 25 mm of mercury or less in a few minutes. Once this level is achieved, the subject does not have to breathe excessively to maintain the low $Paco_2$ so that it is possible to be chronically hypocapnic without appearing to hyperventilate.[8]

Diagnosis and Management. The diagnosis rests on identifying the characteristic associated symptoms in the setting of anxiety dyspnea. It is usually helpful to have the patient voluntarily overbreathe to reproduce their symptoms and to provide insight into the mechanism.[40] In addition to educating the patient, treatment must be directed at the underlying anxiety. We have found that a vigorous exercise program in conjunction with supportive psychotherapy can be very effective for this type of patient. Long-term use of tranquilizers should be avoided because increased tolerance and dependency commonly occur.

Psychophysiologic Dizziness

DEFINITION

A wide range of dizzy sensations are associated with psychiatric illnesses. Feelings of dissociation, as though one has left one's own body, are common. Patients use terms such as "floating," "swimming," and "giddiness" to describe the dizzy sensation. They may report a feeling of imbalance (commonly a rocking or falling sensation) or even of spinning inside the head—sensations that can usually be differentiated from vertigo because they are not associated with an illusion of movement of the environment or with nystagmus.[2] Psychophysiologic dizziness may be constant

or occur in attacks and is typically associated with symptoms of anxiety. Common associated somatic complaints include tension headache, heart palpitations, gastric distress, urinary frequency, backache, and a generalized feeling of weakness and fatigue. Attacks may be provoked by sensory stimuli (driving on a freeway, walking on a brightly polished floor, watching a train go by) or by social situations (eating in a restaurant, shopping in a department store, attending a reception). Symptoms often begin after a period of stress, especially after the death of a loved one or after a patient has been through an illness, and may continue for months or years.

ACUTE ANXIETY

Common causes of anxiety in daily life are circumstances in which one must make a decision that could have major implications for future social and economic status. The symptoms associated with this type of anxiety are usually transitory and completely reversible.[59] Anxiety can also be associated with a number of neurologic and psychiatric disorders. For example, the first sign of dementia or manic depressive illness can be an attack of severe anxiety without obvious cause.

Panic attacks are a distinct form of anxiety which typically occur in a background of persistent apprehension but at times when there appears to be no obviously threatening circumstance.[36] Such attacks often occur when it would be difficult for one to make a rapid exit (e.g., traveling in an airplane or train, driving in the fast lane of the freeway, shopping in a crowded store, or waiting in a supermarket line). The condition typically builds up over 10 to 15 minutes with progressively increasing anxiety associated with dizziness, shortness of breath, sweating, flushing, trembling or shaking, heart palpitations, paresthesias, and a generalized feeling of weakness (Table 4–7). The dizziness can take several forms, from a giddy unsteady sensation to a progressing presyncopal lightheadedness due to the associated hyperventilation. As typically seen with hyperventilation, the person experiences a tightness in the chest as though the lungs cannot be adequately filled. The person

Table 4–7. COMMON SYMPTOMS DURING PANIC ATTACKS

Shortness of breath, smothering, choking
Palpitations, accelerated heart rate
Chest pain or discomfort
Sweating
Dizziness, unsteady feeling, sensory illusions
Nausea or abdominal distress
Depersonalization or derealization
Numbness or tingling sensations (paresthesias)
Flushes (hot flashes) or chills
Trembling or shaking
Fear of dying
Fear of going crazy or doing something uncontrolled

may try to flee and in the future avoid the situation in which the panic attack occurred. There is a clear genetic predisposition to panic disorders, distinguishing them from the more common anxieties that are a response to specific life situations.[4, 18]

AGORAPHOBIA

Agoraphobia, defined as a morbid fear and avoidance of being in public places, is closely linked with anxiety disorders and panic attacks.[59] Often agoraphobia is secondary to panic attacks; the patient restricts outside activities to the point of becoming housebound for fear of having a panic attack. The multiple symptoms of panic attacks (see Table 4–7), including dizziness, are commonly reported by patients with agoraphobia. By contrast, simple phobias—such as fear of flying, heights, and snakes—are usually associated with generalized anxiety rather than panic episodes.[41]

Brandt and Dieterich[11] described a syndrome, which they called phobic postural vertigo, characterized by a frightening feeling of dizziness with subjective postural and gait instability. Although these patients had multiple symptoms of panic attacks, often with a steadily mounting fear of impending death, they felt physically ill and the associated symptoms of anxiety were brought out only after appropriate questions were asked. They described their dizziness as a perception of illusory body motion which could occur in brief bouts lasting seconds or be prolonged over

hours and days. Typically the patients had a fear of falling when sitting or standing, and active body movements provoked unpleasant illusions of body acceleration with simultaneous illusory movement of a stationary environment. With the attack the patients experienced anxiety, psychomotor restlessness with escape reactions, a sudden desire to flee from the place where the attack was provoked, aimless walking, and, if seated, a rigid grasp of the arms of the chair. Anticipatory anxiety led to further attacks of dizziness despite the discrepancy between the subjective fear of falling and the absence of objective unsteadiness. Although some patients developed typical symptoms of agoraphobia, others were able to continue their social and work habits despite symptoms they felt to be dominating their lives.

Marks[41] described a related disorder in which patients developed a profound fear of falling in open spaces where a visuospatial reference was absent. Unlike the fear of public places found with agoraphobia, patients with space phobia feared open spaces where there was no "visual" support nearby. They would crawl on the floor to cross a room or walk close to walls or hedges in streets. The average age of onset of space phobia was later than that of agoraphobia (55 years compared with 24 years), and the former was rarely associated with depression or free-floating anxiety as typically seen with agoraphobia. Marks suggested that many of these patients had an underlying organic disorder of balance, because they were resistant to the exposure treatments that are often successful with agoraphobics. Page and Gresty[51] described a variant of space phobia (the so-called motorist's disorientation syndrome) in which patients experienced an illusion of falling to the side or that the car was turning to the side when they were driving in open spaces, on featureless roads, or on the brows of hills. These abnormal sensations were accompanied by a panic reaction. The authors postulated an underlying vestibular abnormality (peripheral or central), because several patients had abnormalities on electronystagmographic (ENG) testing. Typical of phobias, the patients developed avoidance behavior, either driving at very low speeds in restricted areas or completely stopping driving.

CHRONIC ANXIETY

Unlike acute anxiety, chronic anxiety is often difficult to ascribe to a specific inciting factor.[59] Symptoms are less intense although qualitatively similar to those of acute anxiety. The patient may complain of dizziness and giddiness that persist for years, present from morning to night. The patient appears tense and on edge, and there are often symptoms of associated chronic depression. As with acute anxiety there are typically associated somatic complaints, and on examination there may be several physical signs of chronic tension manifested by a fine tremor of the extended hands, very brisk deep tendon reflexes, chronic tachycardia, and pupillary dilatation.

PATHOPHYSIOLOGY

The pathophysiologic mechanism of psychophysiologic dizziness is poorly understood. Although hyperventilation with its concomitant cerebrovascular vasospasm can explain the presyncopal lightheaded sensation, it cannot explain the many complex sensory distortions such as feelings of dissociation, illusions of body movement, imbalance, and fear of falling. In susceptible patients, panic attacks can be precipitated by a large number of substances including lactate, caffeine, isoproterenol, yohimbine, and benzodiazepine receptor antagonists.[4] All these agents interact with the central noradrenergic neuronal system. A popular hypothesis is that panic attacks result from central dyscontrol of the locus ceruleus, leading to the episodic release of catecholamines.[16] Recent studies using positron-emission tomography (PET) scanning in patients with panic disorder[55] demonstrated an asymmetry of blood flow and oxygen utilization in the parahippocampal gyrus (increased on the right), one of the major projection areas of the locus ceruleus. The parahippocampal region is closely interrelated with the hippocampus, a key multimodal sensory integrative center that receives projections from the association areas of all sensory modalities and projects to other limbic structures and to autonomic centers in the hypothalamus and brainstem. Abnormal activity in this region could account for the sensory illusions, autonomic symptoms, and behavior responses associated with panic attacks.

DIAGNOSIS AND MANAGEMENT

The diagnosis of psychophysiologic dizziness rests on finding the characteristic associated symptoms of acute and chronic anxiety discussed above. One must keep in mind that vestibular disorders can also cause anxiety and fear of further attacks of vertigo.[54] A classic vicious cycle may develop whereby the vestibular disturbance causes anxiety, which in turn causes chronic dizziness that may persist after the vestibular imbalance has been compensated. A negative examination in the face of obvious signs of acute and chronic anxiety will help support the presumed diagnosis based on the history. It can sometimes be difficult to recognize panic attacks because patients will focus on the somatic symptoms, especially the dizziness and autonomic symptoms, rather than the intense anxiety associated with the attack.[35] The physician must ask the right questions.

The first step in management of patients with psychophysiologic dizziness is to explain to them that their symptoms are "real," due to physiologic changes occurring in their bodies and that the pattern of symptoms is commonly reported by other patients. Patients are often convinced that they have a severe neurologic disorder and that the anxiety, which they have recognized, is secondary to the physical disorder. It is important to them that the physician understands that they are suffering from "physical symptoms." An explanation for how the release of catecholamines can produce symptoms such as tachycardia, chest pain, paresthesias, and dizziness may improve their acceptance and provide the groundwork for therapeutic considerations. Recent controlled studies indicate that there are three general classes of medications effective in the treatment of panic attacks: (1) the tricyclic antidepressants (e.g., imipramine and desipramine); (2)

the newer, high-potency benzodiazepines (e.g., alprazolam); and (3) the monoamine-oxidase inhibitors (e.g., phenelzine).[36] Of these, imipramine and alprazolam are most effective with the least bothersome side effects. Increased tolerance and dependency may occur with either drug, however. These medications should be used only in conjunction with supportive psychotherapy and behavioral therapy whereby the patient is repeatedly exposed to the situations that evoke symptoms of panic attack.[56] We strongly encourage patients to enter a progressive exercise program with the goal of gradually improving their diminished physical fitness. It is very important that patients feel responsible for their therapy program.

Dysequilibrium

COMMON CAUSES

Patients often use the term "dizziness" to describe a sensation of imbalance or dysequilibrium that occurs only when they are standing or walking and is unrelated to an abnormal head sensation. Imbalance is common with acute unilateral peripheral vestibular lesions, but it is transient and invariably associated with subjective vertigo. Both the vertigo and imbalance are compensated for within a few days. Patients who slowly lose vestibular function on one side, such as with an acoustic neuroma, may not experience vertigo but often describe a vague feeling of imbalance and unsteadiness on their feet. Bilateral symmetrical vestibular loss results in a more pronounced and persistent unsteadiness, which may be incapacitating in elderly patients.[7] The imbalance due to loss of vestibulospinal and proprioceptive function is typically worse in the dark, when the patient is unable to use vision to compensate for the loss (Fig. 4–1). Patients with cerebellar lesions, on the other hand, show little change in their balance with and without vision (the basis for the Romberg test). Dysequilibrium may be the presenting symptom of lesions involving the motor centers of the basal ganglia and frontal lobes such as with Parkinson's disease, hydrocephalus, and the multiple lacunar infarct syndrome.

FALLS IN THE ELDERLY

Falls in the elderly are a common source of morbidity and mortality.[57] The risk of falls increases linearly with age beyond the

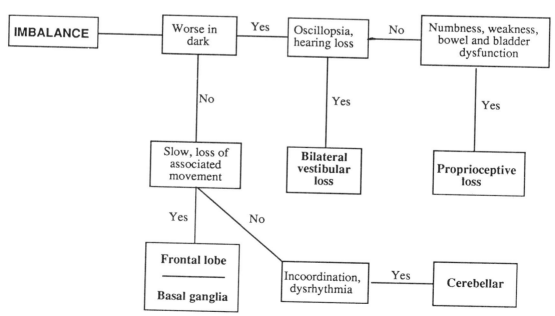

Figure 4–1. Logic for localizing the lesion in patients complaining of dysequilibrium (without vertigo).

Table 4—8. COMMON CAUSES OF FALLS IN THE ELDERLY[57]

Accidental (Falling on stairs, slips, trips)	40–50%
Neurologic (Drop attacks, weakness, ataxia)	20–30%
Dizziness (Orthostatic hypotension, arrhythmia, vertigo)	5–10%
Uncertain	5–10%

age of 60, and it is greater in women than in men. Most falls in the elderly result from an accidental slip or trip (Table 4–8). The cause can often be traced to decreased sensory input, slowing of responses, and weakness of support.[60] Sedating medications are a common contributing factor.[29] Falls can be directly traced to an acute attack of dizziness in less than 10 percent of patients.[57] This low incidence probably can be attributed to the fact that most types of dizziness, including attacks of vertigo, begin slowly enough to allow the patient to sit down or to grab on to a support to avoid falling.

SENILE GAIT

The gradual loss of cells in the sensory and motor centers of the brain with aging is usually a very subtle process that parallels similar slight changes in memory and other cognitive functions, generally considered the normal aging process. The gait of normal elderly men is characterized by slight anteroflexion of the upper torso with flexion of the arms and knees, diminished arm swing, and shorter step lengths;[44] the gait of older women tends to be narrow-based, with a waddling quality.[23] When minor, these changes are not likely to lead to a specific medical complaint. However, a small number of elderly patients develop a progressive deterioration of gait, beginning in the eighth and ninth decades.[1] Their steps shorten and the base widens until their gait is reduced to a shuffle. They turn *en block*, rather than with a normal pivot, and upon arising they have great difficulty in initiating the first step. Once they begin, their arms are held rig-

idly at their sides, and they exhibit a characteristic stooped posture. Walking in tandem is impossible.

On examination, patients are unable to relax their limbs voluntarily. This phenomenon has been described as Gegenhalten or paratonic rigidity. Cortical release signs commonly accompany the diffuse rigidity. The patients attribute their difficulty in walking to a lack of confidence or a fear of falling, and, not surprisingly, major falls frequently occur. In the late stages, patients cannot walk unassisted and may have great difficulty sitting down from a standing position. They land on the edge or side of the chair and fall off. Ultimately they are confined to bed. The neuropathologic basis of the senile gait is poorly understood. Adams[1] suggested that it may be due to a combined frontal lobe and basal ganglia degeneration but cautioned that adequate postmortem examinations do not exist.

DIAGNOSIS AND MANAGEMENT

Considering the many possible loci of dysfunction, the examination of a patient complaining of dysequilibrium must include a careful assessment of gait, strength, coordination, reflexes, and sensory function (particulary of the lower extremities). The broad-based ataxic gait of cerebellar disorders is readily distinguished from the milder gait disorders seen with vestibular or sensory loss. Furthermore, other cerebellar signs (e.g., dysmetria, dysarthria, intention tremor) usually accompany cerebellar ataxia. Bilateral vestibular loss may or may not be associated with hearing loss.[39] The diagnosis rests on finding decreased or absent response to caloric and rotational stimulation (see Chapters 6 and 7).

The deterioration of gait that occurs with aging must be distinguished from that associated with lesions of the cortical and subcortical motor centers.[63] The shuffling, flexed, steppage gait of Parkinson's disease resembles the normal gait of elderly males. The diagnosis of Parkinson's disease rests on finding associated signs, including bradykinesia, cogwheel rigidity, and the characteristic "pill rolling" tremor. Apraxia of gait—characterized by slow, halting, sliding steps as if the patient's feet were adhering to the floor—is caused by bilateral frontal lobe dysfunction.[63] Common causes include multiple subcortical infarcts, infiltrating tumors, and communicating hydrocephalus. High resolution computerized tomography (CT) and magnetic resonance (MR) scanning distinguish these disorders from the nonspecific diffuse atrophy seen in patients with senile gait.

With the exception of communicating hydrocephalus, which can be dramatically reversed with placement of a shunt, most gait disorders in the elderly are not reversible. Some can be helped by improving support with canes or a walker. Tranquilizing medications should be scrupulously avoided, inasmuch as they can further impair the central integration of sensory information.

Ocular Dizziness

COMMON CAUSES

Many patients complain of a vague dizziness when they first wear glasses. They describe a feeling of disorientation, often accompanied by headache. The dizziness most frequently accompanies correction of astigmatism but also occurs after a change in magnification. It is nearly always mild and short-lived. A more persistent and distressing dizziness may occur in patients who are required to use high magnification or who have had a lens implant after cataract removal to correct severe visual loss. In these cases the vestibulo-ocular reflex must adapt if visual objects are to be stabilized during head movements. This compensation process may be slow or inadequate in elderly patients or in subjects who require magnification so high that it is beyond the adaptive range of the vestibulo-ocular reflex.[20]

Dizziness also can result from an imbalance in the extraocular muscles. After an acute ocular muscle paralysis, looking in the direction of the paralyzed muscle causes dizziness (in addition to diplopia). This dizziness results from a mismatch between where the brain "thinks" the eye is, based on its efferent innervation, and where it actually is, based on the visual signal.[10] As with other types of ocular dizziness, the nervous system usually adapts to this altered spatial information and the dizziness is rarely severe or prolonged.

OSCILLOPSIA

The optic illusion that stationary objects are moving back and forth or up and down is called oscillopsia.[9, 62] It is usually a sign of vestibular, brainstem, or cerebellar involvement, although rarely it can result from a lesion in the visual association areas in the cortex (Fig. 4–2). Not surprisingly, oscillopsia is associated with spontaneous nystagmus. If a patient attempts to fixate on an object after an acute unilateral peripheral vestibular lesion, it will appear blurred and seem to be moving in the opposite direction of the slow phase of the spontaneous nystagmus. Some patients will report a flicking back and forth associated with the fast component of nystagmus. The oscillopsia associated with unilateral peripheral vestibular lesions is usually transient, disappearing as the acute vertigo and spontaneous nystagmus disappear. Patients with spontaneous nystagmus due to lesions of the central vestibular pathways report severe persistent oscillopsia, invariably associated with other symptoms and signs of brainstem dysfunction.

Oscillopsia that occurs only with head movement suggests either bilateral symmetrical vestibular or cerebellar dysfunction. Patients with symmetrical loss of vestibulo-ocular reflex function (e.g., due to ototoxic drugs) are unable to fixate on objects when walking because the surroundings appear to be bouncing up and down.[31] The head oscillates in the vertical plane in the frequency range of 2 to 3 Hz. The visual pursuit system cannot compensate for the loss of vestibular function in this frequency range. In order to see the faces of passersby, patients learn to stop and hold their heads still. When reading, they learn to stabilize the head by placing their hand on their chin to prevent even the slightest movements associated with pulsatile cerebral blood flow. Patients with cerebellar lesions cannot suppress their vestibulo-ocular reflex with fixation. They experience a

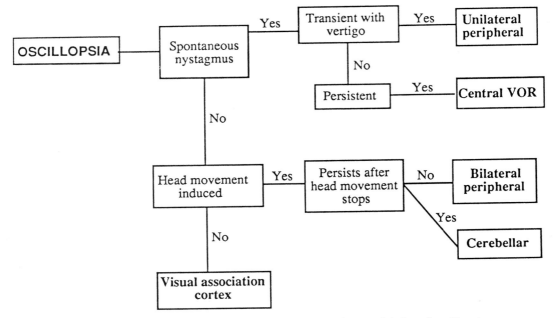

Figure 4–2. Logic for localizing the lesion in patients complaining of oscillopsia.

brief sensation of oscillopsia after each rapid head movement, owing to a transient unwanted vestibular nystagmus. These patients typically have gaze-evoked nystagmus on lateral or vertical gaze, so they may experience oscillopsia with both head and eye movements.

MANAGEMENT

Ocular dizziness due to changes in refraction is rarely severe and usually disappears spontaneously as the patient adjusts to the altered visual environment. Patients should be encouraged to return to normal activities even though the dizziness is initially worse. In the long term this will accelerate the central compensation process. By contrast, oscillopsia is often a severe persistent symptom that can be disabling. The most bothersome type is that associated with an acquired central spontaneous nystagmus[39] (see Chapter 5). With one exception (Baclofen for periodic alternating nystagmus), drugs are not effective in suppressing oscillopsia due to central spontaneous nystagmus.[30] If the nystagmus has a clearly defined null region, prisms fitted in glasses or eye muscle surgery can sometimes be helpful. In patients with head-movement-induced oscillopsia due to bilateral vestibular loss, the visual and neck ocular reflexes can compensate for the loss during low-frequency head movements but not during high-frequency movements.[13, 15] When walking, patients learn to stop and hold their head still in order to see clearly.

Multisensory Dizziness

DEFINITION

Occasionally, one can trace dizziness to disease involving multiple sensory systems, particularly in elderly patients and in patients with systemic disorders, such as diabetes mellitus.[21] A typical combination might include peripheral neuropathy resulting in diminished touch and proprioceptive input, decreased visual acuity (cataracts, glaucoma), and impaired hearing (as in presbycusis). In such patients an added vestibular impairment (from ototoxic drugs, for example) can be devastating, making it impossible for them to walk without assistance. Patients with multisensory dizziness may be unable to adapt to unfamiliar surroundings, such as in the hospital. Not infrequently, their complaint of dizziness will improve when they return to familiar surroundings at home.

MANAGEMENT

Treatment is directed at increasing sensory input wherever possible. This might include improved diabetic control, surgery for cataracts or glaucoma, amplification for presbycusis, and the use of a cane or walker to improve support and increase somatosensory signals. As with other balance disorders, sedating medications should be avoided.

Physiologic Dizziness

Physiologic dizziness refers to a group of phenomena that occur in normal subjects with physiologic stimulation of the vestibular, visual, or somatosensory systems. It typically results from a mismatch in sensory signals, resulting in a feeling of disorientation, imbalance, and vegetative symptoms.[10]

MOTION SICKNESS

Motion sickness refers to the syndrome of dizziness, perspiration, nausea, vomiting, increased salivation, yawning, and generalized malaise induced by motion.[32, 43] It is usually produced by vestibular stimulation but also can occur with visual stimulation (e.g., with prolonged optokinetic stimulation). Both linear and angular head acceleration induce motion sickness if applied for long periods in susceptible subjects. Combinations of linear and angular acceleration or multiplanar angular accelerations are particularly effective. Rotation about the vertical axis, along with either voluntary or involuntary nodding movements in the sagittal plane, rapidly produce motion sickness in nearly everybody. This movement combines linear and angular acceleration (Coriolis effect).

Autonomic symptoms are usually the initial manifestation of motion sickness.[32] Sensitive sweat detectors can identify increased sweating as soon as 5 seconds after onset of motion, and grossly detectable sweating is usually apparent before any noticeable nausea. Increased salivation and frequent swallowing movements occur early. Gastric motility is reduced and digestion is impaired. Hyperventilation is almost always present, and the resulting hypocapnia leads to changes in blood volume with pooling in the lower parts of the body, predisposing the subject to postural hypotension. Motion sickness affects the appetite so that even the sight or smell of food is distressing.

Some people are sensitive to development of motion sickness, but others are highly resistant. Most will adapt to prolonged vestibular stimulation, whereas some never adapt (the chronically seasick ocean voyager). For unknown reasons, babies are highly resistant to motion sickness. Unfortunately, there is no reliable way to predict who will develop motion sickness. Thresholds for vestibular stimulation (rotational or caloric) and the rate of habituation to vestibular stimulation are no different in susceptible and resistant subjects.[19, 33] Patients whose labyrinths have been inactivated by congenital or acquired disease are resistant to motion sickness, whether induced by visual or vestibular stimuli. Such patients can withstand prolonged exposure to wave motion during a heavy storm at sea that would lead to motion sickness in even the most hardened seaman.

Motion sickness seems to result from a visual-vestibular conflict.[43] This theory is supported by the fact that visual influences during body motion have a clear effect on the development of motion sickness. The symptoms are aggravated if one sits in an enclosed cabin on a ship or in the back seat of a moving vehicle. Because the environment is moving with the subject, visual-vestibular conflict occurs. The vestibular system signals movement while the visual system signals a stationary environment. Motion sickness can be alleviated by improving the match between visual and vestibular signals. This can be accomplished on a ship by standing on deck and focusing on the distant horizon or on land, if possible. When riding in a car, the susceptible subject should sit in the front seat to allow ample peripheral vision of the stationary surround. Motion sickness suppressants such as scopolamine and dimenhydrinate are effective, presumably by diminishing activity at the vestibular nucleus and thereby diminishing the potential for visual-vestibular conflict.[64]

SPACE SICKNESS

Space sickness is a kind of motion sickness that is induced by active head movements in space.[38, 48] It has occurred in approximately 50 percent of the astronauts and cosmonauts who have entered space. Most adapt within 2 to 3 days. Because active head movements do not elicit motion sickness within the gravitational conditions on earth, the absence of gravity appears to be a key factor. The leading theory at present is that the symptoms are generated by a mismatch between otolith and semicircular canal signals as well as between otolith and visual signals.[38] On earth, the semicircular canals and otoliths work together, sensing the angular and linear acceleration components of active head movements, but in space the otoliths fail to signal orientation of the head in the absence of gravity. Thus the afferent signals generated by head movements in space are different from the signals expected from prior calibration on earth. The vestibular system must recalibrate to account for the absence of gravity; presumably this recalibration takes about 3 days. Supporting this notion, some astronauts develop transient motion sickness when they return to earth, although it is usually of shorter duration than in space.

HEIGHT VERTIGO

Height vertigo refers to the subjective sensation of instability and imbalance along with a fear of falling and vegetative symptoms that normal subjects experience in high places. More appropriate terms might be height dizziness or height sickness, inasmuch as there is usually no illusion of movement. Brandt and associates[12] demonstrated that height vertigo occurs when the distance between the observer and visible stationary contrasting objects in the environment becomes critically large. Presumably, the normal lateral and fore-aft body sway sensed by the vestibular system conflicts with the visual information of no sway (the greater the distance between the eyes and the nearest stationary object, the smaller the angular displacement on the retina). The symptoms can be reduced by having the subject sit or lie down to increase somatosensory input or by having a nearby stationary object in the visual periphery, such as a railing or window frame. Some subjects develop associated panic attacks and avoidance behavior typical of agoraphobia.

MAL de DEBARQUEMENT SYNDROME

Most of us have experienced the persistent rocking sensation after disembarking from a boat, particularly after a long voyage. This usually subsides gradually over a few hours and seldom is of major significance. Rarely, patients report the persistent rocking sensation of a boat long after returning to land (months to years).[14] These patients are not particularly sensitive to motion sickness; in fact, they frequently report their symptoms are less bothersome back on board a ship. Presumably, they have adapted to the unusual visual-vestibular environment at sea but for some unknown reasons are unable to readapt to an earth-stable environment.

Summary: Distinguishing Between Vestibular and Nonvestibular Types of Dizziness

Although the description alone does not distinguish between vestibular and nonvestibular causes of dizziness, certain words are commonly used to describe each type of dizziness (Table 4–9). A sensation of *spinning* nearly always indicates a vestibular disorder. Patients with nonvestibular dizziness occasionally will report a sensation of spinning inside the head, but the environment remains still and they do not have nystagmus. Patients with vestibular lesions often liken the sensation to that of being *drunk* or *motion sick*. They describe feelings of *imbalance*, as though they are *falling* or *tilting* to one side. Illusions of motion of the environment are rare but illusions of self-motion are common in pa-

Table 4–9. DISTINGUISHING BETWEEN VESTIBULAR AND
NONVESTIBULAR TYPES OF DIZZINESS

	Vestibular	Nonvestibular
Common descriptive terms	Spinning (environment moves), merry-go-round, drunkenness, tilting, motion sickness, off-balance	Lightheaded, floating, dissociated from body, swimming, giddy, spinning inside (environment stationary)
Course	Episodic	Constant
Common precipitating factors	Head movements, position change	Stress, hyperventilation, cardiac arrhythmia, situations
Common associated symptoms	Nausea, vomiting, unsteadiness, tinnitus, hearing loss, impaired vision, oscillopsia	Perspiration, palor, paresthesias, palpitations, syncope, difficulty concentrating, tension headache

tients with nonvestibular dizziness. These patients typically use terms such as *lightheaded, floating, rocking, giddy, or swimming*. The sensation that one has left one's body is characteristic of psychophysiologic dizziness.

Vertigo is an episodic phenomenon, whereas nonvestibular dizziness is often continuous. An exception would be presyncopal lightheadedness caused by postural hypotension or cardiac arrhythmia. Patients with psychophysiologic dizziness often report being dizzy from morning to night without changes for months to years at a time. Vertigo is typically aggravated by head movements, whereas nonvestibular dizziness is often aggravated by movement of visual targets. Episodes of dizziness induced by position change suggest a vestibular lesion if postural hypotension has been ruled out. Although stress can aggravate both vestibular and nonvestibular dizziness, dizziness that is reliably precipitated by stress suggests a nonvestibular cause. Finally, episodes of dizziness occurring only in specific situations (e.g., driving on the freeway, entering a crowded room, or shopping in a busy supermarket) suggest a nonvestibular cause.

The presence of associated symptoms can also help one distinguish between vestibular and nonvestibular causes of dizziness. Nausea and vomiting are usual with vertigo but uncommon with other types of dizziness. Associated auditory or neurologic symptoms suggest a vestibular disorder, presyncopal symptoms and syncope a nonvestibular disorder. Multiple symptoms of acute and chronic anxiety commonly accompany psychophysiologic dizziness.

ILLUSTRATIVE CASES

Vertigo due to an Acute Peripheral Vestibular Lesion

Two weeks after recovering from the flu, a 39-year-old schoolteacher awoke with severe dizziness and nausea. When she attempted to get out of bed the room began to spin; she had to hold on to the bedframe to keep from falling. By holding on to the walls she made her way to the bathroom, where she vomited repeatedly. When returning to bed she felt best with her eyes closed and head perfectly still; any movement aggravated the dizziness. She noted that a clock on the wall seemed to flick back and forth when she tried to read the time.

When seen in the emergency room she had a right-beating spontaneous nystagmus and a tendency to veer or fall to the left when walking. The remainder of the examination, including hearing, was normal. She was sent home on meclizine. The next day the dizziness had improved but she still was unsteady and had difficulty reading. These symptoms gradually resolved over a week, but she did not feel well enough to return to work for 2 weeks.

Presyncopal Lightheadedness due to Orthostatic Hypotension

A 64-year-old man with severe coronary artery disease complained of persistent dizziness dating back about a month. He described the dizziness as a "squeegee," lightheaded sensation along with a feeling of unsteadiness. The dizziness occurred when he was on his feet and was relieved by lying down and raising his legs. He was unable to walk more than a block without experiencing severe dizziness and a feeling that he might black out. He had previously undergone bypass surgery and angioplasty but continued to have severe recurrent angina requiring regular use of nitroglycerin. Other medications included Lanoxin, Inderal, and Procardia. On examination his blood pressure was 100/60 in the sitting position. It did not change immediately on standing, but dropped to 90/40 after standing for 3 minutes.

Presyncopal Lightheadedness due to Hyperventilation

A 43-year-old woman complained of recurrent dizzy spells dating back several years. She described the dizziness as a lightheaded, unsteady feeling that came over her in waves without any apparent precipitating factor. She was never completely free of dizziness, even between the attacks. When the dizziness was pronounced, she experienced associated paresthesias of her hands and feet, tightness in her throat, palpitations, blurring of vision, and difficulty concentrating. Past medical history was of note for frequent faints since her teens and long-standing headaches that she described as a tight bandlike sensation around her head along with pressure at the vertex. She reported being under a great deal of stress in managing her 8-year-old, hyperactive son but did not notice a clear relationship between the stress and her dizziness. She sighed frequently during the interview, and her dizziness was reproduced by 1 minute of hyperventilation. Examination was unremarkable.

Psychophysiologic Dizziness Associated with Acute and Chronic Anxiety

A 31-year-old secretary complained of persistent dizziness for the preceding 2 months. She described the dizziness as a swaying, rocking sensation along with a feeling of unsteadiness. Although con-

stant, the dizziness varied in severity from day to day; when severe it was accompanied by mild nausea, a feeling of dissociation, and difficulty in concentrating. She had had a similar bout of dizziness 4 years before, lasting about 3 to 4 months. Since her teens she had had several panic attacks with hyperventilation without obvious precipitating factors. On examination of gait she lurched from side to side but demonstrated excellent balance to avoid falling. Extraocular movements were full without nystagmus, but she exhibited intermittent convergence spasm.

Psychophysiologic Dizziness Associated with Panic Attacks and Agoraphobia

A 50-year-old attorney complained of intermittent dizziness, gradually increasing in frequency and severity over the previous 2 years. He described the dizziness as a lightheaded, disoriented feeling along with a sensation of falling forward or to either side. At times, he experienced a sensation of swimming or spinning inside of his head even though the surroundings remained still. The dizziness, sometimes accompanied by panic attacks, commonly occurred when he was driving on the freeway (particularly in the fast lane or when there were no other cars nearby), over a brow of a hill, or around a sharp turn, or when he found himself in enclosed spaces (elevators), crowded rooms, or high places. Eventually he stopped driving on the freeway, and would not go above the second floor of buildings. His examination and diagnostic work-up including vestibular function testing, were normal.

Dysequilibrium and Oscillopsia due to Late-Onset Cortical Cerebellar Atrophy

A 69-year-old retired schoolteacher complained of severe dizziness that was becoming progressively worse over the previous 3 years. The dizziness was not a head sensation but rather a feeling of imbalance and unsteadiness when he was on his feet. It completely disappeared when he was sitting or lying. He also noted brief periods (seconds) of oscillopsia after head or eye movements. Family history and review of neurologic symptoms were otherwise negative. On examination he walked with a wide-based, ataxic gait. He could not stand in the Romberg position, even with eyes open. The only finding on cranial nerve examination was a rebound gaze-evoked nystagmus. There was minimal ataxia of the upper extremities. Magnetic resonance imaging documented atrophy of the cerebellar vermis.

Ocular Dizziness after a Lens Implant

An 84-year-old woman complained of constant dizziness since undergoing bilateral cataract surgery with lens implants. She described the dizziness as a lightheaded, off-balance sensation that was most pronounced when she was standing or walking. She noted the dizziness immediately after the patch was removed from her eye after the first surgery and reported that the dizziness became even more bothersome after the second surgery. Because of the dizziness she stopped her daily walks and rarely left home. Examination was unremarkable.

She was encouraged to return to normal activities with the hope that she would adapt to the visual-vestibular conflict. Follow-up 6 months later revealed that the dizziness was still present but that she had "learned to live with it."

Multisensory Dizziness due to Visual, Vestibular, and Somatosensory Loss

A 70-year-old woman with long-standing diabetes mellitus complained of continuous dizziness dating back about 4 years. She described the dizziness as a floating sensation along with a feeling of dysequilibrium and imbalance. There was some associated nausea but no vomiting. The dizziness varied in intensity but never completely disapppeared. She was legally blind because of chronic diabetic retinopathy and had previously received a 3-week

intravenous course of gentamicin for a persistent cellulitis of the foot. On examination she could not stand without assistance and complained of severe "dizziness" when attempting to stand. The only other finding on examination was a moderate peripheral neuropathy with absent deep tendon reflexes in the legs and a stocking-glove-distribution sensory loss. Caloric responses were decreased bilaterally.

REFERENCES

1. Adams, RD: Aging and human locomotion. In Albert, ML (ed): Clinical Neurology of Aging. Oxford University Press, New York, 1984.
2. Afzelius, LE, Henriksson, NG, Wahlgren, L: Vertigo and dizziness of functional origin. Laryngoscope 90:649, 1980.
3. Alford, B: Meniere's disease: Criteria for diagnosis and evaluation of therapy for reporting. Report of subcommittee on equilibrium and its measurements. Trans Am Acad Ophthalmol Otolaryngol 76:1462, 1972.
4. Ballenger, JC: Biological aspects of panic disorder. Am J Psychiatr 143:516, 1986.
5. Baloh, RW and Harker, LA: Central vestibular system disorders. In Cummings, CW, Fredrickson, JM, Harker, LA, Krause, CJ, Schuller, DE (eds): Otolaryngology: Head and Neck Surgery, Vol 4. CV Mosby, St Louis, 1986, p 3313.
6. Baloh, RW, Honrubia, V, Jacobson, K: Benign positional vertigo. Clinical and oculographic features in 240 cases. Neurology (Minneap) 37:371, 1987.
7. Baloh, RW, Jacobson, K, Honrubia, V: Idiopathic bilateral vestibulopathy. Neurology 39:272, 1989.
8. Bass, C and Gardner, WN: Respiratory and psychiatric abnormalities in chronic symptomatic hyperventilation. Br Med J 290:1387, 1985.
9. Bender, MB: Oscillopsia. Arch Neurol 13:204, 1965.
10. Brandt, T and Daroff, R: The multisensory physiological and pathological vertigo syndromes. Ann Neurol 7:195, 1980.
11. Brandt, T and Dieterich, M: Phobischer attackenschwankschwindel ein neues Syndrom. Münch med Wschr 128:247, 1986.
12. Brandt, T, Arnold, F, Bless, W, Kapteyn, TS: The mechanism of physiological height vertigo. I. Theoretical approach and psychophysics. Acta Otolaryngol 89:513, 1980.
13. Bronstein, AM and Hood, JD: Oscillopsia of peripheral vestibular origin. Central and cervical compensatory mechanisms. Acta Otolaryngol 104:307, 1987.
14. Brown, JJ and Baloh, RW: Persistent mal de debarquement syndrome: A motion induced subjective disorder. Am J Otolaryngol 8:219, 1987.

15. Chambers, BR, Mai, M, and Barber, HO: Bilateral vestibular loss, oscillopsia, and the cervico-ocular reflex. Otolaryngol Head Neck Surg 93:403, 1985.
16. Charney, DJ, Heninger, GR, Breier, A: Noradrenergic function in panic anxiety. Arch Gen Psych 41:751, 1984.
17. Chole, RA: Acute and chronic infection of the temporal bone including otitis media with effusion. In Cummings, CW, Fredrickson, JM, Harker, LA, Krause, CJ, Schuller, DE (eds): Otolaryngology-Head and Neck Surgery, Vol 4. CV Mosby, St Louis, 1986, p 2963.
18. Crowe, RR, Pauls, DL, Slymen, DJ, and Noyes, R: A family study of anxiety neurosis. Arch Gen Psychiatr 37:77, 1980.
19. De Witt, G: Seasickness. Acta Otolaryngol (Suppl) 108:1, 1953.
20. Demer, JL, et al: Dynamic visual acuity with telescopic spectacles: Improvement with adaptation. Invest Ophthalmol Vis Sci 29:1184, 1988.
21. Drachman, DA and Hart, CW: An approach to the dizzy patient. Neurology 22:323, 1972.
22. Engel, GL: Psychological stress, vasodepressor (vasovagal) syncope and sudden death. Ann Intern Med 89:403, 1978.
23. Finley, FR, Cody, KA, Finizie, RV: Locomotion patterns in elderly women. Arch Phys Med Rehabil 50:140, 1969.
24. Fisher, CM: Vertigo in cerebrovascular diseases. Arch Otolaryngol 85:529, 1967.
25. Goodhill, V: Leaking labyrinth lesions, deafness, tinnitus and dizziness. Ann Otol Rhinol Laryngol 90:99, 1981.
26. Gotch, F, Meyer, JS, and Yasuyuki, T: Cerebral effects of hyperventilation in man. Arch Neurol 12:410, 1965.
27. Grad, A and Baloh, RW: Vertigo of vascular origin. Clinical and oculographic features. Arch Neurol 46:281, 1989.
28. Hale, WE, Stewart, RB, and Markes, RG: Central nervous system symptoms of elderly subjects using antihypertensive drugs. J Am Geriatr Soc 32:5, 1984.
29. Hale, WE, Stewart, RB, Markes, RG: Antianxiety drugs and central nervous system symptoms in an ambulatory elderly population. Drug Intel Clin Pharm 19:37, 1985.
30. Halmagyi, GM, et al: Treatment of periodic alternating nystagmus. Ann Neurol 8:609, 1980.
31. JC: Living without a balancing mechanism. N Engl J Med 246:458, 1952.
32. Johnson, WH, Jongkees, LBW: Motion sickness. In Kornhuber, HH, (ed): Handbook of Sensory Physiology, Vol VI, Part 2. Springer-Verlag, New York, 1974.
33. Jongkees, LBW: Motion sickness. II. Some sensory aspects. In Kornhuber, HH (ed): Handbook of sensory physiology, Vol VI, Part 2. Springer-Verlag, New York, 1974.
34. Kapoor, WN: Evaluation of syncope in the elderly. J Am Geriatr Soc 35:826, 1987.
35. Katon, W: Panic disorder and somatization. Am J Med 77:101, 1984.
36. Katon, W: Panic disorder: Epidemiology, diagnosis and treatment in primary care. J Clin Psychiatr (Suppl) 47:21, 1986.
37. Kinney, SE: Trauma. In Cummings, CW, Fredrickson, JM, Harker, LA, Krause, CJ, and Schuller, DE (eds): Otolaryngology-Head and Neck Surgery, Vol 4. CV Mosby, St Louis, 1986, p 3033.
38. Lackner, JR and Graybiel, A: Head movements in non-terrestrial force environments elicit motion sickness; Implications for the etiology of space motion sickness. Aviat Space Environ Med 57:443, 1986.
39. Leigh, RJ, et al: Effects of retinal image stabilization in acquired nystagmus due to neurologic disease. Neurology 38:122, 1988.
40. Magarian, GJ: Hyperventilation syndromes: Infrequently recognized common expressions of anxiety and stress. Medicine 61:219, 1982.
41. Marks, I: Space "phobia": A pseudo-agoraphobic syndrome. J Neurol Neurosurg Psychiatry 44:387, 1981.
42. Marks, I: Fears and phobias. Academic Press, New York, 1969.
43. Money, KE: Motion sickness. Physiol Rev 50:1, 1970.
44. Murray, MP, Kory, RC, and Clarkson, BH: Walking patterns in healthy old men. J Gerontol 24:169, 1969.
45. Nadol, JB, Weiss, AD, and Parker, SW: Vertigo of delayed onset after sudden deafness. Ann Otol Rhinol Laryngol 84:841, 1975.
46. Nadol, JB: Positive hennebert's sign in Meniere's disease. Arch Otolaryngol 103:524, 1977.
47. Neely, JG: Complications of temporal bone infection. In Cummings, CW, Fredrickson, JM, Harker, LA, Krause, CJ, Schuller, DE (eds): Otolaryngology: Head and Neck Surgery, Vol 4. CV Mosby, St Louis, 1986, p 2988.
48. Oman, CM, Lichtenberg, BK, Money, KE, McCoy, RK: MIT/Canadian vestibular experiments on the Spacelab-1 mission: 4. Space motion sickness: Symptoms, stimuli, and predictability. Exp Brain Res 64:316, 1986.
49. Onrot, J, et al: Management of chronic orthostatic hypotension. Am J Med 80:454, 1986.
50. Ormerod, AD: Clinical algorithms, Syncope. Br Med J 288:1219, 1984.
51. Page, NGR and Gresty, MA: Motorist's vestibular disorientation syndrome. J Neurol Neurosurg Psychiatry 48:729, 1985.
52. Penfield, W and Kristiansen, K: Epileptic seizure patterns: a study of the localizing value of initial phenomena in focal cortical seizures. Charles C Thomas, Springfield, IL, 1951.
53. Plum, F and Posner, JB: Disturbances of consciousness and arousal. In Wyngarden, JB and Smith, LA (eds); Cecil Textbook of Medicine, ed 18. Harcourt Brace Jovanovich, Philadelphia, 1988, p 2061.
54. Pratt, RTC and McKenzie, W: Anxiety states following vestibular disorders. Lancet 1:347, 1958.
55. Reiman, EM, et al: The application of positron emission tomography to the study of panic disorder. Am J Psychiatry 143:469, 1986.

56. Rohs, RG and Noyes, R: Agoraphobia. Newer treatment approach. J Nerv Ment Dis 166:701, 1978.
57. Rubenstein, LZ, et al: Falls and instability in the elderly. J Am Geriatr Soc 36:266, 1988.
58. Schuknecht, HF and Kitamura, K: Vestibular neuritis. Ann Otol Rhinol Laryngol 90 (Suppl 78): 1, 1981.
59. Tucker, GJ: Psychiatric disorders in medical practice. In Wyngarden, JB, Smith, LH (eds): Cecil Textbook of Medicine, ed 18. Harcourt Brace Jovanovich, Philadelphia, 1988, p 2091.
60. Weiner, WJ, Nora, LM, and Glantz, RH: Elderly inpatients: Postural reflex impairment. Neurology 34:945, 1984.
61. Williams, D and Wilson, TG: The diagnosis of the major and minor syndromes of basilar insufficiency. Brain 85:741, 1962.
62. Wist, ER, Brandt, T, and Krafczyk, S: Oscillopsia and retinal slip. Brain 106:153, 1983.
63. Wolfson, LI, and Katzman, R: The neurologic consultation at age 80. In Katzman, R and Terry, R (eds): The Neurology of Aging. FA Davis, Philadelphia, 1983.
64. Zee, DS: Perspectives on the pharmacotherapy of vertigo. Arch Otolaryngol 111:609, 1985.

Chapter 5

BEDSIDE EXAMINATION OF THE VESTIBULAR SYSTEM

As noted earlier, the vestibular system works in conjunction with the visual and somatosensory systems to achieve ocular and postural stability. To examine the vestibular system adequately, one must isolate it from these other sensory systems. This is a difficult task at the bedside. Vision can be removed with eye-closure, but there is no simple way to eliminate somatosensation. Furthermore, if the eyes are closed, the vestibulo-ocular reflex cannot be observed. Unlike the visual system, in which the optic nerve can be directly visualized and acuity accurately measured, the inner ear is located deep within the temporal bone, and the subjective sensation to vestibular stimulation is ill defined. One can visualize the tympanic membrane and structures within the middle ear, but this provides only indirect information about the status of the inner ear.

EXAMINATION OF THE EAR

The neurotologist must be familiar with the normal anatomy of the external canal and tympanic membrane (see Chapter 2), must be capable of removing cerumen that interferes with visualization of the tympanic membrane, and must be able to recognize certain common disorders on inspection (Fig. 5–1). Otoscopy is performed with the largest speculum that fits comfortably into the external canal; the pinna is gently pulled posterior and superior to straighten the canal. The tympanic membrane is normally translucent; changes in

color indicate middle ear disease (e.g., an amber color with middle ear effusions). Tympanosclerosis, the consequence of a resolved otitis media or trauma, appears as a semicircular crescent or horseshoe-shaped white placque within the tympanic membrane. It is rarely associated with hearing loss but is an important clue to past otitic infections. The pars flaccida region—the area superior to the lateral process of the malleus—should be carefully inspected for evidence of a retraction pocket or attic cholesteatoma. The ossicles and the color of the underlying mucous membrane of the middle ear can often be assessed through a normal translucent tympanic membrane. Pneumatoscopy allows one to determine the mobility of the tympanic membrane. Lack of mobility may indicate an unsuspected perforation (usually under an anterior overhang), fluid in the middle ear, or severe scarring of the tympanic membrane or middle ear.

Fistula Test

A fistula test is performed by transiently increasing and decreasing the pressure in the external canal with a pneumatoscope. A positive fistula sign (a transient burst of nystagmus and vertigo) occurs in patients with a perforated tympanic membrane and erosion of the bony labyrinth (from chronic infection, surgery, trauma). The change in pressure is transmitted directly to the perilymph, compressing the membranous labyrinth and stimulating the

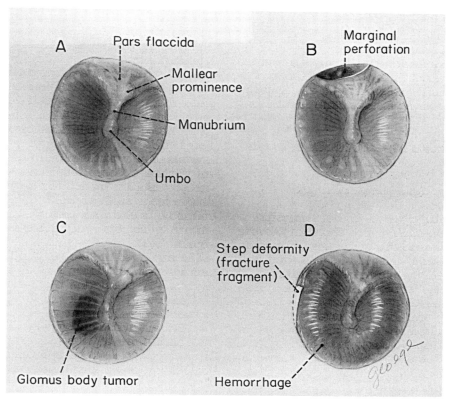

Figure 5—1. Appearance of the tympanic membrane in *(A)* a normal subject and in patients with *(B)* a superior marginal perforation and cholesteatoma, *(C)* a tympanic glomus body tumor, and *(D)* a step deformity caused by a longitudinal temporal bone fracture.

semicircular canal crista. The resulting nystagmus usually lasts from 10 to 20 seconds. The direction of the nystagmus may be toward or away from the involved ear and is often the same for both positive and negative pressure changes.

Lesser ocular and subjective responses may occur in patients with an intact tympanic membrane (Hennebert's sign). Hennebert[47] first described this sign in patients with congenital syphilis and subsequent investigators[62] reported its occurrence in patients with Meniere's syndrome and other labyrinthine disorders. The response is a slow ocular deviation (toward or away from the affected ear) that may be followed by, at most, a few beats of nystagmus even with sustained pressure. Hennebert's sign has been reported in patients with ruptures of the oval and/or round windows, but most investigators agree that it neither establishes nor excludes the diagnosis.[60, 76] Furthermore, Hennebert's

sign can occasionally be elicited during routine pneumatoscopy in normal subjects. In these cases it is usually present bilaterally, however. How pressure changes in the external auditory canal result in a pressure gradient across any of the vestibular receptor organs is unclear (see Perilymph Fistula, Chapter 14). In the case of endolymphatic hydrops (idiopathic or secondary to infection), fibrous adhesions between the medial surface of the stapedial footplate and the membranous labyrinth could result in displacement of endolymph when the footplate moves. A similar mechanism could explain the production of dizziness by loud noises (Tulio phenomenon).

TESTS OF VESTIBULOSPINAL REFLEXES

As discussed in Chapter 3, the labyrinths influence spinal cord motoneurons through the lateral vestibulospinal tract, the reticulospinal tract, and the descending medial longitudinal fasciculus (MLF). Labyrinthine stimulation of the spinal cord increases extensor tone and decreases flexor tone, resulting in a facilitation of the antigravity muscles. Both otolith and semicircular canal signals influence spinal cord anterior horn cells, but the former are more important in maintaining posture.

Pastpointing

Pastpointing refers to a reactive deviation of the extremities caused by an imbalance in the vestibular system (Fig. 5–2). The test is performed by having the patient place his or her extended index finger on that of the examiner's, close his or her eyes, raise the extended arm and index finger to a vertical position, and attempt to return the index finger to the examiner's. Consistent deviation to one side is pastpointing.

Pastpointing tests represent one of the earliest attempts to clinically assess vestibular function. In 1910, Bárány[12] published a review of pointing deviation and emphasized the importance of having patients sit with their eyes closed to avoid confusion with other orienting information. Bárány showed that caloric stimulation consistently induced pastpointing in the direction of the slow component of induced nystagmus. Cold caloric irrigation (inhibiting the horizontal ampullary nerves' spontaneous firing rate) resulted in pastpointing toward the stimulated ear, and warm caloric irrigation induced the opposite effect. As expected, patients with acute unilateral loss of vestibular function pastpointed toward the damaged side. Bárány and numerous others emphasized that repeated testing shows a large variability, occasionally with drift in the wrong direction. Subsequent investigators tried to improve test accuracy by eliminating tactile feedback and using small finger lamps that could be photographed, but the large variability

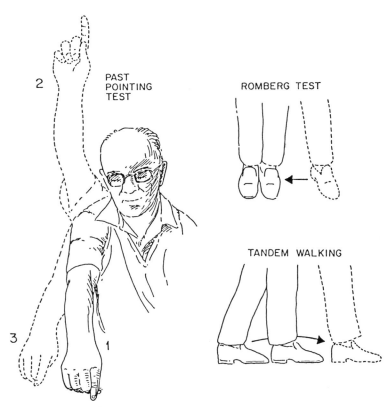

Figure 5–2. Bedside tests of vestibulospinal function.

among normal subjects and patients remained. Fukuda[34] introduced a vertical writing test to identify pastpointing, but subsequent evaluation of his test suggests that it was no more reliable than the more standard test.[17]

It is apparent that results from a single pointing test can be misleading and should not be considered in isolation. Extralabyrinthine influences should be eliminated as much as possible by having the patient seated with eyes covered and arms and index fingers extended throughout the test. The standard finger-to-nose test will not identify pastpointing, inasmuch as joint and muscle proprioceptive signals permit accurate localization even when vestibular function is lost. Although patients with acute peripheral vestibular damage usually pastpoint toward the side of loss, compensation rapidly corrects the pastpointing and can even produce a drift to the other side. The cortical and subcortical pathways to the spinal anterior horn cells, illustrated in Fig. 3–25, apparently account for the compensation.

Static Posture

Patients with damage to the vestibular system often suffer instability of the trunk and lower limbs so that they sway back and forth or even fall to one side. In 1846, Romberg[68] noted that patients with proprioceptive loss from tabes dorsalis were unable to stand with feet together and eyes closed. Bárány[12] first emphasized the importance of vestibular influences in maintaining the Romberg position (see Fig. 5–2). As with pastpointing, he noted that patients with acute unilateral labyrinthine lesions swayed and fell toward the diseased side, that is, in the direction of the slow component of nystagmus. However, like the pastpointing test, the Romberg test was found to be rather insensitive for detecting chronic unilateral vestibular impairment, and sometimes the patient would fall toward the intact ear. The so-called sharpened Romberg test is a more sensitive indicator of vestibular impairment.[31] For this test the patient stands with feet aligned in the tandem heel-to-toe position with eyes closed and arms folded

against the chest. Most normal subjects under the age of 70 can stand in this position for 30 seconds; older normal subjects and patients with unilateral or bilateral vestibular impairment usually cannot sustain the position.

Although lower mammals consistently develop ipsilateral hypotonia of extensor muscles after labyrinthectomy, one rarely finds this in human patients. Occasionally slight asymmetry in posture is found with the ipsilateral upper extremity slightly flexed and abducted compared to the contralateral upper extremity. The clinically elicited deep tendon reflexes are also unaffected by vestibular lesions. Apparently other supraspinal influences on the anterior horn cells rapidly compensate for the loss of tonic vestibular signals.

Walking Tests

Unterberger[78] was the first to systematically study the tendency of vestibular stimulation or unilateral vestibular lesions to induce blindfolded subjects to turn in the earth's vertical axis when walking. The direction of turning coincided with the direction of pastpointing and falling (in the direction of the slow component of nystagmus). Fukuda[33] obtained similar results by having subjects take 50 to 100 steps on the same spot and recording the angle of rotation as well as forward and backward movements. Both of these tests were performed with arms extended parallel and horizontal in front of the subject, so upper extremity deviation (pastpointing) may have added to the tendency to rotate in a given direction. Peitersen[67] further modified the stepping test so that the blindfolded subjects stepped with the arms folded and tried to stay in the center of two concentric circles drawn on the floor. The tests were performed in a quiet darkened room to exclude orientation from auditory and visual clues. Despite these attempts to improve test precision he found marked variability in the rotation angle from one subject to another and in the same subject on repeated testing.

Tandem gait tests (see Fig. 5–2) are widely used as part of the routine neurologic examination, and most clinicians recognize normal and abnormal performances. When performed with eyes open, tandem walking is primarily a test of cerebellar function, because vision compensates for chronic vestibular and proprioceptive deficits. Acute vestibular lesions, however, may impair tandem walking, even with the eyes open. Tandem walking with the eyes closed provides a better test of vestibular function as long as cerebellar and proprioceptive functions are intact. The blindfolded subject is asked to start with feet in the tandem position and arms folded against the chest and to make 10 tandem steps, at a comfortable speed, beyond the first 2 starting steps. The number of steps without sidestepping is scored on three trials.[67] Most normal subjects can make a minimum of 10 accurate tandem steps in three trials. Patients with acute or chronic vestibular disease fail the test, but the direction of falling is not a reliable indicator of the side of the lesion. The test sensitivity can be increased by having the patient walk on a rail a few inches above the floor, but, again, the results are nonspecific and some normal subjects may not be able to perform the task.

TESTS OF THE VESTIBULO-OCULAR REFLEXES

The Doll's Eye Test (Oculocephalic Response)

The doll's eye test induces reflex eye movements by rapidly moving the head back and forth in the horizontal or vertical plane. In an alert human these eye movements result from combined visual and vestibular stimulation. Therefore, a patient with complete loss of vestibular function will have compensatory eye movements on the test if the visuomotor system is intact. The doll's eye test is a useful bedside test of the vestibulo-ocular reflex in a comatose patient, however, inasmuch as in this case the pursuit system is not functioning.[57] Conjugate compensatory eye movements indicate normally functioning vestibulo-ocular pathways (those shown in Fig. 3–5). Disconjugate eye movements may indicate a lesion of the MLF, the oculomotor neurons, or the ocular muscles

(depending on the abnormal pattern). Absence of reflex eye movements in a comatose patient is usually an ominous sign, indicating massive brainstem damage if acute drug intoxication or metabolic disorders can be ruled out.[61]

Head-Shaking Nystagmus

Patients with a compensated vestibular imbalance due to either peripheral or central lesions may develop a transient spontaneous nystagmus after vigorous head shaking.[42] The test is performed by having the patient shake the head back and forth in the horizontal plane as fast as possible for approximately 10 cycles. Spontaneous nystagmus after head shaking is abnormal, indicating an imbalance within the vestibulo-ocular pathways. With unilateral peripheral vestibular lesions the abnormal side is in the direction of the slow phase. Hain and colleagues[42] suggested that head-shaking nystagmus results from asymmetric velocity storage within the central vestibulo-ocular pathways. Rotation toward the intact side results in greater velocity storage than rotation toward the abnormal side (a result of Ewald's second law, see Characteristics of Primary Afferent Neurons, Chapter 2). Vertical head shaking also can be performed, although the results are more difficult to interpret because some normal subjects will have transient vertical nystagmus after vertical head shaking.

Dynamic Visual Acuity

The dynamic visual acuity test is performed by having the patient shake the head rapidly back and forth in the horizontal plane at approximately 2 Hz while reading a Snellen visual acuity chart at the standard distance. Inasmuch as the smooth pursuit system functions best below 1 Hz and almost not at all at 2 Hz, this is primarily a test of the horizontal vestibulo-ocular reflex. A drop in acuity of more than one line on the Snellen chart suggests an abnormal vestibulo-ocular reflex, usually due to bilateral symmetrical damage.

Cold Caloric Test

Because of its ready availability, ice water (approximately 0°C) is commonly used for bedside caloric testing.[29, 64] To bring the horizontal canal into the vertical plane the patient lies in the supine position with the head tilted 30 degrees forward or in the sitting position with the head tilted 60 degrees backward (see Fig. 2–6). Infusion of ice water induces a burst of nystagmus with slow phase toward the side of infusion, usually lasting from 1 to 3 minutes. The volume of ice water recommended for this test varies from 50 ml to less than 1 ml. Regardless of the volume used, however, it is critical that the stimulus reaches the eardrum (i.e., not injected into the canal wall or cerumen). Direct visualization of the eardrum is mandatory. We suggest using 2 ml of ice water infused directly against the tympanic membrane through a small rubber hose. The ear being infused is turned uppermost for approximately 30 seconds after the infusion to be certain that the water stays against the drum. In an alert subject a burst of nystagmus will develop within 30 seconds to 1 minute after infusion and last from 1 to 3 minutes. In a comatose patient only a slow tonic deviation toward the side of stimulation is observed. In normal subjects duration and speed of induced nystagmus varies greatly, but greater than 20 percent asymmetry in nystagmus duration suggests the possibility of a lesion on the side of the decreased response. This should always be confirmed, however, with standard bithermal caloric testing and electronystagmography (see Chapter 6).

Rotational Testing

Qualitative rotational testing of the horizontal vestibulo-ocular reflex can be performed at the bedside by using a swivel chair. Bárány[11] introduced a rotatory test in which the chair on which the patient was seated was manually rotated 10 times in 20 seconds and then suddenly stopped with the patient facing the observer. The duration of postrotatory nystagmus in each direction was then measured. In normal subjects an average of 22 seconds was required for cessation of postrotatory nystagmus, but intersubject variability was large. Much of this variability could be traced to the difficulty in manually maintaining constant velocity and then a uniform sudden deceleration. Furthermore, the vestibular response to the initial acceleration was often not completed before deceleration began, resulting in interaction between the two responses. As with the ice water caloric testing, this type of qualitative testing can provide only gross information about the presence and symmetry of vestibular function. One aspect of rotational testing that is useful at the bedside is the *fixation-suppression test*. With this test the subject extends the arm rigidly and attempts to fixate on the extended thumb while the entire body is rotated back and forth *en bloc*. Normal subjects can completely suppress their vestibulo-ocular reflex, keeping their eyes fixed in the center of the orbits (as shown in Fig. 1–9). Abnormal fixation-suppression (nystagmus) indicates a central lesion, often involving the cerebellum (see Visual-Vestibular Interaction, Chapter 7).

TESTS FOR PATHOLOGIC NYSTAGMUS

Definitions

Nystagmus can be defined as a nonvoluntary rhythmic oscillation of the eyes. It usually has clearly defined fast and slow components alternating in opposite directions. By convention, the direction of the fast component defines the direction of nystagmus. Physiologic nystagmus refers to nystagmus that occurs in normal subjects, whereas pathologic nystagmus implies an underlying abnormality (Table 5–1). Spontaneous nystagmus refers to nystagmus that occurs with the patient

Table 5–1. TYPES OF NYSTAGMUS

Physiologic	Pathologic
Rotational-induced	Spontaneous
Caloric-induced	Gaze-evoked
Optokinetic	Positional
End-point	

seated, eyes in the primary position, and without external stimulation such as movement of the head or surroundings. Gaze-evoked nystagmus is induced by changes in gaze position. Nystagmus that is not present in the sitting position but is present in some other head and body position is called positional nystagmus. This definition excludes nystagmus present in the sitting position that is modified by a change in position.

Methods of Examination

The clinical examination for pathologic nystagmus should include a systematic study of changes in (1) fixation, (2) eye position, and (3) head position. Omission of any of these three maneuvers may lead to overlooking the presence of nystagmus or misinterpreting its type.

Spontaneous nystagmus may be present with fixation, or it may occur only when fixation is inhibited. There are several simple methods for achieving the latter at the bedside. Frenzel glasses consist of +30 lenses mounted in a frame that contains a light source on the inside so that the patient's eyes are easily visualized (Fig. 5–3). The light can be powered by a battery, making the entire system portable. Frenzel glasses should be used only in a darkened room, because the patient can fixate (at least partially) through the lenses in a lighted room. An ophthalmoscope can also be used to block fixation and bring out a

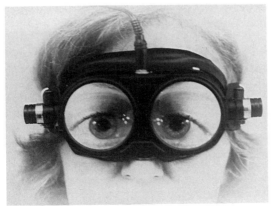

Figure 5–3. Frenzel glasses.

spontaneous nystagmus. While the fundus of one eye is being visualized the patient is asked to lightly cover the other eye with one hand. Nystagmus appears as a slow drift of the retina in one direction interrupted by flicking movements in the opposite direction (the direction of the nystagmus is reversed, inasmuch as one is visualizing the back pole of the eye). Occasionally nystagmus can be seen even through closed lids. This can be misleading, however, because lid-twitch movements often mimic nystagmus.

The effect of change in eye position is evaluated by having the patient fixate on a target 30 degrees to the right, left, up, and down. Because horizontal eye deviation beyond 40 degrees may result in a low-amplitude high-frequency torsional nystagmus in normal subjects (so-called end-point nystagmus), extreme eye positions should be avoided. Each eye position is held for at least 20 seconds. First-degree nystagmus refers to nystagmus that is present only on gaze in the direction of the fast component. Second-degree nystagmus is present in the midposition and on gaze in the direction of the fast component, and third-degree nystagmus is present even on gaze away from the fast component. These terms are not applicable to all varieties of nystagmus and, therefore, can lead to confusion. A simple description can be rapidly summarized with a box diagram as illustrated in Figure 5–4. The size, shape, and direction of the arrows provide information about the amplitude and direction of the fast component of nystagmus in each eye position.

Routinely, two types of positional testing are used: slow and rapid. With the first the patient slowly moves into the supine, right lateral, and left lateral positions. Positional nystagmus induced by slow positioning is persistent, low in frequency, and often present only when fixation is inhibited. Paroxysmal positional nystagmus, however, is best induced by a rapid change from the erect sitting to the supine headhanging left, center, or right positions. It is typically high in frequency and persists even when the patient is attempting to fixate. It depends on both the positioning maneuver and the final head-hanging position (see Chapter 10).

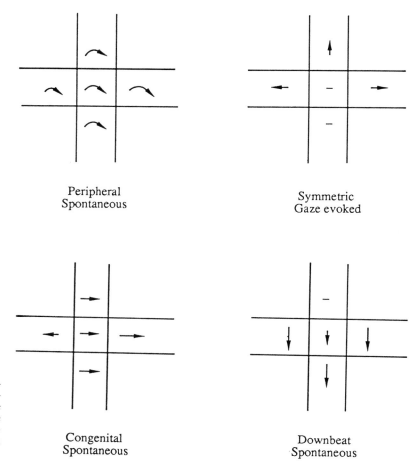

Peripheral
Spontaneous

Symmetric
Gaze evoked

Congenital
Spontaneous

Downbeat
Spontaneous

Figure 5–4. Method for describing the effect of eye position on nystagmus amplitude and direction. *Arrows* indicate direction of nystagmus (direction of fast component) in each eye position.

TYPES OF PATHOLOGIC NYSTAGMUS

Spontaneous Nystagmus

MECHANISM

Spontaneous nystagmus results from an imbalance of tonic signals arriving at the oculomotor neurons. Because the vestibular system is the main source of oculomotor tonus, it is the driving force of most types of spontaneous nystagmus (tonic signals arising in the pursuit and optokinetic systems may also play a role, particularly with congenital nystagmus).[56] A vestibular imbalance results in a constant drift of the eyes in one direction interrupted by fast components in the opposite direction. If the imbalance results from a

peripheral vestibular lesion, patients can use their pursuit system to cancel it. If it results from a central vestibular lesion, their pursuit system cannot suppress it (because central vestibular and pursuit pathways are highly integrated—see Visual-Vestibular Interaction, Chapter 3). The features that separate peripheral from central varieties of spontaneous nystagmus are summarized in Table 5–2.

PERIPHERAL SPONTANEOUS NYSTAGMUS

Lesions of the peripheral vestibular system (labyrinth or VIII nerve) typically interrupt tonic afferent signals originating from all of the receptors of one labyrinth so that the resulting nystagmus has com-

Table 5–2. DIFFERENTIATION BETWEEN SPONTANEOUS
NYSTAGMUS OF PERIPHERAL AND CENTRAL ORIGIN

	Appearance	Fixation	Gaze	Mechanism	Localization
Peripheral	Combined torsional, horizontal	Inhibited	Unidirectional (Alexander's law)	Asymmetric loss of peripheral vestibular tone	Labyrinthine or vestibular nerve
Central	Often pure vertical, horizontal, or torsional	Usually little effect	May change direction	Imbalance in central oculomotor tone; usually central vestibular, may be pursuit or OKN	CNS, usually brainstem or cerebellum

bined torsional, horizontal, and vertical components. The horizontal component dominates, because the tonic activity from the intact vertical canals and otoliths partially cancels out. Gaze in the direction of the fast component increases the frequency and amplitude, whereas gaze in the opposite direction has the reverse effect (Alexander's law). The slow phase is linear, resulting in a sawtoothed waveform. As noted above, peripheral spontaneous nystagmus is strongly inhibited by fixation. Unless the patient is seen within a few days of the acute episode, spontaneous nystagmus will not be present when fixation is permitted.

CENTRAL SPONTANEOUS
NYSTAGMUS

Central spontaneous nystagmus is prominent with and without fixation. It may be purely vertical, horizontal, torsional, or have some combination of torsional and linear components. As with peripheral spontaneous nystagmus, gaze in the direction of the fast component usually increases nystagmus frequency and amplitude, but unlike peripheral spontaneous nystagmus, gaze away from the direction of the fast component will often change the direction of the nystagmus. There is typically a null region several degrees off center in the direction opposite to that of the fast component where nystagmus is minimal or absent. Gaze beyond this null region results in reversal of nystagmus direction. The slow phase of central spontaneous nystagmus may be linear, exponentially increasing, or exponentially decreasing.[56]

With spontaneous downbeat nystagmus

the vertical amplitude increases with horizontal gaze deviation.[3] Downward gaze also increases the amplitude in about two thirds of cases, but in the other one third it decreases it. Upward gaze may reverse the direction to upbeat. Downbeat nystagmus has been produced in monkeys after lesions of the uvula and flocculonodular lobes of the cerebellum.[75, 84] In the human it is localizing to the cervicomedullary junction. Common causes of downbeat nystagmus include cerebellar atrophy, vertebrobasilar ischemia, multiple sclerosis, and Arnold-Chiari malformation.[4, 44] The latter produces downbeat nystagmus, presumably by pressure on the flocculonodular region of the cerebellum; in some cases it may be reversed by decompression of the foramen magnum region.[71] Spontaneous upbeat nystagmus usually results from lesions of the dorsal central medulla in the region of the medial vestibular and prepositus hypoglossi nuclei.[4, 30, 53] Common causes include infarction, infiltrating tumors, and multiple sclerosis. Pure torsional spontaneous nystagmus is frequently associated with syringomyelia and syringobulbia. A high-frequency small-amplitude pendular spontaneous nystagmus is commonly seen in the late stages of multiple sclerosis.[2] This pendular nystagmus converts to a sawtooth pattern on lateral gaze to either side. Lesions involving the vestibular nuclear region can produce a horizontal torsional nystagmus similar to that seen with peripheral lesions, but, unlike the latter, the direction of nystagmus does not reliably indicate the side of lesion and the nystagmus persists with fixation due to damage of visual-vestibular interaction pathways.[9]

CONGENITAL NYSTAGMUS

Congenital spontaneous nystagmus is almost always highly dependent on fixation, disappearing or decreasing with loss of fixation.[20] In some instances a slow nystagmus in the reverse direction is recorded with eyes closed. One common variety, so-called latent congenital nystagmus, occurs only when either eye is covered, permitting monocular fixation. The resulting nystagmus beats toward the fixating eye. Latent congenital nystagmus is usually associated with other congenital ocular defects such as concomitant squint and alternating hyperphoria.[25]

Several characteristic clinical features help distinguish congenital from acquired spontaneous nystagmus. It is usually purely horizontal and may diminish or disappear with convergence. The waveform may be pendular to sawtooth, with many variations in between.[24, 82] Different waveforms occur in the same patient in different eye positions. Gaze in the direction of the fast component converts a pendular nystagmus to a jerk nystagmus; often there is a null region where the nystagmus is minimal. Several different waveforms may be seen in members of the same family with congenital nystagmus. The frequency of congenital nystagmus is usually greater than 2 beats/sec and at times reaches 5 to 6 beats/sec. Nystagmus of this high frequency is unusual other than on a congenital basis. Of course, most patients are aware that the nystagmus has been present since infancy.

The pathophysiologic mechanism of congenital nystagmus is only partially understood.[26] Convincing evidence exists that the slow component causes the target to slip from the fovea, and the fast component brings the target back to the fovea. The slow component is not the result of, but the cause of, decreased vision. Maneuvers designed to decrease the target slippage (fitting glasses with prisms and extraocular muscle surgery) improve visual acuity. Patients with congenital nystagmus can make normal velocity saccades, indicating that the extraocular muscles and orbital mechanics are normal. The vestibular system also appears to be normal in most of these patients.[81] Abnormali-

ties in smooth pursuit and optokinetic slow phases are uniformly present, but it is difficult to know whether these abnormalities are due to a superimposition of the spontaneous nystagmus on attempted tracking eye movements or to an underlying abnormality.[80]

PERIODIC ALTERNATING NYSTAGMUS (PAN)

PAN is a spontaneous nystagmus that periodically changes direction without a change in eye or head position.[8] Cycle length varies between 1 and 6 minutes with null periods between each half cycle varying from 2 to 20 seconds. The nystagmus slowly builds in intensity and reaches a peak slow component velocity near the center of each half cycle before slowly decreasing. PAN has been reported in association with such varied conditions as encephalitis, brainstem ischemia, demyelinating disease, syringobulbia, syphilis, trauma, and as a congenital disorder.[8, 23] Unlike patients with other forms of congenital nystagmus, patients with congenital PAN frequently complain of oscillopsia because they are unable to adapt to the constantly changing direction of nystagmus. PAN is usually present with fixation, although cases have been reported in which PAN occurs only with loss of fixation.

Necropsy studies from three patients with acquired PAN revealed diffuse brainstem involvement, with a predilection for the caudal brainstem.[52] Three reported cases have been associated with downbeat nystagmus, further suggesting caudal brainstem dysfunction.[52] The pathophysiologic mechanism for production of PAN is unknown. PAN cycles can be altered in both phase and magnitude by a vestibular stimulus (rotatory or caloric), suggesting that the PAN rhythm is not the result of an independent central nervous system (CNS) pacemaker but, rather, a response pattern of the central vestibulo-ocular reflex arc.[8, 58] It is important to recognize this unusual form of spontaneous nystagmus because the acquired variety is markedly diminished by baclofen, a gamma-aminobutyric acid (GABA) agonist.[45] Unfortunately, congenital PAN does not respond to baclofen.

Gaze-Evoked Nystagmus

MECHANISM

Patients with gaze-evoked nystagmus are unable to maintain stable conjugate eye deviation away from the primary position. The eyes drift back toward the center with an exponentially decreasing waveform; corrective saccades (fast components) constantly reset the desired gaze position. Gaze-evoked nystagmus is therefore always in the direction of gaze. The site of abnormality can be anywhere from the neuromuscular junction to the multiple brain centers controlling conjugate gaze (Table 5–3). Dysfunction of the so-called oculomotor integrator (see Chapter 3) may be a common mechanism for several types of gaze-evoked nystagmus.[56]

SYMMETRIC

Symmetric gaze-evoked nystagmus (equal amplitude to the left and right) is most commonly produced by ingestion of drugs such as phenobarbital, phenytoin, alcohol, and diazepam. With these agents, high-frequency small-amplitude nystagmus (less than 2 degrees) is found in all directions of gaze. A rough correlation exists between nystagmus amplitude and blood drug level.[36] The nystagmus initially appears at extreme horizontal gaze positions and moves toward the midposition with higher drug levels. In addition to its association with drug ingestion, symmetric gaze-evoked nystagmus commonly occurs in patients with myasthenia gravis, multiple sclerosis, and cerebellar atrophy.

ASYMMETRIC

Asymmetric horizontal gaze-evoked nystagmus always indicates a structural brain lesion. When it is caused by a focal lesion of the brainstem or cerebellum, the larger amplitude nystagmus is usually directed toward the side of the lesion.[5] Large cerebellopontine angle tumors commonly produce asymmetric gaze-evoked nystagmus from compression of the brainstem and cerebellum (Bruns' nystagmus). Some patients with large acoustic neuromas develop a combination of asymmetric gaze-evoked nystagmus from brainstem compression and peripheral spontaneous nystagmus from VIII nerve damage. Asymmetric gaze-evoked nystagmus may be present during the recovery from gaze paralysis (either cortical or subcortical in origin), in which case it is large in amplitude and low in frequency and present only in one direction of gaze (the direction of the previous gaze paralysis).

REBOUND

Rebound nystagmus is a type of gaze-evoked nystagmus that either disappears or reverses direction as the lateral gaze position is held.[49, 50] When the eyes return to the primary position, another burst of nystagmus occurs in the direction of the return saccade. Thus, the patient may have a transient primary position nystagmus in either direction. Rebound nystagmus occurs in patients with cerebellar atrophy and focal structural lesions of the cerebellum; it is the only variety of nystagmus thought to be specific for cerebellar involvement.

DISSOCIATED

Dissociated or disconjugate gaze-evoked nystagmus commonly results from lesions

Table 5–3. CAUSES OF GAZE-EVOKED NYSTAGMUS

	Localization	Common Causes
Symmetric	Nonlocalizing	Drugs, metabolic disorders
Asymmetric	Unilateral brainstem and/or cerebellum	Tumor, infarction
Rebound	Cerebellum	Tumor, infarction, atrophy
Dissociated	MLF, extraocular nerve, or muscle	Multiple sclerosis, myasthenia gravis

of the medial longitudinal fasciculus (MLF), so-called internuclear ophthalmoplegia. With early MLF lesions the eyes appear to move conjugately, but the abducting eye on the side opposite the MLF lesion develops a regular small amplitude high-frequency nystagmus in the direction of gaze. With more extensive MLF lesions the adducting eye lags behind and develops a low-amplitude nystagmus while the abducting eye overshoots the target and develops large-amplitude nystagmus that has a characteristic "peaked waveform."[10] MLF nystagmus can be bilateral or unilateral, depending on the extent of MLF involvement. Bilateral MLF nystagmus is most commonly seen with demyelinating disease, whereas unilateral MLF nystagmus most often accompanies vascular disease of the brainstem.[19] Patients with myasthenia gravis develop dissociated gaze-evoked nystagmus similar to MLF nystagmus (pseudo MLF nystagmus) because of unequal impairment of neuromuscular transmission in adducting and abducting muscles. Unlike MLF nystagmus, the dissociated nystagmus with myasthenia progressively increases in amplitude as the gaze position is maintained.[72] An edrophonium test should be administered to patients with isolated MLF nystagmus to exclude myasthenia gravis.

Positional Nystagmus

MECHANISM

Since the time of Bárány, positional nystagmus has been attributed to lesions of the otoliths and their connections in the vestibular nuclei and cerebellum, inasmuch as these are the receptors that are sensitive to changes in the direction of gravity.[12, 51, 65] Recently, other mechanisms for the production of positional nystagmus have been proposed, forcing reexamination of traditional concepts. If the semicircular canal cupula is altered so that its specific gravity no longer equals that of the surrounding endolymph, the organ would become sensitive to changes in the direction of gravity and could produce positional nystagmus. Several types of evidence suggest that both structural and metabolic factors can alter the specific gravity of the cupula and cause positional nystagmus (see Acute Effects of Alcohol, Chapter 15 and Pathophysiology of Benign Positional Vertigo, Chapter 10).

Traditional classifications of positional nystagmus are often confusing and can be difficult to apply in clinical practice. Some classifications have been based on clinical observations obtained while the patient is fixating, whereas others have been based on electronystagmography (ENG) recordings with eyes closed or with eyes open in darkness. Some investigators use slow positioning maneuvers, but others employ only rapid positioning. These different methods make it difficult to compare classifications. Nylen[65] initially described three types of positional nystagmus based on visual inspection of nystagmus direction and regularity. Type I—direction-changing—and type II—direction-fixed—remained constant as long as the position was maintained. Type III was less clearly defined, comprising all paroxysmal varieties of positional nystagmus and some persistent varieties that did not fit into types I and II. Numerous modifications of Nylen's original classification have subsequently been proposed, and the definition of each type has changed. Most investigators do agree that two general categories of positional nystagmus can be identified: paroxysmal and static.

PAROXYSMAL POSITIONAL NYSTAGMUS

Paroxysmal positional nystagmus is induced by a rapid change from erect sitting to the supine head-hanging left, center or right position (Fig. 5–5). It is initially high in frequency but dissipates rapidly within 30 seconds to a minute. The most common variety (so-called benign paroxysmal positional nystagmus) usually has a 3- to 10-second latency before onset and rarely lasts longer than 30 seconds.[7] The nystagmus has combined torsional and linear components (see Fig. 6–9). Although infrequent bilateral cases have been reported, the nystagmus is usually prominent only in one head-hanging position, and a burst

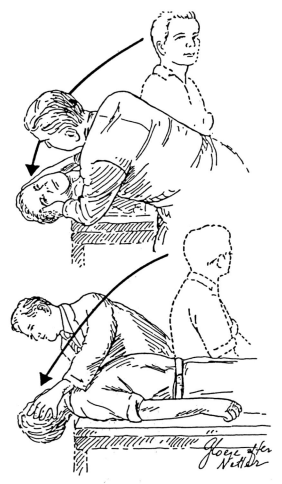

Figure 5–5. Technique for inducing paroxysmal positional nystagmus (Hallpike maneuver). Patient is taken rapidly from the sitting to head-hanging position.

of nystagmus occurs in the reverse direction when the patient moves back to the sitting position. Another key feature is that the patient experiences severe vertigo with the initial positioning, but with repeated positioning vertigo and nystagmus rapidly disappear (so-called fatigability).

Benign paroxysmal positional nystagmus is a reliable sign of vestibular end-organ disease (see Chapter 10). It can be the only finding in an otherwise healthy individual or it may be associated with other signs of peripheral vestibular damage, such as peripheral spontaneous nystag-

mus and unilateral caloric hypoexcitability. In those instances in which an abnormality is identified on caloric testing, the nystagmus will usually occur when the patient is positioned with the damaged ear down. Benign paroxysmal positional nystagmus is a common sequela of head injury, viral labyrinthitis, and occlusion of the vasculature of the inner ear. In the majority of cases, however, it occurs as an isolated sign of unknown cause.

Paroxysmal positional nystagmus can also result from brainstem and cerebellar lesions. The central type does not decrease in amplitude or duration with repeated positioning, does not have a clear latency, and usually lasts longer than 30 seconds.[18] The direction is unpredictable and may be different in each position. It is often purely vertical with fast phase directed downward (i.e., toward the cheeks). The presence or absence of associated vertigo is not a reliable differential feature. Central paroxysmal positional nystagmus can be the initial presenting sign of a posterior fossa tumor such as a medulloblastoma or cerebellar glioma.[38, 39] It is, therefore, critical to distinguish it from the benign peripheral variety (Table 5–4).

STATIC POSITIONAL NYSTAGMUS

This type of positional nystagmus remains as long as the position is held, although it may fluctuate in frequency and amplitude. It may be in the same direction in all positions or change directions in different positions. Not infrequently, patients with paroxysmal positional nystagmus will have static positional nystagmus after the paroxysmal positional nystagmus has disappeared, or if the position is reached very slowly. Despite earlier reports to the contrary,[65] it is now generally accepted that direction-changing and direction-fixed static positional nystagmus are most commonly associated with peripheral vestibular disorders, although both occur with central lesions.[13, 59] Their presence indicates only a dysfunction in the vestibular system without localizing value. As with spontaneous nystagmus, however, lack of suppression with fixation and signs of associated brainstem dysfunction suggest a central lesion.

Table 5–4. DIFFERENTIATION BETWEEN PERIPHERAL AND
CENTRAL PAROXYSMAL POSITIONAL NYSTAGMUS

	Appearance	Latency	Duration	Fatigability	Mechanism	Localization
Peripheral	Torsional, upbeat, disconjugate	Usual	<30 sec	Usual	Change in cupula specific gravity	Labyrinth
Central	Conjugate, pure horizontal or vertical	Unusual	>30 sec	Unusual	Damage to central otolith-ocular pathways	Brainstem or cerebellum

OTHER OCULAR OSCILLATIONS

Dissociated Spontaneous Nystagmus

Several different lesions of the posterior fossa can result in a spontaneous nystagmus with torsional, horizontal, and vertical components varying in each eye. The nystagmus is usually synchronized, however, in that the fast component occurs at exactly the same time in both eyes. Tumors, vascular disease, and demyelinating disease of the brainstem produce this form of dissociated nystagmus.[21] Frequently the eye on the side of the lesion shows the largest amplitude oscillation. Monocular nystagmus results from similar posterior fossa lesions; this unusual form of dissociated nystagmus also has been reported with such varied entities as congenital syphilis, meningitis, optic nerve glioma, cerebral trauma, unilateral amblyopia, and high refractive error.[28, 63] As expected, these patients are typically bothered by severe oscillopsia.

Seesaw nystagmus is an unusual type of dissociated nystagmus in which one eye rhythmically rises and intorts and the other eye falls and extorts. It may be congenital but most often is produced by acquired lesions near the optic chiasm, particularly those producing a bitemporal field defect and decreased central visual acuity.[1, 22] Lesions associated with seesaw nystagmus include craniopharyngiomas, syringobulbia, brainstem infarction, and diffuse choroiditis; compression of the interstitial nucleus of Cajal in the midbrain tegmentum may be the common denominator.[69]

Voluntary Ocular Oscillations (Voluntary Nystagmus)

Some normal subjects are able to produce rapid oscillations of the eyes at will, apparently by producing rapid sequenced saccades back and forth.[70] The main significance of these ocular gymnastics is that they may be mistaken for pathologic nystagmus. High in frequency (90 to as high as 1380 cycles/min), low in amplitude (2 to 5 degrees), these rapid horizontal movements cannot be maintained for more than 20 to 30 seconds before fatigue sets in.[14] Several siblings in the same family may have the ability to produce voluntary ocular oscillations, and Keyes[54] reported two generations of the same family who could produce the eye movements suggesting a dominant mode of inheritance.

Convergence Retraction Nystagmus

This dramatic ocular motor disorder results from lesions involving the diencephalic-midbrain junction. When the patient attempts to make voluntary upward saccades or when involuntary upward saccades (fast components) are induced by an optokinetic or vestibular stimulus, the patient develops co-contraction of all extraocular muscles and the eyes rhythmically retract and converge.[37] In other cases convergence nystagmus occurs without retraction, apparently due to asynchronous adducting saccades.[66] Convergence retraction nystagmus is usually associated with other signs of midbrain dysfunction (impaired upward gaze, pupillary abnormalities, accommodative spasm, retraction of the lids, and skew deviation), constituting the dorsal midbrain syndrome.[6] This syndrome is most frequently produced by dysgerminomas of the pineal region but is also associated with other tumors and vascular lesions involving the tectal or pretectal area.

Saccadic Intrusions

Included under this category are square wave jerks, macrosquare wave jerks, macrosaccadic oscillations, ocular flutter, and opsoclonus. The common feature is that unwanted saccades disrupt steady fixation. *Square wave jerks* refer to small-amplitude involuntary saccades that take the eyes off the target followed after a normal intersaccadic interval (130 to 200 msec) by a corrective saccade bringing the eyes back to the target. Infrequent small square wave jerks can be seen in normal subjects, especially the young and elderly.[48] Persistent large-amplitude square wave jerks (1 to 5 degrees) are abnormal but nonlocalizing. They are prominent with cerebellar lesions and with progressive supranuclear palsy and have been reported with diffuse cerebral lesions, Huntington disease, and schizophrenia.[32, 77] So-called *macrosquare wave jerks* (10 to 50 degrees) have been observed in multiple sclerosis and olivopontocerebellar atrophy. *Macrosaccadic oscillations* are typically seen in patients with saccade overshoot dysmetria (i.e., those with cerebellar lesions). After refixation, patients make a series of hypermetric saccades, apparently because they are unable to make a small enough saccade to bring the target onto the fovea. *Ocular flutter* refers to a burst of to-and-fro horizontal saccades occurring either spontaneously or after a saccade to a target. This burst of saccades lacks the characteristic delay normally present between serial saccades. Ocular flutter is typically seen with diffuse involvement of brainstem-cerebellar pathways, being particularly prominent in such varied disorders as Friedreich's ataxia and brainstem encephalitis.[35]

The most prominent saccadic oscillations are seen with *opsoclonus*.[27] With this rare eye movement disorder the eyes are constantly making random conjugate saccades of unequal amplitude in all directions. As with ocular flutter, there is typically no intersaccade interval. The phenomenon occurs with several different types of CNS disease and probably represents a mixed group of eye movement disorders. The inappropriate saccades are most prominent immediately before or after a refixation and are only slightly affected by loss of fixation. One variety of opsoclonus probably represents a continuum with square wave jerks and ocular flutter. Other more dramatic varieties of opsoclonus have been reported in patients with brainstem encephalitis, as a remote effect of tumors (e.g., neuroblastoma), and in association with toxins (e.g., the pesticide kepone).

These saccade disorders probably represent a release of the brainstem saccade burst neurons from supranuclear control. Zee and Robinson[83] suggested that dysfunction of the pontine omnipause neurons might be a common underlying mechanism.

Ocular Bobbing

Ocular bobbing consists of abrupt, non-rhythmic, conjugate, downward jerks of the eyes, followed by slow return to midposition. The abnormal movements are classically seen in comatose patients with intrinsic pontine lesions that also produce absent reflex horizontal eye movements, but they have also been reported with posterior fossa lesions that compress the pons and with metabolic encephalopathy.[15, 56] Inverse ocular bobbing or ocular dipping refers to a slow downward movement of the eyes followed by a rapid return to midposition.[55] Reverse bobbing consists of a rapid deviation of the eyes upward followed by a slow return to the primary position. These latter phenomena may be variations of ocular bobbing because all can be seen in the same subject at different times.[73] As with typical ocular bobbing, they are usually seen with metabolic disorders or structural lesions of the pons.

Palato-Ocular Myoclonus

This is a rhythmic oscillation of the eyes associated with synchronous oscillation of the palate. An associated rhythmic oscillation of the pharynx, larynx, mouth, tongue, diaphragm, extremities, and intercostal muscles may also occur.[41, 74] The eye movements are typically pendular oscillations that are often vertical but may have a horizontal or torsional component. The frequency varies from 1 to 3 per second, and the movements may continue with loss of fixation. Ocular myoclonus often disappears during sleep even though the palatal movements continue.[74] Palato-ocular myoclonus is seen in association with lesions disrupting the connections between the cerebellar dentate nucleus, the red nucleus, and the inferior olivary nucleus (Guillain-Mollaret triangle). It most commonly accompanies vascular lesions but also occurs with tumors and degenerative disease. When seen in association with vascular lesions, it often develops months after the brainstem or cerebellar infarction. Intravenous scopolamine has been reported to abolish the ocular oscillations temporarily, but there is no good long-term treatment.[40]

OCULAR TILT REACTION

If a subject is tilted in the frontal plane (about the nasal occipital axis), the head reflexly tilts and the eyes counter-roll and skew toward the opposite side. The functional role of this reflex in visual stabilization during natural body movements is minimal, however, inasmuch as the magnitude of the compensatory head tilt and ocular counter-rolling is only about 10 percent of angular displacement of the head. The ocular tilt reaction is principally a labyrinthine reflex; it is independent of the position of the head, relative to the body (indicating that neck position is not important). Westheimer and Blair[79] first elicited the ocular tilt reaction by electrical stimulation of the rostral midbrain tegmentum in the region of the interstitial nucleus of Cajal. Clinically, the ocular tilt reaction has been seen in patients with peripheral labyrinthine lesions (a complication of stapedectomy), lesions of the lateral medulla (particularly Wallenberg's syndrome), and with lesions of the rostral midbrain.[16, 43, 46] Based on the animal and clinical data, Halmagyi and colleagues[43] proposed that the excitatory ocular tilt reaction arises in the utricle of the dependent ear, passes through or synapses in the vestibular nuclei of the same side, and then projects to the opposite side of the upper brainstem. Therefore, stimulation of the utricular nerve or the region of the vestibular nuceli results in a contralateral ocular tilt reaction, whereas stimulation of the midbrain results in an ipsilateral ocular tilt reaction (as observed by Westheimer and Blair).[79] Lesions in these regions would, of course, result in an ocular tilt reaction in the opposite direction. Paroxysmal tonic ocular tilt reactions have been reported in patients with multiple sclerosis and in a patient with a focal brainstem abscess.[46] Such patients may respond to carbamazepine or baclofen.

REFERENCES

1. Arnott, FJ and Miller, SJH: See-saw nystagmus. Trans Ophthalmol Soc UK 90:483, 1970.
2. Aschoff, JC, Conrad, B, and Kornhuber, HH: Acquired pendular nystagmus with oscillopsia in multiple sclerosis: A sign of cerebellar nuclei disease. J Neurol Neurosurg Psychiatr 37:570, 1974.
3. Baloh, RW and Spooner, JW: Downbeat nystagmus: A type of central vestibular nystagmus. Neurology 31:304, 1981.
4. Baloh, RW and Yee, RD: Spontaneous vertical nystagmus. Rev Neurol (Paris) (in press).
5. Baloh, RW, et al: Cerebellar-pontine angle tumors. Results of quantitative vestibulo-ocular testing. Arch Neurol 33:507, 1976.
6. Baloh, RW, Furman, JM, and Yee, RD: Dorsal midbrain syndrome: Clinical and oculographic findings. Neurology 35:54, 1985.
7. Baloh, RW, Honrubia, V, and Jacobson, K: Benign positional vertigo: Clinical and oculographic features in 240 cases. Neurology 37:371, 1987.
8. Baloh, RW, Honrubia, V, and Konrad, HR: Periodic alternating nystagmus. Brain 99:11, 1976.
9. Baloh, RW, Yee, RD, and Honrubia, V: Eye movements in patients with Wallenberg's syndrome. Ann NY Acad Sci 374:600, 1981.
10. Baloh, RW, Yee, RD, and Honrubia, V: Internuclear ophthalmoplegia. I. Saccades and

dissociated nystagmus. Arch Neurol 35:484, 1978.

11. Bárány, R: Physiologie and Pathologie des Bogengangsapparates beim Menschen. Deuticke, Vienna, 1907.

12. Bárány, R: Neue Untersuchungsmethoden, die Beziehungen zwischen Vestibularapparat, Kleinhirn, Grosshirn and Rückenmark betreffend. Wien med Wschr 60:2033, 1910.

13. Barber, HO: Positional nystagmus: Testing and interpretation. Ann Otol Rhinol Laryngol 73:838, 1964.

14. Blair, CJ, Goldberg, MF, and von Norden, GK: Voluntary nystagmus. Arch Ophthalmol 77:349, 1976.

15. Bosch, EP, Kennedy, SS, and Aschenbrener, CA: Ocular bobbing: The myth of its localizing value. Neurology 25:949, 1975.

16. Brandt, T and Dieterich, M: Pathological eye-head coordination in roll: Tonic ocular tilt reaction in mesencephalic and medullary lesions. Brain 110:649, 1987.

17. Brunia, CHM and Hoppenbrouwers, T: In search of tonic cervical reflexes. An evaluation of Fukuda's vertical writing test. Acta Otolaryngol 61:547, 1966.

18. Cawthorn, T and Hinchcliffe, R: Positional nystagmus of the central type as evidence of subtentorial metastases. Brain 84:415, 1961.

19. Cogan, DG, Kubik, SC, and Smith, WL: Unilateral internuclear ophthalmoplegia: Report of eight clinical cases and one post-mortem study. Arch Ophthalmol 44:783, 1950.

20. Cogan, DG: Congenital nystagmus. Can J Ophthalmol 2:4, 1967.

21. Cogan, DG: Dissociated nystagmus with lesions in the posterior fossa. Arch Ophthalmol 70:121, 1963.

22. Daroff, RB: See-saw nystagmus. Neurology 15:874, 1965.

23. Davis, DG and Smith, JL: Periodic alternating nystagmus. Am J Ophthalmol 72:757, 1971.

24. Dell'Osso, LF and Daroff, RB: Congenital nystagmus waveforms and foveation strategy. Doc Ophthalmol 19:155, 1975.

25. Dell'Osso, LF, Schmidt, D, and Daroff, RB: Latent, manifest latent, and congenital nystagmus. Arch Ophthalmol 97:1877, 1979.

26. Dell'Osso, LF: Congenital nystagmus. Basic aspects. In Lennerstrand, G, Zee, DS, Keller, EL (eds): Functional Basis of Ocular Motility Disorders. Pergamon Press, Oxford, 1982.

27. Digre, KR: Opsoclonus in adults. Arch Neurol 43:1165, 1986.

28. Donin, JF: Acquired monocular nystagmus in children. Can J Ophthalmol 2:212, 1967.

29. Eviator, A and Eviator, L: A critical look at "cold calorics." Arch Otolaryngol 99:361, 1974.

30. Fisher, A, Gresty, M, Chambers, B, and Rudge, P: Primary position upbeat nystagmus: A variety of central positional nystagmus. Brain 106:949, 1983.

31. Fregly, AR: Vestibular ataxia and its measurement in man. In Kornhuber, HH (ed): Handbook of Sensory Physiology, Vol VI, Part 2. Springer-Verlag, New York, 1974.

32. Fukazawa, T, Tashiro, K, Hamada, T, and Kase, M: Multisystem degeneration: Drugs and square wave jerks. Neurology 36:1230, 1986.

33. Fukuda, T: The stepping test: Two phases of the labyrinthine reflex. Acta Otolaryngol 50:95, 1959.

34. Fukuda, T: Vertical writing with eyes covered: A new test of vestibulospinal reaction. Acta Otolaryngol 50:26, 1959.

35. Furman, JM, Perlman, S, and Baloh, RW: Eye movements in Friedreich's ataxia. Arch Neurol 40:343, 1983.

36. Gallagher, BB, et al: Primidone, dipenylhydantoin and phenobarbital. Aspects of acute and chronic toxicity. Neurology 23:145, 1973.

37. Gay, AJ, Brodkey, J, and Miller, JE: Convergence retraction nystagmus: An electromyographic study. Arch Ophthalmol 70:456, 1963.

38. Grand, W: Positional nystagmus: An early sign of medulloblastoma. Neurology 21:1157, 1971.

39. Gregorius, FK, Crandall, PH, and Baloh, RW: Positional vertigo in cerebellar astrocytoma. Report of two cases. Surgical Neurol 6:283, 1976.

40. Gresty, MA, Ell, JJ, and Findley, LJ: Acquired pendular nystagmus: Its characteristics, localizing value and pathophysiology. J Neurol Neurosurg Psychiatr 45:431, 1982.

41. Guillain, G: The syndrome of synchronous and rhythmic palato-pharyngo-laryngo-oculo-diaphragmatic myoclonus. Proc Roy Soc Med 31:1031, 1938.

42. Hain, TC, Fetter, M, and Zee, DS: Head-shaking nystagmus in patients with unilateral peripheral vestibular lesions. Am J Otolaryngol 8:36, 1987.

43. Halmagyi, GM, Gresty, MA, and Gibson, WPR: Ocular tilt reaction with peripheral vestibular lesions. Ann Neurol 6:80, 1979.

44. Halmagyi, GM, Rudge, P, Gresty, MA, and Sanders, MD: Downbeating nystagmus. Arch Neurol 40:777, 1983.

45. Halmagyi, GM, et al: Treatment of periodic alternating nystagmus. Ann Neurol 8:609, 1980.

46. Hedges, TR and Hoyt, WF: Ocular tilt reaction due to an upper brain stem lesion: Paroxysmal skew deviation, torsion, and oscillation of the eyes with head tilt. Ann Neurol 11:537, 1982.

47. Hennebert, C: A new syndrome in hereditary syphilis of the labyrinth. Presse Med Belg Brux 63:467, 1911.

48. Herishanu, YO and Sharpe, JA: Normal square wave jerks. Invest Ophthalmol Vis Sci 20:268, 1981.

49. Hood, JD, Kayan, A, and Leech, J: Rebound nystagmus. Brain 96:507, 1973.

50. Hood, JD: Further observations on the phenomenon of rebound nystagmus. Ann NY Acad Sci 374:352, 1981.

51. Jongkees, LBW: On positional nystagmus. Acta Otolaryngol (Suppl)159:78, 1961.

52. Keane, JR: Periodic alternating nystagmus with downward beating nystagmus. A clinico-anatomical case study of multiple sclerosis. Arch Neurol 30:399, 1974.

53. Keane, JR and Itabashi, HH: Upbeat nystagmus: Clinicopathologic study of two patients. Neurology 37:491, 1987.

54. Keyes, MJ: Voluntary nystagmus in two generations. Arch Neurol 29:63, 1973.

55. Knobler, RL, Somasundaram, M, and Schutta, HS: Inverse ocular bobbing. Ann Neurol 9:194, 1981.

56. Leigh, RJ and Zee, DS: The Neurology of Eye Movements. FA Davis, Philadelphia, 1983.

57. Leigh, RJ, Hanley, DF, Munschauer, FE, and Lasker, AG: Eye movements induced by head rotation in unresponsive patients. Ann Neurol 15:465, 1984.

58. Leigh, RJ, Robinson, DA, and Zee, DS: A hypothetical explanation for periodic alternating nystagmus: Instability in the optokinetic-vestibular system. Ann NY Acad Sci 374:619, 1981.

59. Lin, J, Elidan, J, Baloh, RW, and Honrubia, V: Direction changing positional nystagmus: Incidence and meaning. Am J Otolaryngol 7:306, 1986.

60. Mattox, DE: Perilymph fistulas. In Cummings, CW, Fredrickson, JM, Harker, LA, Krause, CJ, Schuller, DE (eds): Otolaryngology: Head and Neck Surgery. CV Mosby, St Louis, 1986.

61. Mueller-Jensen, A, Neunzig, H-P, and Emskötter, TH: Outcome prediction in comatose patients: Significance of reflex eye movement analysis. J Neurol Neurosurg Psych 50:389, 1987.

62. Nadol, JB: Positive Hennebert's sign in Meniere's disease. Arch Otolaryngol 103:524, 1977.

63. Nathanson, M, Bergman, PS, and Berker, MB: Monocular nystagmus. Am J Ophthalmol 40:685, 1955.

64. Nelson, JR: The minimal ice water test. Neurology 19:577, 1969.

65. Nylen, CO: Positional nystagmus. A review and future prospects. J Laryngol Otol 64:295, 1950.

66. Ochs, AL, Stark, L, Hoyt, WF, and D'Amico, D: Opposed adducting saccades in convergence-retraction nystagmus. Brain 102:497, 1979.

67. Peitersen, E: Measurement of vestibulo-spinal responses in man. In Kornhuber, HH (ed): Handbook of Sensory Physiology, Vol VI, Part 2. Springer-Verlag, New York, 1974.

68. Romberg, MH: Lehrbuch der Nervenkrankheiten des Menschen. A Dunker, Berlin, 1946.

69. Sano, K, et al: Stimulation and destruction of the region of the interstitial nucleus in cases of torticollis and see-saw nystagmus. Confinia Neurologica (Basel) 34:331, 1972.

70. Shults, WT, Stark, L, Hoyt, WF, and Ochs, AL: Normal saccadic structure of voluntary nystagmus. Arch Ophthalmol 95:1399, 1977.

71. Spooner, JW and Baloh, RW: Arnold-Chiari malformation: Improvement in eye movements after surgical treatment. Brain 104:51, 1981.

72. Spooner, JW and Baloh, RW: Eye movement fatigue in myasthenia gravis. Neurology 29:29, 1979.

73. Stark, SR, Masucci, EF, and Kurtzke, JF: Ocular dipping. 34:391, 1984.

74. Tahmoush, AJ, Brooks, JE, and Keltner, JL: Palatal myoclonus associated with abnormal ocular and extremity movements. Arch Neurol 27:431, 1972.

75. Takemori, S and Susuki, M: Cerebellar contribution to oculomotor function. OLR 39:209, 1977.

76. Thompson, JN and Kohut, MRI: Perilymph fistulae: Variability of symptoms and results of surgery. Otolaryngol Head Neck Surg 87:898, 1979.

77. Troost, BT and Daroff, RB: The ocular motor defects in progressive supranuclear palsy. Ann Neurol 2:397, 1977.

78. Unterberger, S: Neue objectiv registrierbare Vestibularis—Körperdrehreaktion, erhalten durch Treten auf der Stelle: Der "Tretversuch." Arch Ohr-Nas-u-Kehlk-Heilk 145:478, 1938.

79. Westheimer, G and Blair, M: The ocular tilt reaction—a brain stem oculomotor routine. Invest Ophthalmol 14:833, 1975.

80. Yee, RD, Baloh, RW, and Honrubia, V: A study of congenital nystagmus: Optokinetic nystagmus. Br J Ophthalmol 64:926, 1980.

81. Yee, RD, Baloh, RW, Honrubia, V, and Kim, YS: A study of congenital nystagmus: Vestibular nystagmus. J Otolaryngol 10:89, 1981.

82. Yee, RD, et al: A study of congenital nystagmus: Waveforms. Neurology 26:326, 1976.

83. Zee, DS and Robinson, DA: A hypothetical explanation of saccadic oscillations. Ann Neurol 5:405, 1979.

84. Zee, DS, Yamazaki, A, Batter, PH, and Gücer, G: Effects of ablation of flocculus and paraflocculus on eye movements in primates. J Neurophysiol 46:878, 1981.

Chapter 6

ELECTRONYSTAG-MOGRAPHY

METHOD OF RECORDING EYE MOVEMENTS

Electro-oculography (EOG) is the simplest and most readily available system for recording eye movements. With this technique, a voltage surrounding the orbit is measured, the magnitude of which is proportional to the amplitude of the eye movement. When used for evaluating vestibular function, the technique has been termed electronystagmography (ENG), and often the terms EOG and ENG are used interchangeably.[18, 23] ENG provides a permanent record for comparison with nystagmus reports in other patients. Because of the transient nature of many types of nystagmus, a permanent record is invaluable. By comparing clinical observations with paper recordings, both students and experienced clinicians become more efficient in recognizing different varieties of nystagmus. With ENG, one can quantify the slow component velocity, frequency, and amplitude of spontaneous or induced nystagmus, and the changes in these measurements brought about by loss of fixation (either with eyes closed or eyes open in darkness). In addition, visually controlled eye movements (saccade, smooth pursuit, and optokinetic nystagmus) can be recorded and quantitatively assessed.

Principle of ENG

The principle of ENG is illustrated in Figure 6–1. The pigmented layer of the retina maintains a negative potential with regard to the surrounding tissue by means of active ion transport. The potential difference between the cornea and the retina, known as the corneal-retinal potential, acts as an electric dipole, oriented in the direction of the long axis of the eye. In relation to a remote location, an electrode placed in the vicinity of the eye becomes more positive when the eye rotates toward it and less positive when it rotates in the opposite direction. Recordings are usually made with a three-electrode system, using differential amplifiers. Two of the (active) electrodes are placed on each side of the eye, and the reference (ground) electrode is placed somewhere remote from the eye. The two active electrodes measure a potential change of equal amplitude but opposite direction. The difference in potential between these electrodes is amplified and used to control the displacement of a pen-writing recorder or similar device to produce a permanent record. Because the differential amplifiers monitor the difference in voltage between the two active electrodes, remote electrical signals (electrocardiographic or electroencephalographic, for example) arrive at the electrodes with approximately equal amplitude and phase and are cancelled out.

The corneal-retinal potential on which the ENG is based varies with the amount of light striking the retina, with a maximum light-adapted potential being approximately twice that of the dark-adapted potential. Therefore, the ENG signal must be calibrated frequently, and major shifts in room lighting should be avoided.

The sensitivity and frequency response of the ENG equipment can vary markedly from one laboratory to another.[23, 41] With properly designed amplification, ENG can consistently record eye rotations of 0.5

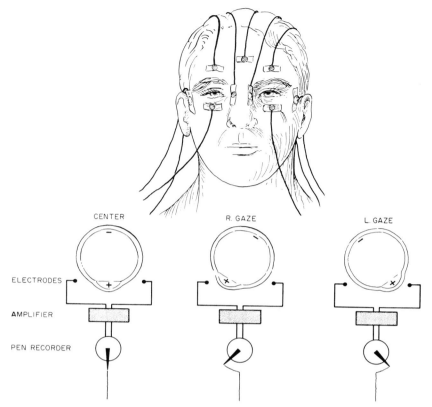

CENTER   R. GAZE   L. GAZE

ELECTRODES

AMPLIFIER

PEN RECORDER

Figure 6–1. Recording of eye movements with electronystagmography (ENG). See text for details.

degrees, although one occasionally encounters a patient with a high noise-to-signal ratio (particularly elderly patients), limiting the sensitivity to 1 to 2 degrees. Even at its best, the sensitivity of ENG is less than that of direct visual inspection (approximately 0.1 degree), and therefore visual inspection for small-amplitude eye movements (e.g., gaze-evoked nystagmus) remains an important part of the examination. With all electronic equipment, one must tailor the frequency response so that interfering signals (for example, 60 cycle hum and muscle potentials) are removed with the least possible interference with the desired event. In order to reproduce the high-frequency transients of eye movement recordings accurately (nystagmus fast components and saccades), we have found that the upper-frequency cutoff must be at least 25 Hz, and preferably above 40 Hz.[10]

Electrode Placement

The plane of the recording electrodes defines the plane of recorded eye movements. Electrodes attached medial and lateral to the eye will record the horizontal components of eye movement; those above and below the eye, the vertical components (see Fig. 6–1). A ground electrode is placed on the center of the forehead or on the auricle. The horizontal component of both eyes is summed by placing an electrode lateral to each eye (bitemporal recording). This has the advantage of increasing the signal-to-noise ratio but the disadvantage of camouflaging disconjugate eye movements. Bitemporal recordings should be used only after monocular recordings have verified conjugacy. The vertically aligned electrodes sense the voltage associated with both eye and lid movement, so that the recording represents a summation of these two movements.[20] For this reason, ENG cannot be used for quantitative analysis of vertical eye movements. In most instances, however, it is adequate for qualitative clinical assessment of vertical eye movement disorders. Vertical recordings also provide a valuable monitor of eye blinks.

Interpreting the Recording

By convention, for horizontal recordings, eye movements to the right are displayed so that they produce upward pen deflection and those to the left produce downward pen deflection. For vertical recordings, upward and downward eye movements produce upward and downward deflections, respectively. In order to interpret ENG recordings, calibration must be performed so that a standard angle of eye deviation is represented by a known amplitude of pen deflection. The patient is asked to look at a series of dots or lights 10 to 15 degrees on each side of, above, and below the central fixation point. Once this relationship is established, the amplitude, duration, and velocity of recorded eye movements can be easily calculated. Figure 6–2 illustrates the relationship between components of a typical beat of nystagmus as recorded with ENG.

Values chosen for each component are those commonly seen with vestibular nystagmus recorded in the dark. The fast component moves to the left, so by convention the nystagmus is to the left. A 10-degree fast component would have an average velocity (a/fd) of approximately 100 deg/sec. The slow component velocity (a/sd) is usually much slower; in this case, 10-deg/sec. It is approximately the product of the amplitude times frequency as long as the fast duration is small compared with the slow duration. Although the magnitude of each nystagmus measurement shown in Figure 6–2 can be calculated directly from the polygraph recording, such a procedure is tedious and therefore subject to error. Digital computers are ideally suited for making such measurements. After analog to digital conversion of the data, a digital computer, using a programmed algorithm, calculates the amplitude, duration, and velocity of each of the slow and fast components.[10] Plots of the nystagmus slow component velocity versus time are particularly useful for quantifying the magnitude of induced nystagmus (as will be shown later).

In order to interpret ENG recordings properly, one must be able to recognize common artifacts (Fig. 6–3). Eye blinks are readily identified in the vertical chan-

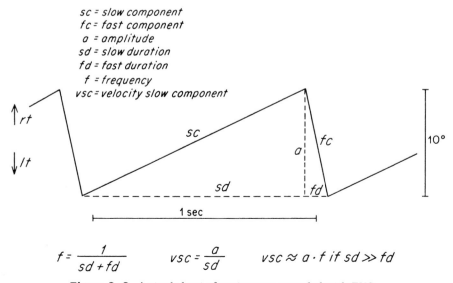

sc = slow component
fc = fast component
a = amplitude
sd = slow duration
fd = fast duration
f = frequency
vsc = velocity slow component

$$f = \frac{1}{sd + fd} \qquad vsc = \frac{a}{sd} \qquad vsc \approx a \cdot f \text{ if } sd \gg fd$$

Figure 6–2. A single beat of nystagmus recorded with ENG.

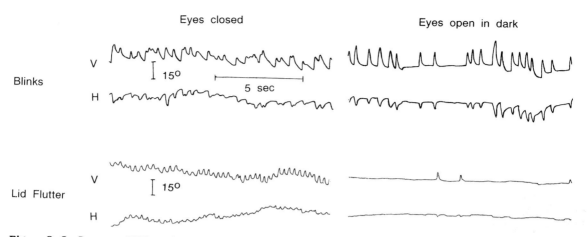

Figure 6–3. Common ENG artifacts caused by frequent blinking (*upper traces*) or lid flutter (*lower traces*). Note stable baseline between blinks with eyes open in darkness. *V*, vertical monocular; *H*, horizontal bitemporal.

nel because of their peaked waveform and short duration. Their appearance in the horizontal channel varies; they can mimic saccades or even nystagmus (see Fig. 6–3, *upper traces*). Large blink artifacts in the horizontal channel can often be decreased or even eliminated by repositioning the electrodes. Many patients exhibit a constant lid flutter with eye closure that looks like nystagmus (in both the horizontal and vertical channels) (see Fig. 6–3, *lower traces*). For this reason, recordings should always be made with eyes open in the dark as well as with eyes closed. Tremors of the face and head also produce a nystagmus-like waveform due to mechanical displacement of the electrodes.

Standard Test Battery

ENG can be used to evaluate any type of eye movement disorder, and the testing procedure should be flexible enough to deal with any such abnormality encountered. It is useful, however, to have a standard test battery that will at least screen all areas of potential abnormality (Table 6–1). In most clinical laboratories, the test battery includes (1) recording for pathologic nystagmus, (2) the bithermal caloric test, and (3) tests of visual ocular control.

Table 6–1. STANDARD ENG TEST BATTERY

A. Recording for pathologic nystagmus
 1. Fixation at midposition
 2. Fixation inhibited with eyes open in darkness (constant mental alerting)
 3. Gaze held 30 degrees right, left, up, and down
 4. Rapid and slow positional changes

B. Bithermal caloric test
 1. 30°C and 44°C water infused into each ear, eyes open in darkness, continuous mental alerting, allow at least 5 minutes between each

C. Visual tracking tests
 1. Saccades: 5–40 degrees, target can be series of dots or lights
 2. Smooth pursuit: target velocity 20–40 deg/sec
 3. Optokinetic nystagmus (OKN): stripe velocity 20–40 deg/sec
 4. Optokinetic after nystagmus (OKAN): lights turned off after 1 minute constant velocity OKN in each direction

RECORDING PATHOLOGIC NYSTAGMUS

The same systematic search for pathologic nystagmus outlined in the previous chapter should be conducted during the ENG examination. Recording with eyes closed or with eyes open in darkness is more effective than Frenzel glasses for identifying peripheral spontaneous and positional nystagmus. Approximately 20 percent of normal subjects have spontaneous nystagmus and as many as 75 percent have positional nystagmus when tested with eyes closed or with eyes open in darkness.[19, 39] Apparently the vestibular system is unable to stabilize the position of the eyes when visual signals are removed. If the average slow component velocity of the spontaneous or positional nystagmus exceeds 4 deg/sec, however, it is a sign of vestibular impairment.[46, 57]

Spontaneous Nystagmus

The effect of change in ocular position and fixation on peripheral spontaneous nystagmus is illustrated with the ENG recordings in Figure 6–4. The patient was tested three days after and again two weeks after a left labyrinthectomy. On the initial recording, nystagmus was present with fixation, although it was more prominent without fixation. On the subsequent recording, nystagmus occurred only when eye closure removed fixation. This pattern is typical of an acute peripheral vestibulopathy of any cause. The nystagmus is exaggerated with gaze in the direction of the

fast component (Alexander's law). As a general rule, nystagmus with fixation (nystagmus seen on routine neurologic examination) disappears within one to two weeks after the occurrence of an acute peripheral vestibular lesion. By contrast, spontaneous nystagmus can be recorded with eyes closed for as long as 5 to 10 years after an acute peripheral vestibular lesion.[60] In some patients, the spontaneous nystagmus emerges only when they are mentally alerted (for example, when performing serial seven subtractions from 100).

Changes in head position with respect to gravity may alter the direction and magnitude of peripheral spontaneous nystagmus. A patient tested 4 weeks after the onset of an acute left-sided labyrinthitis did not have nystagmus with eyes open, but with eyes closed he developed a right-beating spontaneous nystagmus in the sitting position (Fig. 6–5). In the supine position, the nystagmus increased in frequency and amplitude, beating down and to the right. The right lateral position (affected ear up) accentuated the vertical component, and the left lateral position (affected ear down)

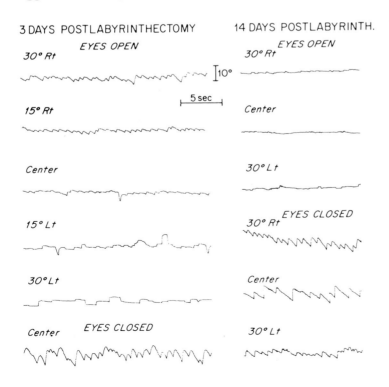

Figure 6–4. Peripheral spontaneous nystagmus (bitemporal horizontal recording) taken 3 days and 14 days after the patient underwent a left labyrinthectomy. Nystagmus with eyes open disappears by 14 days, but nystagmus with eyes closed remains prominent.

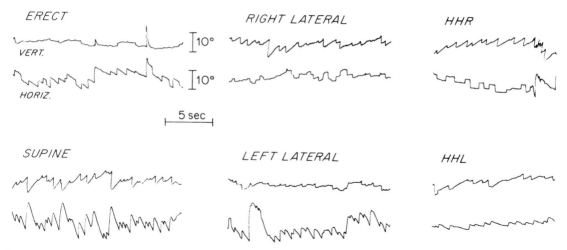

Figure 6–5. Effect of changes in position on spontaneous peripheral nystagmus. Vertical component is accentuated in the right lateral position (affected ear up), and horizontal component is accentuated in the left lateral position (affected ear down). All recordings (bitemporal horizontal and monocular vertical) are with eyes closed.

increased the horizontal component. The head-hanging positions had similar effects. This pattern of positional change with peripheral spontaneous nystagmus frequently occurs after an acute unilateral vestibulopathy and can be explained on the basis of otolith-canal interaction on the remaining intact side[32] (see Interactions of Semicircular Canal and Otolith-Induced Eye Movements, Chapter 3). The effects of positional change on long-standing spontaneous nystagmus of peripheral

and central origin are less predictable, however, and one cannot consistently identify the abnormal side on the basis of positional information alone.

ENG recordings can help differentiate congenital and central varieties of spontaneous nystagmus from peripheral varieties. The downbeat nystagmus shown in Figure 6–6a increases in frequency and amplitude with downward gaze, but it reversed direction with upward gaze. Loss of fixation did not change the nystagmus fre-

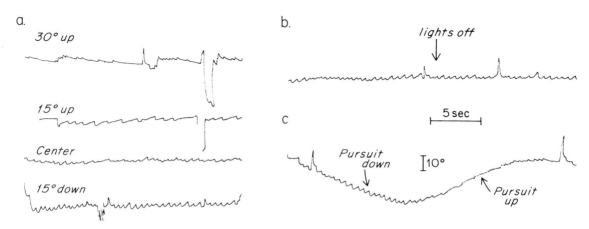

Figure 6–6. Spontaneous downbeat nystagmus (monocular vertical recordings). (a) Nystagmus increased on downward gaze and changed direction on upward gaze. (b) Loss of fixation had little effect. (c) Nystagmus was superimposed on attempted vertical pursuit.

a.

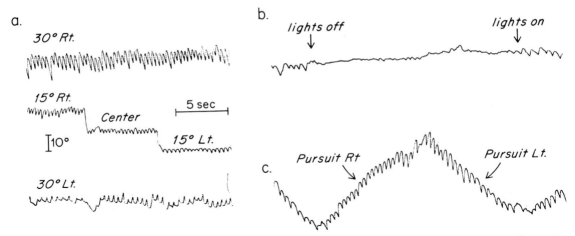

b.

c.

Figure 6—7. Congenital nystagmus (bitemporal horizontal recordings). (*a*) Waveform changed in different gaze positions. (*b*) Nystagmus decreased with loss of fixation. (*c*) Nystagmus was superimposed on attempted horizontal pursuit.

quency or amplitude (Fig. 6—6*b*). The spontaneous vertical nystagmus was superimposed on attempted vertical pursuit (Fig. 6—6*c*).[3] The waveform of the congenital nystagmus illustrated in Figure 6—7*a* changed in different horizontal gaze positions (from pendular to near sawtooth).[68] When fixation is inhibited by darkness, the nystagmus almost disappeared (Fig. 6—7*b*). Horizontal smooth pursuit was markedly impaired in both directions (Fig. 6—7*c*). By comparison, peripheral spontaneous nystagmus does not change direction with change in gaze position, increases with loss of fixation, and usually does not impair smooth pursuit. The slow component with acquired spontaneous nystagmus is typically linear, producing a sawtooth pattern, whereas the slow com-

ponent with congenital nystagmus is usually exponentially increasing.[27]

Gaze-Evoked Nystagmus

The most common type of gaze-evoked nystagmus (drug-induced) is small in amplitude, so it is readily seen on neurologic examination but difficult to record with ENG. A large-amplitude asymmetric gaze-evoked nystagmus is often seen with lesions of the CP angle (so-called Bruns' nystagmus).[5] The lesion is usually on the side of the larger-amplitude nystagmus. Rebound gaze-evoked nystagmus decays as the lateral gaze position is held (Fig. 6—8, *upper trace*) and recurs transiently after returning to the primary position with fast

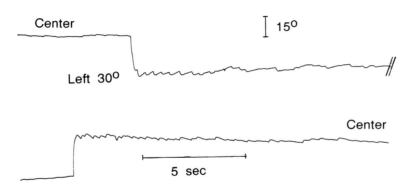

Figure 6—8. Rebound nystagmus (horizontal bitemporal recording). Nystagmus decays as the lateral gaze position is held and recurs on return to the primary position. The reverse occurred with gaze to the right.

components in the direction of the return saccade (Fig. 6—8, *lower trace*).[38]

Positional Nystagmus

Although benign positional nystagmus can be readily identified on routine physical examination, recording the nystagmus documents its stereotyped profile (Fig. 6—9). For this reason, we include rapid positional testing as part of our ENG examination; the technician also observes the nystagmus while it is being recorded. Although ENG does not record the torsional component of the nystagmus, there is nearly always a large vertical component (upbeat) and a smaller horizontal component (beating away from the down ear).[11] The vertical component is larger in the eye uppermost after the head-hanging position has been achieved. The nystagmus in the undermost eye is more torsional;

smaller vertical and horizontal components are recorded (see Chapter 10, for explanation of nystagmus profile).

As suggested earlier, static positional nystagmus is a common finding on ENG when recordings are made with eyes closed or with eyes open in darkness. When the average slow phase velocity exceeds 4 deg/sec, it is abnormal but nonlocalizing; both direction-fixed and direction-changing static positional nystagmus occur with peripheral and central vestibular lesions.[46] Lack of suppression with fixation indicates a central lesion.

THE BITHERMAL CALORIC TEST

Mechanism of Stimulation

The caloric test uses a nonphysiologic stimulus (water or air) to induce endolym-

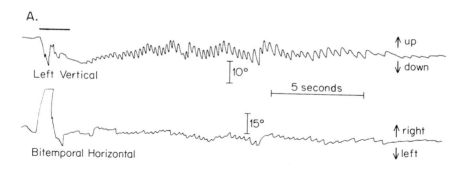

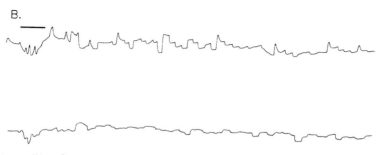

Figure 6—9. Benign positional nystagmus induced in the head-hanging-right position (vertical monocular and horizontal bitemporal recording). (*A*) Sitting to head hanging. (*B*) Head hanging to sitting. *Solid bar* indicates duration of rapid positioning maneuver. (From Baloh, RW, et al: Benign positional vertigo: Clinical and oculographic features in 240 cases. Neurology 37:371, 1987, with permission.)

phatic flow in the semicircular canals by creating a temperature gradient from one side of the canal to the other (Fig. 6–10).[50, 55] Irrigation of the external auditory canal with water or air that is below or above body temperature transfers a temperature gradient from the external auditory canal to the inner ear by conduction. The horizontal semicircular canal develops the largest temperature gradient because it lies closest to the source of temperature change. Because the vertical canals are relatively remote from the external ear, caloric stimulation of the vertical canals is unreliable. The endolymph circulates because of the difference in its specific gravity on the two sides of the canal when the semicircular canal being investigated is in the vertical plane. Caloric testing of horizontal semicircular canal function is usually performed with the patient in the supine position, head tilted 30 degrees up (placing the horizontal semicircular canals in the vertical plane—see Fig. 2–6). With the warm caloric stimulus illustrated in Figure 6–10, the column of endolymph nearest the middle ear rises because of its decreased density. This causes the cupula to deviate toward the utricle (ampullopetal flow) and

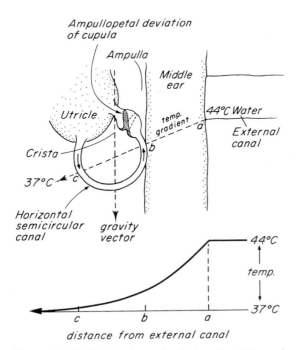

Figure 6–10. Mechanism of caloric stimulation of the horizontal semicircular canal (see text for details).

produces horizontal nystagmus with the fast component directed toward the stimulated ear. A cold stimulus produces the opposite effect on the endolymph column, causing ampullofugal endolymph flow and nystagmus directed away from the stimulated ear (COWS—cold opposite, warm same). If the same test is repeated with the patient lying on the abdomen, so that the horizontal canal is reversed in the vertical plane (i.e., the direction of the gravity vector with relation to the head is reversed), the direction of nystagmus induced by warm and cold stimulation is reversed.[21]

Robert Bárány received the Nobel Prize for proposing the above described mechanism of caloric stimulation. There probably are others. Monkeys who have had their horizontal semicircular canals blocked with paraffin still have caloric-induced nystagmus, although lesser in magnitude than prior to surgery.[51] Presumably, the spontaneous afferent nerve activity increases and decreases due to heating and cooling of the afferent nerve, respectively. Consistent with this interpretation, the caloric-induced nystagmus in canal-blocked animals does not reverse direction when the gravity vector is reversed.[51] This mechanism could also explain the unexpected finding of caloric-induced nystagmus in space, outside of earth's gravity.[54] Other mechanisms, including differential pressure effects from the temperature gradient and central otolith-canal interactions, have also been proposed to account for caloric responses in space.[53] From a clinical point of view, however, gravity is the main driving force for the caloric response. The response can be effectively shut off (in instances in which the patient becomes extremely uncomfortable) simply by positioning the head so that the horizontal canals are horizontal (i.e., approximately 30 degrees tilted downward while sitting).[21]

The caloric test is the most widely used clinical test of the vestibulo-ocular reflex for two major reasons: (1), each labyrinth can be stimulated individually, and (2), the stimulus is easy to apply without requiring complex equipment. Several limitations of the test must be appreciated if one is to assess the results properly, however. The slow component velocity and duration of caloric-induced nystagmus are dependent not only on the relationship between the temperature gradient vector and the gravity vector but also on the blood flow to the skin, length of transmission pathway from the tympanic membrane to the horizontal canal, and heat conductivity of the temporal bone.[1, 53, 70] If local blood flow to the skin is decreased (from vasoconstriction due to pain or to anxiety), the maximum slow component velocity of the response decreases (from decreased heat conductivity through skin), but its duration is prolonged (from delayed heat transfer). Patients with infection or fluid in the middle ear and mastoid air cells may have an increased caloric response (increased maximum slow component velocity) because of the increased heat conductivity from the external ear to the inner ear. Similarly, patients who have undergone mastoid surgery and reconstruction of their middle ear may have increased responses due to a shortening of the conduction pathway. A thickened temporal bone, on the other hand, would produce the opposite effect, because of decreased bone heat conductivity. Some of these factors no doubt underlie the large variability of caloric responses measured in normal subjects and explain the occasional unexpected increase or decrease in caloric response found in patients with temporal bone disease.

Test Methodology

With the bithermal caloric test introduced by Fitzgerald and Hallpike,[30] each ear is irrigated for a fixed duration (30 to 40 seconds) with a constant flow rate of water that is 7 degrees below body temperature (30°C) and 7 degrees above body temperature (44°C). One must wait a minimum of 5 minutes from the end of one response to the next stimulus to avoid additive effects. The major advantages of this test methodology are (1) both ampullopetal and ampullofugal endolymph flow are serially induced in each horizontal semicircular canal, (2) the caloric stimulus is highly reproducible from patient to patient, and (3) the test is tolerated by most patients. The major limitation is the need for constant temperature baths and plumbing to maintain continuous circulation of water through the infusion hose.

The magnitude of caloric-induced nystagmus is highly dependent on the degree of fixation permitted during the test procedure. Four different fixation conditions have been used for caloric testing: (1) eyes open, fixating; (2) eyes open, Frenzel glasses; (3) eyes open, total darkness; and (4) eyes closed. Without eye movement recording devices, obviously only the first two conditions can be used. Comparison of these four conditions in normal subjects reveals a consistently lower coefficient of variation (standard deviation/mean) for response measurements when the test is performed with eyes open, either behind Frenzel glasses or in total darkness.[4]

When caloric testing is performed with fixation (as initially described by Fitzgerald and Hallpike), two separate systems are being evaluated: the vestibulo-ocular reflex and the smooth pursuit system (see Visual Vestibular Interaction, Chapter 3). Some normal subjects are very good at suppressing caloric-induced nystagmus with fixation,[4] others are not. Patients with impaired smooth pursuit (such as patients with cerebellar atrophy) may show no difference in caloric-induced nystagmus with or without fixation.[61] When measured with fixation the responses in these patients will appear hyperactive when compared with those of subjects with a normal smooth pursuit system. Eye closure and the associated upward deviation of the eyes can lead to suppression of both spontaneous and induced nystagmus.[4] It can also alter the nystagmus waveform, making it more difficult to quantify with ENG. Patients with central nervous system (CNS) lesions often have a horizontal deviation of the eyes on closure, which can also change the waveform of induced nystagmus.[24] To avoid these uncontrollable variables, we recommend that caloric testing be performed with eyes open, preferably in total darkness. For a brief period during the test, fixation can be permitted to evaluate the functional status of the smooth pursuit system.

Normative Data

The response to caloric stimulation can be assessed in several ways. The simplest method is to measure the duration of nystagmus after each infusion, using a stopwatch. Prior to the development of ENG this was the only practical way to quantify the bithermal caloric test. Now, however, it is possible to record multiple response measurements accurately. Figure 6–11 illustrates an ENG recording of a normal caloric response. The subject was supine, head elevated 30 degrees, and eyes open behind Frenzel glasses in a darkened room. Two hundred fifty ml of 44°C water was infused into the left ear during the 40 seconds marked on the figure, resulting in ampullopetal endolymph flow in the left horizontal semicircular canal, producing left-beating horizontal nystagmus. The nystagmus began just before the end of stimulation, reached a peak approximately 60 seconds poststimulus, and then slowly decayed over the next minute. Next to the ENG tracing, nystagmus slow component velocity, slow component amplitude, and frequency are plotted versus time. Each measurement demonstrates beat-to-beat variability, but the velocity of the slow components shows the least variability. Furthermore, a decrease in slow component velocity is the most sensitive indicator of vestibular damage.[13]

As suggested earlier, the absolute magnitude of caloric response depends on several physical factors unique to each subject that are unrelated to actual semicircular canal function. The maximum slow component velocity (MSCV) after a caloric stimulus can be as low as 5 deg/sec and as high as 75 deg/sec and still be within the 95 percent confidence interval for normal subjects.[57] Because of this large intersubject variability, intrasubject measurements have been found to be more useful clinically (Fig. 6–12). The vestibular paresis formula

$$\frac{(R30° + R44°) - (L30° + L44°)}{R30° + R44° + L30° + L44°} \times 100$$

compares the MSCV of right-sided responses with that of left-sided responses, and the directional preponderance formula

$$\frac{(R30° + L44°) - (R44° + L30°)}{R30° + L44° + R44° + L30°} \times 100$$

compares the MSCV of nystagmus to the right with that of nystagmus to the left in the same subject. Dividing by the total response normalizes the measurements to remove the large variability in absolute magnitude of normal caloric responses.

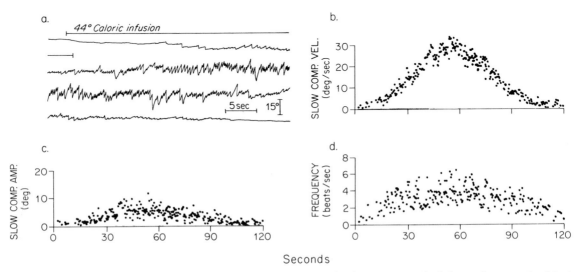

Figure 6–11. Caloric response produced by infusion of 250 ml of 44°C water into the left ear of a normal subject (a). Bitemporal ENG recording. *Horizontal bar* indicates duration of infusion. Plots of slow component velocity (b), slow component amplitude (c) and frequency (d) versus time generated by a digital computer.

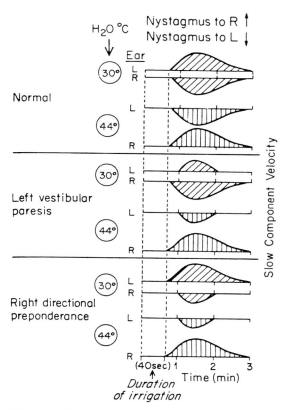

Figure 6–12. Normal and two common patterns of abnormal response to bithermal caloric testing. With a vestibular paresis, the responses to cold (30°C) and warm (44°C) water are decreased on the same side. With a directional preponderance the responses to warm water on one side and cold on the opposite side are decreased.

A caloric fixation suppression index is obtained by having the patient fixate on a target during the middle of the response. Because the slow component velocity of caloric-induced nystagmus is constantly changing, it is important that the fixation period occurs near the time of maximum response to obtain the best estimate of fixation suppression. The fixation suppression index is defined as (MSCV with fixation $\div$ MSCV without fixation) $\times$ 100. With each of these formulas, the result is reported as a percentage of the total response.

In our laboratory, a vestibular paresis is defined as greater than 25 percent asymmetry between left- and right-sided responses, and a directional preponderance as greater than 30 percent asymmetry between left- and right-beating nystagmus, and a fixation suppression index greater than 70 percent is abnormal. These values are comparable to those reported by other investigators, but it must be emphasized that each laboratory should establish its own normal range because of the many methodologic variables discussed earlier.

Results in Patients

Table 6–2 summarizes the abnormalities found in caloric testing, their meaning in terms of location of lesion, and the mechanism by which each abnormality is produced.

PERIPHERAL LESIONS

The finding of a significant vestibular paresis with bithermal caloric stimulation suggests damage to the peripheral vestibular system that can be located anywhere from the end-organ to the vestibular nerve root entry zone in the brainstem. It is almost certainly a sign of unilateral peripheral vestibular disease if there are no associated brainstem signs. Animal studies

Table 6–2. INTERPRETING THE RESULTS OF BITHERMAL CALORIC TESTING

	Location of Lesion	Mechanism
Vestibular paresis	Labyrinth, 8th nerve	Decreased peripheral sensitivity
Directional preponderance	Not localizing	Tonic bias in vestibular system
Hyperactive responses	Cerebellum	Loss of inhibitory influence on vestibular nuclei
Dysrhythmia	Cerebellum	Loss of inhibitory influence on pontine nuclei
Impaired fixation suppression	CNS pursuit pathways	Interruption of visual signals on way to oculomotor neurons
Perverted nystagmus	4th ventricular region	Disruption of vestibular commissural fibers

support this clinical impression. Uemura and Cohen[63] studied caloric responses after various focal lesions in and around the vestibular nuclear complex in monkeys and found that a vestibular paresis occurred only with lesions involving the eighth nerve root entry zone. Focal lesions in different vestibular nuclei did not produce a vestibular paresis. A directional preponderance on caloric testing occurs with peripheral end-organ and eighth nerve lesions and with CNS lesions (from brainstem to cortex).[13] It indicates an imbalance in the vestibular system and is usually associated with spontaneous nystagmus; the velocity of the slow components of the spontaneous nystagmus adds to that of the caloric-induced nystagmus in the same direction and subtracts from that of the caloric-induced nystagmus in the opposite direction.[22] Occasionally, a directional preponderance will occur in patients without spontaneous nystagmus; in this case a central lesion is more likely.

The need to distinguish between end-organ and eighth nerve lesions is a common clinical problem. Partial lesions of the eighth nerve should not, in theory, affect the duration of induced nystagmus, inasmuch as it is related to the time course of cupular deflection and not to the ability of the nerve fibers to transmit action potentials. On the other hand, end-organ lesions involving the cupula and hair cells should affect both the MSCV and duration of the responses. Unfortunately, this turns out not to be a reliable way of differentiating end-organ from eighth nerve lesions. Lesions involving the eighth nerve can reduce the duration of nystagmus, whereas end-organ lesions (particularly in the early stages) frequently result only in decreased MSCV (the duration of response remains unaffected). The magnitude of loss is of some help in differentiating nerve from end-organ lesions. A complete or nearly complete unilateral paralysis is more commonly associated with nerve lesions than with labyrinthine lesions.

The vestibular paresis and directional preponderance formulas are of little use in evaluating patients with bilateral peripheral vestibular lesions, inasmuch as caloric responses are symmetrically depressed. Because of the wide range of normal values

for MSCV, the patient's value may decrease severalfold before falling below the normal range. Serial measurements in the same patient are needed if one hopes to identify early bilateral vestibular impairment such as that produced by ototoxic drugs.

CENTRAL LESIONS

As suggested earlier, patients with CNS lesions may exhibit a vestibular paresis on caloric testing if the lesion involves the root entry zone of the vestibular nerve. The most common neurologic disorders associated with this finding are multiple sclerosis, lateral brainstem infarction, and infiltrating gliomas. Each disease produces other brainstem signs so that the finding of a vestibular paresis is not likely to be misinterpreted as a sign of a peripheral vestibular disorder. In rare cases, a massive brainstem infarction or diffusely infiltrating glioma leads to bilateral decreased caloric responses.

Lesions of the cerebellum can lead to increased caloric responses, possibly because of loss of the normal inhibitory influence of the cerebellum on the vestibular nuclei. Because of the wide range of normal caloric responses, however, it is unusual for any of the responses to exceed the upper normal range. Patients with the cerebellar atrophy syndromes demonstrate a wide range of caloric responses.[9] Those with Friedreich's ataxia often have bilaterally decreased responses because of associated atrophy of the vestibular nerve and ganglia, whereas those with olivopontocerebellar atrophy have decreased, normal, or even increased responses, depending on which areas of the medulla and pons are involved. Increased caloric responses, when they do occur, are usually found in patients with clinically pure cerebellar atrophy.

An abnormal fixation suppression index on caloric testing typically occurs with lesions involving the smooth pursuit system (from the parietal-occipital cortex to the pons and cerebellum).[61] Lesions of the midline cerebellum produce the most profound impairment of fixation suppression. When asymmetric, pursuit deficits in one direction correlate with suppression deficits in the opposite direction.[16]

Dysrhythmia refers to a marked beat-to-beat variability in caloric-induced nystagmus amplitude without any change in the slow component velocity profile. The cerebellum is important for controlling the amplitude of nystagmus fast components, and loss of this control with cerebellar lesions may lead to a disorganized nystagmus pattern. Unfortunately, from a diagnostic point of view, caloric dysrhythmia also occurs in normal subjects when they are tired and inattentive. As will be shown in the next chapter, rotatory stimuli are better suited than caloric stimuli for examining the pattern of induced nystagmus.

Vertical or oblique nystagmus produced by caloric stimulation of the horizontal semicircular canals is called perverted nystagmus. Normal subjects commonly exhibit a small vertical component on ENG recordings of caloric-induced nystagmus, but vertical components larger than the horizontal components are clearly abnormal.[29] Perverted nystagmus with caloric stimulation has been reported with both peripheral and central lesions, the latter usually in the region of the floor of the fourth ventricle (near the vestibular nuclei).[33, 49] Uemura and Cohen[63] found perverted caloric nystagmus in rhesus monkeys after producing unilateral focal lesions in the rostral/medial vestibular nucleus. Warm caloric stimulation on the intact side produced downward nystagmus, and cold stimulation produced upward diagonal nystagmus. The investigators attributed their findings to a disturbance of the commissural fibers between the vestibular nuclei.

TESTS OF VISUAL-OCULAR CONTROL

The central vestibulo-ocular connections are highly integrated with the visual-ocular stabilizing pathways, and both systems share the final common pathway of the oculomotor neurons (see Comparison of Vestibular and Visual Induced Eye Movements, Chapter 3). If the efferent limb of the vestibulo-ocular reflex arc is damaged, visually controlled eye movements are also abnormal; but if the afferent limb of the reflex is damaged, visually controlled eye movements are usually normal. Because ENG techniques used for quantifying the vestibulo-ocular reflex can also be used to quantify visually controlled eye movements, an important "bonus" of information is obtained with little increased effort. Table 6–3 summarizes the types of saccade, smooth pursuit, and optokinetic abnormalities commonly associated with focal lesions of the nervous system.

Saccadic Eye Movements

METHODS OF TESTING AND RESULTS IN NORMAL SUBJECTS

One can induce saccadic eye movements with a series of dots or lights separated by known angular degrees, or with a dot of light generated on a screen and moved through a series of stepwise jumps of different amplitudes. The ENG recording in Figure 6–13, *top*, illustrates the high speed and accuracy of saccadic eye move-

Table 6–3. SUMMARY OF VISUAL OCULAR CONTROL ABNORMALITIES PRODUCED BY FOCAL NEUROLOGIC LESIONS

Location of Lesion	Saccades	Smooth Pursuit and OKN Slow Phase
Cerebellopontine (CP) angle	Ipsilateral dysmetria*	Progressive ipsilateral impairment
Diffuse cerebellar	Bilateral dysmetria	Bilateral impairment
Intrinsic brainstem	Marked slowing, increased delay time	Ipsilateral or contralateral impairment
Basal ganglia	Mild slowing, hypometria,† increased delay time	Bilateral impairment
Frontoparietal cortex	Difficulty inhibiting reflex saccades	Ipsilateral impairment

*Under and overshoots.
†Undershoots only.

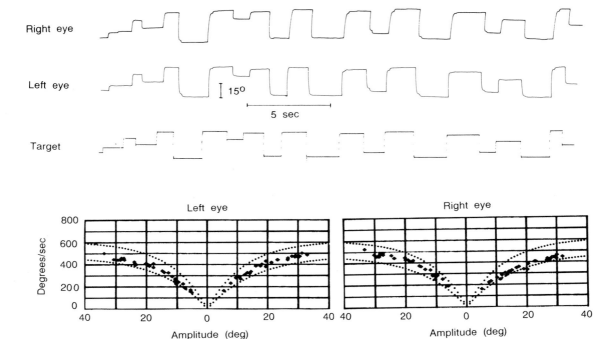

Figure 6—13. Saccadic eye movements induced in a normal subject by a target moving in steps of random amplitude (3–36 degrees) and changing intervals between jumps (0.5 to 2.5 seconds). (*Upper*) monocular horizontal ENG recordings. (*Lower*) computer generated plots of peak velocity versus amplitude for entire sequence (*dotted lines* represent normal mean ± 1 standard deviation).

ments induced in a normal subject by a target moving in steps of random amplitude. Normal subjects consistently undershoot the target for jumps larger than 20 degrees, requiring a small corrective saccade to achieve the final position. Overshoots of the target are rare. A characteristic delay time of approximately 200 milliseconds occurs between each target jump and induced saccade.

Computer algorithms have been developed to rapidly quantify these saccade parameters.[10] Saccades are easily identified based on their characteristic velocity profile. The relationship between peak velocity and amplitude (the so-called main sequence) is nonlinear, with decreasing peak velocities at higher amplitudes (Fig. 6–13, *bottom*). For example, the average peak velocity for a 15-degree saccade is 400 deg/sec, whereas that for a 30-degree saccade is 550 deg/sec. Saccade accuracy is defined as the ratio of the saccade amplitude divided by the target displacement amplitude times 100. The mean saccade accuracy for normal subjects on the random

saccade test is 88 percent. Overshooting of the target rarely occurs in normal subjects. The mean delay time on the same test is 186 seconds.[17]

RESULTS IN PATIENTS

Slowing of saccadic eye movements can occur with lesions anywhere in the diffuse central pathways involved in generating saccades. The most pronounced slowing occurs with lesions of the pretectal and paramedian pontine gaze centers, the oculomotor neurons, and the extraocular muscles. Lesions involving these pathways impair both voluntary and involuntary saccades. Damage to the oculomotor neurons, oculomotor nerves, and extraocular muscles cause a slowing of saccades when the paretic muscle is the agonist required to generate the sudden force necessary to move the globe rapidly. Saccade slowing identified on ENG examination can occur before clinical examination reveals the presence of strabismus.[48, 58] ENG has been particularly helpful for identifying early lesions of the medial longitudinal fasciculus (MLF), manifested by slowing of adducting saccades made by the medial rectus on the side of the lesion (Fig. 6–14).[25, 47] A characteristic saccade abnormality is seen with myasthenia gravis. Saccades begin with normal velocity, but within a short time the transmitters at the myoneural junction are depleted, and the remainder of the saccade is markedly slow.[67] In some patients with severe oculomotor dysfunction, only brief bursts of oculomotor firing are possible before a complete block occurs. This results in the unusual situation in which a patient with almost complete absence of sustained eye movements can have small-amplitude, high-velocity saccades followed by a quick return to the primary position (so-called ocular quiver). These saccade abnormalities are usually rapidly reversed with intravenous Tensilon.[2]

Reversible saccade slowing is produced by fatigue and by ingestion of alcohol or tranquilizers.[12, 35, 65] This results from impaired synaptic transmission through the multineuronal networks needed to generate the high-frequency firing for horizontal and vertical saccades. Patients with Huntington's disease and progressive supranuclear palsy develop slowing of saccades apparently due to diffuse degeneration of supranuclear pathways.[45, 62] Focal disease of the pretectum or paramedian pontine reticular formation produces selective slowing of vertical and horizontal saccades, respectively.[6, 7] Lesions of one paramedian pontine center produce ipsilateral saccade slowing. The pretectal centers for upward and downward saccades are separate (downward ventral dorsal to the upward center) but are so close together that lesions usually involve both. Destruction of the pretectal and pontine supranuclear saccade centers results in complete absence of saccadic eye movements (voluntary and involuntary). Patients with such a dysfunction produce only a slow tonic deviation of the eyes with vestibular or optokinetic stimuli because of the absence of fast components (see Fig. 7–6c).[7]

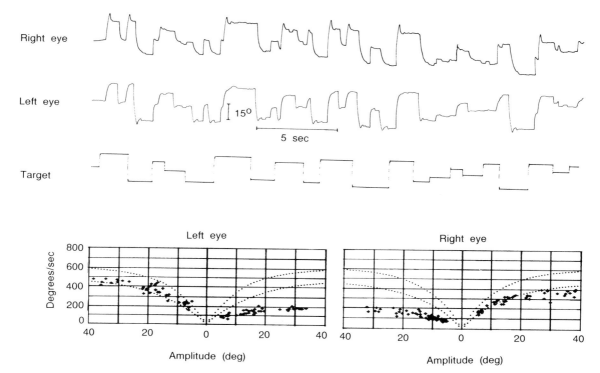

Figure 6–14. Saccadic eye movements in a patient with a bilateral MLF lesion caused by multiple sclerosis. Recordings as in Figure 6–13. Adducting saccades are markedly slow; abducting saccades have normal velocity but overshoot the target.

Impaired saccade accuracy is most commonly seen with cerebellar disorders.[9, 72] Overshooting of the target (saccade overshoot dysmetria) is most apparent, inasmuch as overshoots rarely occur in normal subjects. The velocity of these inaccurate saccades is normal unless the brainstem is also involved. Of the cerebellar atrophy syndromes, saccade dysmetria is most prominent with Friedreich's ataxia.[34] Monocular overshoots in the abducting eye are characteristic of MLF lesions (see Fig. 6–14). Disorders of the cortical and subcortical supranuclear centers also affect the accuracy of saccades.[26, 64] Patients with Parkinson's disease exhibit delayed saccade reaction time and hypometria of voluntary saccades. Complete removal of one hemisphere or the presence of a large frontal parietal lesion results in hypometria of horizontal saccades made in the contralateral direction.[56] Vertical saccades are unaffected. Animals with lesions of the frontal eye fields may have normal-appearing saccade metrics but have difficulty inhibiting reflex saccades.[28] Patients with lesions of the frontal cortex and basal ganglia have similar difficulties.[36, 43] This can be demonstrated with the so-called antisaccade test, whereby a fixation target is illuminated in the periphery and the patient is instructed to make a saccade in the exact opposite direction. Normal subjects can reliably perform this task, but patients with lesions involving cortical and subcortical presaccade structures often make unwanted saccades to the fixation target before refixating in the desired location.

Patients with acquired and congenital oculomotor apraxia[73] and ataxia telangiectasia[14] exhibit prolonged reaction time for the initiation of voluntary saccades and use a series of hypometric saccades to produce refixations. Nystagmus fast components (involuntary saccades) are also abnormal, such that the eyes deviate in the direction of the slow component rather than in the direction of the fast component. To compensate for impaired voluntary saccades these patients often use head thrusts to perform refixation. Because their vestibulo-ocular reflex is intact, the head thrusts produce controversive deviation of the eyes, necessitating an overshoot of the head thrusts in order to obtain fixation. Fixation is then maintained as the head is slowly returned on line with the target. The site of the anatomic defect that produces these abnormalities in voluntary saccades is unknown.

Smooth Pursuit

METHODS OF TESTING AND
RESULTS IN NORMAL SUBJECTS

The examining physician can test smooth pursuit eye movements by slowly moving his finger or a pencil back and forth and asking the patient to follow it as well as possible. The target should be moved as smoothly as possible and the movement should not be too fast (about ½ cycle/sec is an ideal rate). A more exact relationship between the velocity of the target and the eye is determined by using precise targets and ENG. A pendulum hanging from the ceiling or a metronome provides an inexpensive reproducible sinusoidally moving target. Precise control of the target can be achieved over a series of velocities by projecting a dot onto a screen with a motor-controlled device. Figure 6–15b illustrates a polygraph recording of horizontal smooth pursuit in a normal subject as he follows a sinusoidally moving dot on a white screen (0.3 Hz, maximum amplitude 18 degrees). The accuracy of smooth pursuit is quantified by repeatedly sampling eye and target velocity and plotting the two velocities against each other (see Fig. 6–15d). A computer algorithm makes the comparison between eye and target velocity after saccade waveforms have been removed.[10] The slope of this eye-target velocity relationship (in this case, 0.95) represents the gain of the smooth pursuit system. The mean gain determined from similar plots in 25 normal young subjects was 0.95 ± 0.07. Elderly normal subjects (more than 70 years of age) show marked variability in pursuit ability, and therefore pursuit testing must be interpreted with caution in elderly patients.[59, 69] Also, smooth pursuit gain decreases both with increasing frequency and increasing velocity of the target. Each

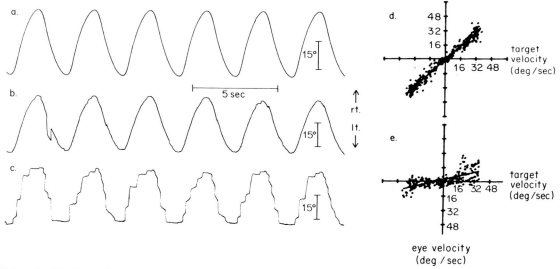

Figure 6–15. Smooth pursuit of a target (*a*) moving with a sinusoidal waveform in a normal subject (*b*) and a patient with cerebellar atrophy (*c*). Bitemporal horizontal recording. In *d* and *e* eye velocity is plotted against target velocity (both sampled 10 times per second) after saccades have been removed for the normal subject and patient, respectively.

laboratory must establish normative data for their standard test protocol.

RESULTS IN PATIENTS

Patients with impaired smooth pursuit require frequent corrective saccades to keep up with the target, producing so-called cogwheel or saccadic pursuit (see Fig. 6–15c). As expected, the gain (given by the slope of the eye velocity–target velocity plot) of the smooth pursuit system is markedly decreased in such patients (see Fig. 6–15e). It must be emphasized, however, that normal subjects may intermix saccades with smooth pursuit movements, particularly if they are inattentive or fatigued, or if the target velocity exceeds the limit of their smooth pursuit system.[40] Therefore, quantitative analysis of intersaccadic eye velocity is a more reliable way of assessing the accuracy of smooth pursuit than simply observing the frequency of superimposed saccades.

Abnormalities of smooth pursuit are of limited localizing value, inasmuch as they occur with disorders throughout the CNS. Acute lesions of the peripheral labyrinth or vestibular nerve transiently impair smooth pursuit contralateral to the lesion when the eyes are moving against the slow component of spontaneous nystagmus.[8] This asymmetry in smooth pursuit disappears within a few weeks despite the continued presence of spontaneous nystagmus in darkness. Just as they affect saccadic eye movements, tranquilizing drugs, alcohol, and fatigue also impair smooth pursuit eye movements.[37, 52] Rashbass[52] found that barbiturates impaired smooth pursuit before affecting saccadic eye movements, suggesting an increased sensitivity of the smooth pursuit system. Patients with diffuse cortical disease[31] (degenerative or vascular), basal ganglia disease[26, 45] (Parkinson's and Huntington's disease), and diffuse cerebellar disease[9, 72] consistently have bilaterally impaired smooth pursuit eye movements. Focal disease of one cerebellar hemisphere or one side of the brainstem usually produces ipsilateral impairment of smooth pursuit, although large cerebellar pontine angle tumors are frequently associated with bilaterally impaired smooth pursuit.[5] Focal cortical lesions in the parieto-occipital region impair ipsilateral smooth pursuit (Fig. 6–16a).[16, 44]

A

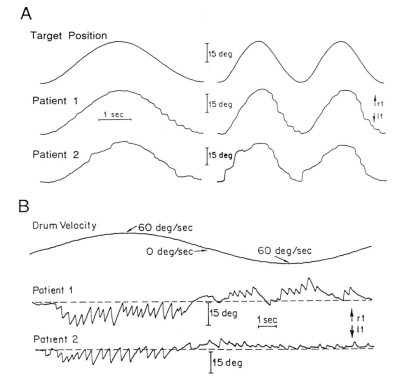

B

Figure 6–16. Horizontal smooth pursuit (*A*) and optokinetic nystagmus (*B*) from two patients with left parietal lobe lesions.[16] In *A* the patients tracked a laser dot moving in a sinusoidal fashion (*left*: 0.2 Hz, peak velocity 22.5 degrees/second; *right*: 0.4 Hz, peak velocity 45 degrees/second). In *B* a surrounding optokinetic drum moved in a sinusoidal pattern (0.05 Hz, peak velocity 60 degrees/sec). Right monocular recordings. Pursuit and OKN slow phases to the left were markedly impaired.

Optokinetic Nystagmus

METHODS OF TESTING AND RESULTS IN NORMAL SUBJECTS

The simplest optokinetic stimulus is a striped cloth that can be moved across the patient's visual field in each direction. While the patient stares at the cloth, the amplitude of induced nystagmus in each direction is compared. This type of test permits identification of absent or markedly asymmetric optokinetic nystagmus (OKN). The test sensitivity is improved by using an optokinetic stimulus of known velocity and ENG recording of the induced nystagmus. Figure 6–17 shows such a recording of OKN induced by a striped drum completely surrounding a subject and moving at a constant velocity of 30 deg/sec. At the arrow, the lights were turned off and optokinetic-after-nystagmus (OKAN) was recorded. A plot of slow component velocity is provided beneath the tracing. Typically, the OKN slow component velocity approaches that of the drum velocity as long as the drum velocity does not exceed 30 to 40 deg/sec. As with smooth pursuit gain, the gain of OKN (slow component velocity/drum velocity) drops off with increasing frequency and drum velocities in normal subjects (Fig. 6–18).[15] OKAN velocity is more variable than OKN velocity even in young normal subjects. There is a rapid exponential drop-off followed by a gradual decay as shown in Figure 6–17. The mean OKAN slow component velocity (after the initial rapid drop-off) and the mean OKAN duration in 20 normal subjects after 1 minute of 30 deg/sec optokinetic stimulation was 6.3 deg/sec ± 4.5 deg/sec and 23.75 seconds ± 23.1 seconds, respectively.[71]

RESULTS IN PATIENTS

As a general rule, abnormalities of optokinetic slow components parallel abnormalities in smooth pursuit and abnormalities of fast components correlate with abnormalities of voluntary saccades.[15] Symmetrically decreased slow component

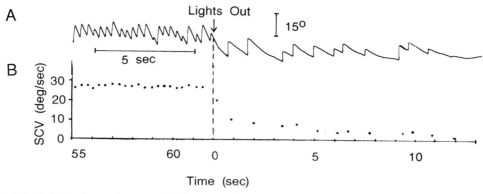

Figure 6–17. Optokinetic nystagmus (OKN) induced by a surrounding striped drum moving at a constant velocity of 30 degrees/sec. At the *arrow* the lights were turned off, and optokinetic after nystagmus (OKAN) was recorded. (*A*) Bitemporal ENG recording. (*B*) Plot of slow phase velocity versus time.

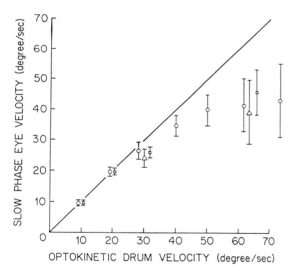

Figure 6–18. Normal mean ± 1 standard deviation for horizontal OKN slow phase velocity at different drum velocities. ○, ramp acceleration from 0 to 70 deg/sec in 1 minute; □, constant velocity for 30 seconds; △, sinusoidal (0.05 Hz.). (From Baloh et al,[15] with permission.)

velocity is produced by diffuse disease of the cortex, diencephalon, brainstem, and cerebellum.[9, 31, 45, 64, 72] As with smooth pursuit, focal lateralized disease of the parietal occipital region, brainstem, and cerebellum result in impaired optokinetic nystagmus when the stimulus moves toward the damaged side (see Fig. 6–16b).[16, 44] Lesions of the occipital lobe, although associated with a hemianoptic visual field defect, are not associated with impaired smooth pursuit or optokinetic nystagmus, presumably because each parietal lobe receives oculomotor signals from each occipital lobe. Some patients with severely impaired smooth pursuit exhibit a gradual buildup in OKN slow component velocity (Fig. 6–19).[66] This is a feature of OKN normally seen in afoveate animals that have only a subcortical OKN system (see Optokinetic Nystagmus, Chapter 3). Presumably, in normal humans the cortical pursuit system dominates the subcortical OKN system, so normal OKN exhibits features of normal pursuit. When the cortical pursuit system is lesioned, however, the remaining OKN may exhibit features of the subcortical system.

Patients who are unable to produce saccadic eye movements produce only a slow tonic deviation of the eyes in the direction of an optokinetic stimulus. Although patients with slow saccades produce optokinetic nystagmus, the waveform is rounded, and the amplitude and slow component velocity are decreased. The delayed ending of the impaired fast component subtracts from the initial part of the slow component in the opposite direction. The many causes of saccade slowing were outlined in detail in the previous section.

Abnormalities of OKAN are typically seen with peripheral vestibular lesions.[42] Unilateral lesions result in asymmetric OKAN (present only in the direction of the spontaneous nystagmus), whereas bilateral le-

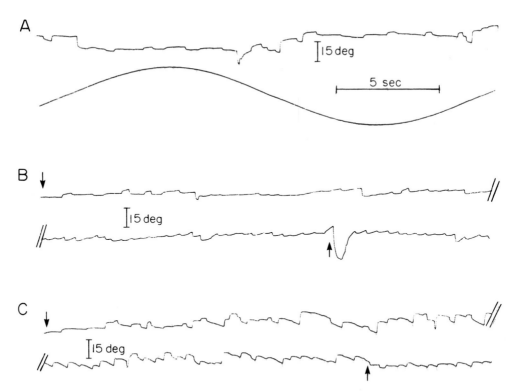

Figure 6–19. Optokinetic nystagmus (OKN) induced by sinusoidal (0.05 Hz, peak velocity 30 deg/sec) (*A*) and constant velocity (30 deg/sec) (clockwise, *B*; counterclockwise, *C*) drum rotation in a patient with midline cerebellar atrophy. In *B* and *C* the *downward arrows* mark the onset of drum rotation and the *upward arrows* indicate when the lights were turned off; 25 seconds elapsed between the *upper* and *lower traces*. Bitemporal horizontal ENG recordings. The patient had minimal response to sinusoidal stimulation (*A*) but exhibited a gradual buildup in OKN and normal OKAN with constant velocity stimulation (*B* and *C*). (From Baloh, RW, et al: Late onset cerebellar atrophy. Brain 109:159, 1986, with permission.)

sions (e.g., due to ototoxic drugs) result in diminished or absent OKAN in both directions.[71]

REFERENCES

1. Baertschi, AJ, Johnson, RN, and Hanna, GR: A theoretical and experimental determination of vestibular dynamics in caloric stimulation. Biol Cybern 20:175, 1975.
2. Baloh, RW and Keesey, JC: Saccade fatigue and response to edrophonium for the diagnosis of myasthenia gravis. Ann NY Acad Sci 274:631, 1976.
3. Baloh, RW and Spooner, JW: Downbeat nystagmus: A type of central vestibular nystagmus. Neurology 31:304, 1981.
4. Baloh, RW, et al: Caloric testing. I. Effect of different conditions of ocular fixation. Ann Otol Rhinol Laryngol (Suppl 43) 86:1, 1977.
5. Baloh, RW, et al: Cerebellar-pontine angle tumors. Results of quantitative vestibulo-ocular testing. Arch Neurol 33:507, 1976.
6. Baloh, RW, Furman, J, and Yee, RD: Dorsal midbrain syndrome: Clinical and oculographic findings. Neurology 35:54, 1985.
7. Baloh, RW, Furman, J, Yee, RD: Eye movements in patients with absent voluntary horizontal gaze. Ann Neurol 17:283, 1985.
8. Baloh, RW, Honrubia, V, and Sills, A: Eye-tracking and optokinetic nystagmus. Results of quantitative testing in patients with well-defined nervous system lesions. Ann Otol Rhinol Laryngol 86:108, 1977.
9. Baloh, RW, Konrad, HR, and Honrubia, V: Vestibulo-ocular function in patients with cerebellar atrophy. Neurology 25:160, 1975.
10. Baloh, RW, Langhofer, L, Honrubia, V, and Yee, RD: On-line analysis of eye movements using a digital computer. Aviat Space Environ Med 51:563, 1980.
11. Baloh, RW, Sakala, SM, and Honrubia, V: Benign

paroxysmal positional nystagmus. Am J Otolaryngol 1:1, 1979.

12. Baloh, RW, Sharma, S, Moskowitz, H, and Griffith, R: The effect of alcohol and marijuana on eye movements. Aviat Space Environ Med 50:18, 1979.

13. Baloh, RW, Sills, AW, and Honrubia, V: Caloric testing. III. Patients with peripheral and central vestibular lesions. Ann Otol Rhinol Laryngol (Suppl. 43) 86:24, 1977.

14. Baloh, RW, Yee, RD, and Boder, E: Ataxia-telangiectasia. Quantitative analysis of eye movements in six cases. Neurology 28:1099, 1978.

15. Baloh, RW, Yee, RD, and Honrubia, V: Clinical abnormalities of optokinetic nystagmus. In Lennerstrand, G, Zee, D (eds): Functional Basis of Ocular Motility Disorders. Pergamon Press, New York, 1982, p 311.

16. Baloh, RW, Yee, RD, and Honrubia, V: Optokinetic nystagmus and parietal lobe lesions. Ann Neurol 7:269, 1980.

17. Baloh, RW and Honrubia, V: Reaction time and accuracy of the saccadic eye movements of normal subjects in a moving-target task. Aviat Space Environ Med 47:1165, 1976.

18. Barber, HO and Stockwell, CW: Manual of electronystagmography. CV Mosby, St Louis, 1976.

19. Barber, HO and Wright, G: Positional nystagmus in normals. Adv Otol Rhinol Laryngol 19: 276, 1973.

20. Barry, W and Melvill Jones, G: Influence of eye lid movement upon electro-oculographic recording of vertical eye movements. Aerospace Med 36:855, 1965.

21. Coats, AC and Smith, SY: Body position and the intensity of caloric nystagmus. Acta Otolaryngol 63:515, 1967.

22. Coats, AC: Directional preponderance and spontaneous nystagmus. Ann Otol Rhinol Laryngol 75:1135, 1966.

23. Coats, AC: Electronystagmography. In Bradford, L (ed): Physiological Measures of the Audio-Vestibular System. Academic Press, New York, 1975.

24. Cogan, DG: Neurologic significance of lateral conjugate deviation of the eyes on forced closure of the lids. Arch Ophthalmol 39:37, 1948.

25. Crane, TB, Yee, RD, Baloh, RW, and Hepler, RS: Analysis of characteristic eye movement abnormalities in internuclear ophthalmoplegia. Arch Ophthalmol 101:206, 1983.

26. Dejong, JD and Melvill Jones, G: Akinesia, hypokinesia and bradykinesia in the oculomotor system of patients with Parkinson's disease. Exp Neurol 32:58, 1971.

27. Dell'Osso, LF and Daroff, RB: Congenital nystagmus waveforms and foveation strategy. Doc Ophthalmol 19:155, 1975.

28. Deng, S-Y, et al: The effect of unilateral ablation of the frontal eye fields of saccadic performance in the monkey. In Keller, EL, Zee, DS (eds): Adaptive Processes in Visual and Oculomotor Systems. Pergamon Press, Oxford, 1986, p 201.

29. Elidan, J, Gay, I, and Lev, S: On the vertical calo-

ric nystagmus. J Otolaryngol 14:287, 1985.

30. Fitzgerald, G and Hallpike, CS: Studies in human vestibular function: I. Observations of the directional preponderance of caloric nystagmus resulting from cerebral lesions. Brain 65:115, 1942.

31. Fletcher, WA and Sharpe, JA: Smooth pursuit dysfunction in Alzheimer's disease. Neurology 38:272, 1988.

32. Fluur, E: Interaction between the utricles and the horizontal semicircular canals. IV. Tilting of human patients with acute unilateral vestibular neuritis. Acta Otolaryngol 76:349, 1973.

33. Fredrickson, JM and Fernández, C: Vestibular disorders in fourth ventricle lesions. Arch Otolaryngol 80:521, 1964.

34. Furman, JM, Perlman, S, and Baloh, RW: Eye movements in Friedreich's ataxia. Arch Neurol 40:343, 1983.

35. Gentles, W and Llewellyn-Thomas, E: Effect of benzodiazepines upon saccadic eye movements in man. Clin Pharmacol Ther 12:563, 1971.

36. Guitton, O, Buchtel, HA, Douglas, RM: Frontal lobe lesions in man cause difficulties in suppressing reflexive glances and in generating goal-directed saccades. Exp Brain Res 58: 455, 1985.

37. Holzman, PS, et al: Smooth-pursuit eye movements, and diazepam, CPZ, and secobarbital. Psychopharmacologia 44:111, 1975.

38. Hood, JD, Kayan, A, and Leech, J: Rebound nystagmus. Brain 96:507, 1973.

39. Kamei, T and Kornhuber, HH: Spontaneous and head shaking nystagmus in normals and in patients with central lesions. Can J Otolaryngol 3:372, 1974.

40. Kaufman, SR and Abel, LA: The effects of distraction on smooth pursuit in normal subjects. Acta Otolaryngol 102:57, 1986.

41. Ktonas, PY, Black, FO, and Smith, JR: Effect of electronic filters on electronystagmographic recordings. Arch Otolaryngol 101:413, 1975.

42. Lafortune, S, Ireland, DJ, Jell, RM, and Duval, L: Human optokinetic after nystagmus. Acta Otolaryngol 101:183, 1986.

43. Lasker, AG, et al: Saccades in Huntington's disease: Initiation defects and distractibility. Neurology 37:364, 1987.

44. Leigh, RJ and Tusa, RJ: Disturbance of smooth pursuit caused by infarction of parieto-occipital cortex. Ann Neurol 17:185, 1985.

45. Leigh, RJ, et al: Abnormal ocular motor control in Huntington's chorea. Neurology 33:1268, 1983.

46. Lin, J, Elidan, J, Baloh, RW, and Honrubia, V: Direction-changing positional nystagmus: Incidence and meaning. Am J Otolaryngol 7:306, 1986.

47. Meienberg, O, Muri, R, and Rabineau, PA: Clinical and oculographic examinations of saccadic eye movements in the diagnosis of multiple sclerosis. Arch Neurol 43:438, 1986.

48. Metz, HS, et al: Ocular saccades in lateral rectus palsy. Arch Ophthalmol 84:453, 1970.

49. Norre, ME: Caloric vertical nystagmus: The verti-

cal semicircular canal in caloric testing. J Otolaryngol 16:1, 1987.
50. O'Neill, G: The caloric stimulus. Temperature generation within the temporal bone. Acta Otolaryngol 103:266, 1987.
51. Paige, G: Caloric vestibular responses despite canal inactivation. Invest Ophthalmol Vis Sci 25 (Suppl):229, 1984.
52. Rashbass, C: The relationship between saccadic and smooth tracking eye movements. J Physiol 159:326, 1961.
53. Scherer, H and Clarke, AH: The caloric vestibular reaction in space. Physiological considerations. Acta Otolaryngol 100:328, 1985.
54. Scherer, H, et al: European vestibular experiments on the spacelab-1 mission: 3. Caloric nystagmus in microgravity. Exp Brain Res 64:255, 1986.
55. Schmaltz, G: The physical phenomena occurring in the semicircular canals during rotatory and thermic stimulation. Proc Roy Soc Med 25:359, 1932.
56. Sharpe, JA, Lo, AW, and Rabinovitch, HE: Control of the saccadic and smooth pursuit systems after cerebral hemidecortication. Brain 102:387, 1979.
57. Sills, AW, Baloh, RW, and Honrubia, V: Caloric testing. II. Results in normal subjects. Ann Otol Rhinol Laryngol 86 (Suppl. 43): 7, 1977.
58. Solingen, LD, et al: Subclinical eye movement disorders in patients with multiple sclerosis. Neurology 27:614, 1977.
59. Spooner, JW, Sakala, SM, and Baloh, RW: Effect of aging on eye tracking. Arch Neurol 37:575, 1980.
60. Stahle, J: Electronystagmography—its value as a diagnostic tool. In Wolfson, RJ (ed): The Vestibular System and Its Diseases. University of Pennsylvania Press, Philadelphia, 1968.
61. Takemori, S: Visual suppression test. Ann Otol Rhinol Laryngol 86:80, 1977.

62. Troost, BT and Daroff, RB: The ocular motor defects in progressive supranuclear palsy. Ann Neurol 2:397, 1977.
63. Uemura, T and Cohen, B: Effects of vestibular nuclei lesions on vestibulo-ocular reflexes and posture in monkeys. Acta Otolaryngol (Suppl) 315:1, 1973.
64. White, OB, Saint-Cyr, JA, Tomlinson, RD, and Sharpe, JA: Ocular motor deficits in Parkinson's disease. II. Control of the saccadic and smooth pursuit systems. Brain 106:925, 1983.
65. Wilkinson, IMS, Kime, R, and Purnell, M: Alcohol and human eye movement. Brain 97:785, 1974.
66. Yee, RD, et al: Slow build-up of optokinetic nystagmus associated with downbeat nystagmus. Invest Ophthalmol Vis Sci 18:622, 1979.
67. Yee, RD, et al: Rapid eye movements in myasthenia gravis. II. Electro-ocular analysis. Arch Ophthalmol 94:1465, 1976.
68. Yee, RD, Wong, EK, Baloh, RW, and Honrubia, V: A study of congenital nystagmus: Waveforms. Neurology 26:326, 1976.
69. Zackon, DH and Sharpe, JA: Smooth pursuit in senescence: Effects of target velocity and acceleration. Acta Otolaryngol 104:290, 1987.
70. Zangemeister, WH and Bock, O: The influence of pneumatization of mastoid bone on caloric nystagmus response. Acta Otolaryngol 88:105, 1979.
71. Zasorin, NL, Baloh, RW, Yee, RD, and Honrubia, V: Influence of vestibulo-ocular reflex gain on human optokinetic responses. Exp Brain Res 51:271, 1983.
72. Zee, DS, et al: Ocular motor abnormalities in hereditary cerebellar ataxia. Brain 99:207, 1976.
73. Zee, DS, Yee, RD, and Singer, HS: Congenital ocular motor apraxia. Brain 100:581, 1977.

Chapter 7

ROTATIONAL AND OTHER NEWER DIAGNOSTIC TESTS

Current quantitative tests of vestibular function concentrate on the horizontal semicircular canal ocular reflex because it is the easiest reflex to stimulate and record. Tests of the other vestibulo-ocular reflexes (vertical semicircular canal and otolith) and of the vestibulospinal reflexes are still in the developmental stage and have yet to be shown useful in the clinical setting.

EOG VERSUS OTHER METHODS FOR RECORDING EYE MOVEMENTS

As indicated in the prior chapter, electro-oculography (EOG) is the simplest and most readily available system for recording eye movements. It is relatively inexpensive, easily administered, noninvasive, does not interfere with vision, and does not require head restraint. Furthermore, it is reasonably accurate even for the large-amplitude horizontal eye movements that are encountered during routine rotational testing. The disadvantages of EOG include the inability to measure vertical eye movements accurately, interference of eye blink artifacts, poor signal-to-noise ratio, and dependence upon lighting conditions in the test room.[35, 57] Table 7–1 compares the characteristics of EOG with three other eye movement recording techniques that are used primarily in the research setting.[25, 39, 63, 70] These other techniques are more sensitive than EOG but at the present time are not practical for routine patient testing. Direct video recording of eye movements is the newest and most promising of these techniques. It uses a video camera that is interfaced with a digital computer. At regular intervals images are stored by the computer for subsequent data analysis. Specialized digital signal processing algorithms are then used to determine horizontal and vertical eye positions. With the rapid advances that are occurring in this area it is reasonable to expect that the technical difficulties will be solved and the costs will decrease in the near future.

ROTATIONAL TESTING OF THE HORIZONTAL SEMICIRCULAR CANAL

Rotational testing of the horizontal semicircular canal offers several advantages over caloric testing. Multiple graded stimuli can be applied in a relatively short period of time, and the testing is usually well tolerated by patients. Unlike caloric testing, a rotational stimulus to the semicircular canals is unrelated to physical features of the external ear or temporal bone, so a more exact relationship between stimulus and response is possible. However, rotational stimuli affect both labyrinths simultaneously, as opposed to the selective stimulation of one labyrinth possible with caloric testing.

According to the pendulum model introduced in Chapter 2 (and expanded in the Appendix), the slow component velocity of rotational-induced nystagmus should be proportional to the deviation of the cupula which, in turn, is proportional to the intensity of stimulation. As will be demon-

Table 7–1. IMPORTANT FEATURES OF DIFFERENT EYE MOVEMENT RECORDING TECHNIQUES

	EOG	IR	SCC	Video
Recording device	Paste-on electrodes	Photovoltaic diodes on glasses	Coil inside contact lens	Video camera
Principle	Corneo-retinal potential	Differential reflection of iris and sclera	Electrical current induced in coil	Digital processing of video image
Range of horizontal eye movement	±40°	±10–15°	Unlimited	Unlimited
Range of vertical eye movement	±30°	± 5–10°	Unlimited	Unlimited
Range of torsional eye movement	—	—	Unlimited	Unlimited
Approximate accuracy	1–2°	0.5°	0.01°	0.5°
Approximate cost (including electronic amplifiers if needed)	$2,000	$8,000	$20,000	$100,000
Ability to record with eyes closed	+	—	+	—
Ability to record during normal vision	+	+	+	+
Ability to record during head movement	+	—	+	+
Susceptibility to eye blink artifacts	+	+	+	+
Sensitivity to changes in room lighting	+	—	—	—
Sensitivity to electrical interference	+	+	+	—
Sensitivity to electromyographic interference	+	—	—	—

Key: EOG = electrooculography; IR = infrared reflection; SCC = scleral search coil; Video = computer analyzed video recordings.

strated in the following sections, this model's applicability to different forms of stimulation is remarkably consistent and provides a rational approach to the evaluation of clinical rotational testing.

Background

Three types of angular acceleration have been used clinically to evaluate the horizontal canal ocular reflex: (1) impulsive, (2) constant, and (3) sinusoidal. Historically, each type of stimulation has been popular at different times for different reasons. In 1907, Bárány[18] introduced an impulsive rotational test in which the chair in which the patient was seated was manually rotated 10 times in 20 seconds and then suddenly stopped with the patient facing the observer. The function of the horizontal semicircular canals was assessed by measuring the duration of visually monitored nystagmus after clockwise and counterclockwise rotation. As indicated earlier,

the results from this qualitative rotational test were variable, primarily because of the imprecise nature of the stimulus. Van Egmond, Groen, and Jongkees[66] attempted to improve the reliability of impulsive rotational testing by slowly bringing the patient to different constant velocities with subliminal acceleration and then suddenly stopping the rotating chair with a brake. They introduced the term *cupulometry* for the plot of the duration of postrotatory turning sensation and nystagmus versus the magnitude of the sudden step change in velocity (see Psychophysical Studies, Chapter 3). For the range of impulses used (up to 60 deg/sec) the duration of postrotatory nystagmus was proportional to the log of the impulse intensity.

As electronystagmography (ENG) techniques became available for recording nystagmus during rotation (per rotatory nystagmus), rotational tests using constant and sinusoidal acceleration became popular in several clinical laboratories. Montandon[50] introduced a constant acceleration test in which the patient was slowly brought to a constant angular velocity (90 deg/sec) and then, after a period of constant speed (3 minutes), slowly decelerated to 0 velocity. The nystagmus threshold was determined (the rate of acceleration and deceleration at which nystagmus was first observed) for a series of different constant accelerations (0.5 to 9 deg/sec^2). In normal subjects this value was approximately 1 deg/sec^2 whereas in patients with vestibular disease, values of 6 to 7 deg/sec^2 or more were obtained. Subsequent investigation suggested that the difference in nystagmus threshold between acceleration and deceleration could be more accurately determined by presenting a constant acceleration stimulus just above threshold (2 deg/sec^2) and measuring the delay before the onset of nystagmus in each direction. This type of testing permitted a rapid assessment of the symmetry in nystagmus threshold between clockwise and counterclockwise stimulation.

Nystagmus threshold measurements relied on the identification of the first beat of nystagmus (first fast component) after the beginning of the constant acceleration stimulus. As discussed in Chapter 3, several factors determine the threshold of fast components. Particularly important is the eye position in the orbit when the slow movement of the vestibulo-ocular reflex begins. Threshold measurements, therefore, are not simply an assessment of the reflex threshold but, rather, an assessment of the interaction of the vestibular signal with the fast component generating centers in the pontine reticular formation.

Several investigators[27, 49, 55] have suggested that a sinusoidal rotational stimulus is a more useful stimulus than an impulse rotational stimulus. The sinusoidal stimulus is defined by two simple variables: (1) the period of oscillation and (2) the amplitude of oscillation, both of which can be controlled with relatively simple mechanical devices. The torsion swing test was popularized in France as a simple reproducible method of generating sinusoidal acceleration in a clinic setting. With this test, the patient was seated in a chair, the rotation of which was mechanically controlled by the action of a calibrated spring.[65] When the chair was deviated from its equilibrium position, it returned to that position with a damped sinusoidal oscillation. This stimulus alternately deviates the cupula in ampullopetal and ampullofugal directions, producing nystagmus that alternates direction with each half cycle of rotation. The torsion swing provides a reproducible stimulus in that responses to clockwise and counterclockwise rotation can be compared in a given subject. The stimulus intensity, however, is dependent on the weight and distribution of mass in the chair and so varies from subject to subject.

Relationship between Stimulus and Response

With modern motorized rotational chairs the angular acceleration can be precisely controlled and multiple response measurements can be accurately monitored. Figure 7–1 illustrates the nystagmus responses of a normal subject to the three basic types of angular acceleration. The subject was rotated in the plane of the horizontal semicircular canals with the eyes open in complete darkness while he performed continuous mental arithmetic to maintain alertness. Each stimulus produced a peak angular velocity of 120 deg/sec.

The slow component velocity profiles (Fig. 7–1, *right side*) for each stimulus can be predicted by the pendulum model discussed in Chapter 2. Note the similarity between these profiles and the time course of cupula deviation illustrated in Figure 2–11. An important feature not addressed by the simple pendulum model is the adaptation phenomena (see Characteristics of Primary Afferent Neurons, Chapter 2). The impulsive response best illustrates the effect of adaptation on induced nystagmus. Instead of slowly returning to the base line as would be predicted by the pendulum model, the velocity of the slow component reverses direction and then slowly returns to the base line (as shown in Fig. 7–1a,d). Reversals of this type consistently occur in normal subjects when the step change in angular velocity is greater than 100 deg/sec.[59]

Two types of measurements are typically used to quantify the response to rotational

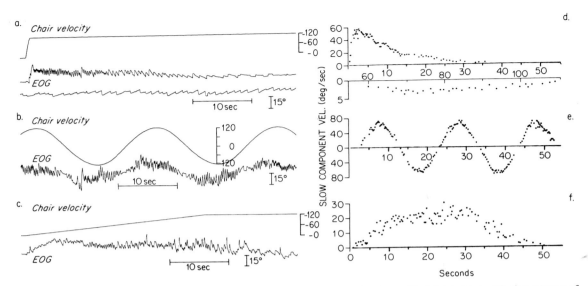

Figure 7–1. Nystagmus recording *(left side)* and slow component velocity profile *(right side)* with three types of angular acceleration, each resulting in a maximum velocity of 120 deg/sec. With the impulse stimulus *(a)* the change in velocity occurs in less than 1 second, with an acceleration of 140 deg/sec². The sinusoidal stimulus *(b)* has a frequency of 0.05Hz (20 sec/cycle) and a maximum acceleration of 38 deg/sec². The constant acceleration stimulus *(c)* is 4 deg/sec² for 30 seconds (horizontal bitemporal EOG recordings).

stimulation: a magnitude (gain) and a timing (time constant or phase shift) measurement. The gain is traditionally defined as the peak slow phase eye velocity divided by the peak stimulus velocity. The time constant of the impulse response is defined as the time required for the response to decay to $\frac{1}{e}$ or to 37 percent of the maximum value (see Appendix for further discussion). For a sinusoidal test, the phase is typically measured by comparing the time of the maximum head velocity with the time of the maximum slow phase eye velocity. Consistent with models of the canal-ocular reflex, the maximum slow phase eye velocity leads the maximum head velocity at low frequencies of sinusoidal rotation in normal subjects (see Figure 3, Appendix). The time constant (T_{COR}) of the canal-ocular reflex measured after a step change in angular velocity is inversely related to the phase lead at low frequencies of sinusoidal rotation by[5]

$$T_{COR} = \frac{1}{\omega \tan \theta}$$

where $\omega = 2\pi F$.

Test Methodology

For rotational testing of the horizontal canal-ocular reflex in our laboratory, the patient is seated on a chair mounted on a motorized rotating platform placed inside a dark electrically shielded room.[9, 11] An array of three light-emitting diodes (LEDs) spaced at the center and 15 degrees to the right and left is attached to the chair directly in front of the patient. Frequent EOG calibrations are interspersed throughout the testing procedure to correct for any fluctuations in corneal-retinal potential. Subjects are constantly questioned to maintain mental alertness. Of the three basic types of angular acceleration, impulsive and sinusoidal acceleration have been most popular for clinical testing. As will be shown below, each provides different kinds of information, and each has advantages and disadvantages. For sinusoidal testing the computer generates stimulus signals at frequencies ranging from 0.0125 to 1.6 Hz and peak velocities of 15 to 120 deg/sec. Impulse changes in velocity (32 to 256 degrees per second) occur with an acceleration of 140 degrees per second². For screening purposes, we routinely use the sinusoidal frequency of 0.05 Hz and a peak velocity of 60 deg/sec, and a step change in velocity of 100 deg/sec.

Results in Normal Subjects

As with caloric testing, maximum slow component velocity is the response measurement most useful for quantifying testing. The coefficient of variation (standard deviation divided by the mean) for maximum slow component velocity after a rotational stimulus is about one half the coefficient of variation after a caloric stimulus.[12] Even with this increased precision, however, there is still large variation in the rotational responses of normal subjects. Factors such as stress, fatigue, level of mental alertness, and habituation all contribute to the variability (see Nystagmus, Chapter 3).

IMPULSE ROTATIONAL TESTS

The main advantage of the impulse stimulus is that it provides a rapid assessment of the gain and the time constant of the canal-ocular reflex independently in each direction. Because the stimulus is so brief, however, if the subject is not maximally alert or if he or she attempts to suppress the response, the initial peak will be blunted and the estimate of gain, inaccurate. For this reason, several measurements should be averaged in each direction. The results of a typical impulse response in a normal subject are shown in Figure 7–2A. Slow component velocity (logarithmic scale) is plotted versus time; each dot represents the average slow component velocity over a 25-millisecond interval. Fast components have been removed. The gain (peak slow component velocity ÷ change in chair velocity) can be read directly from these plots. The time constant (T_{COR}) represents the time required for the slow component velocity to fall to 37 percent of its initial value given by the slope of a regression line fitted to the data. The normal mean gain and T_{COR} values calculated from similar plots in 20 normal subjects was 0.63 ± 0.18 and 12.2 ± 3.6 seconds, respectively.[5] These values are relatively stable over a wide range of step

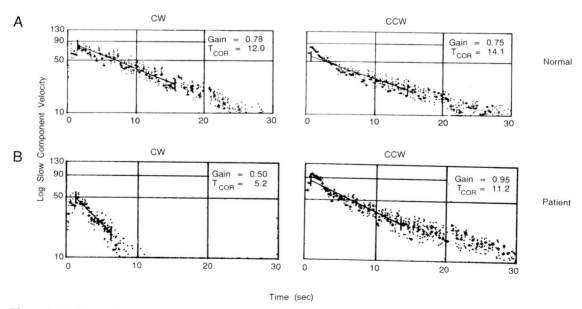

Figure 7–2. Plots of nystagmus slow component velocity (log scale) versus time after a step change in angular velocity (100 deg/sec, acceleration 140 deg/sec^2) in a normal subject *(A)* and a patient with an acute right peripheral vestibular lesion *(B)*. T_{COR} is the slope of a regression line best fit to the data. *CW,* clockwise; *CCW,* counterclockwise.

changes in velocity (0 to 250 deg/sec) but both show a gradual decrease with larger magnitude impulses (greater than 120 deg/sec).[12, 59]

The variance associated with measurements comparing clockwise and counterclockwise responses in the same subject is less than the variance in response between subjects. A normalized difference formula [(clockwise − counterclockwise) ÷ (clockwise + counterclockwise)] × 100 is analogous to the directional preponderance formula used with caloric testing. Greater than 20% asymmetry on this normalized difference formula is abnormal in our laboratory.

SINUSOIDAL ROTATIONAL TESTS

With sinusoidal rotational testing the gain of the canal-ocular reflex can be measured at multiple discrete frequencies after the subject has attained a "steady state" response. It usually provides a more accurate assessment of gain than is obtained with the impulse test. The main disadvan-

tage is the lengthy procedure required to test a broad frequency range. Also, unlike the impulse test, sinusoidal testing measures only a single time constant (the low-frequency phase lead reflects the average time constant in both directions).

Two standard computer plots generated during sinusoidal rotational testing in a normal subject are shown in Figure 7–3A. The subject was rotated at 0.05 Hz (peak velocity 60 deg/sec) with eyes open in the dark while performing continuous mental alerting tasks. As with the impulsive data shown in Figure 7–2, each dot represents the average slow component velocity over a 25-millisecond interval. The gain (peak slow component velocity ÷ peak chair velocity) in each direction can be read directly from these plots, or an average gain can be calculated by performing a frequency analysis (Fourier analysis) on the data. From this analysis, one obtains the gain, dc bias, and phase relationship between the fundamental of the slow component velocity and the chair velocity.[9] If the slow component velocity data are symmet-

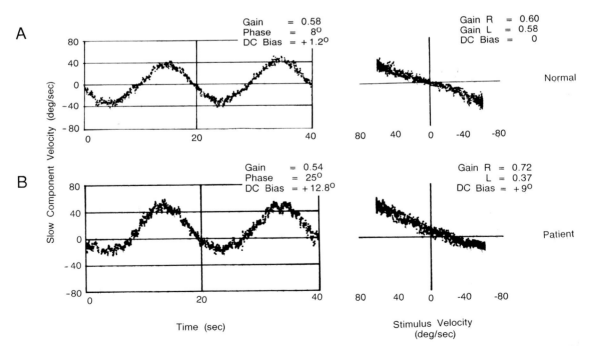

Figure 7–3. Plots of nystagmus slow component velocity versus time *(left side)* and versus chair velocity *(right side)* during sinusoidal angular rotation (0.05 Hz, 60 deg/sec peak velocity) in a normal subject *(A)* and a patient with an acute right peripheral vestibular lesion *(B)* (same patient as Figure 7–2). The gain, phase (lead) and DC bias (+ rightward bias) were determined from frequency analysis (Fourier analysis) of the data.

rical (as in normal subjects) the phase can be read directly from these plots by comparing the time of the maximum or the zero eye velocity with that of the chair velocity. However, if the responses are asymmetric (as in Fig. 7–3B), an accurate assessment of phase can be obtained with a Fourier analysis of the data. The plot of slow component velocity versus stimulus velocity (Fig. 7–3, *right*) provides a rapid visual assessment of dc bias and facilitates measurement of an average gain in each direction (i.e., the slope of the line in each direction). As with impulsive rotational stimuli, more than 20 percent asymmetry on the standard directional preponderance formula is abnormal for all frequencies and amplitudes of stimulation.

The gain and phase of the canal-ocular reflex vary with frequency in normal subjects (Fig. 7–4)[5] consistent with the pendulum model (see Fig. A–1, Appendix). Normal subjects exhibit an approximate 45 degrees phase lead of eye velocity relative to chair velocity at 0.01 Hz, but this phase lead is near zero by 0.2 Hz.

PSEUDORANDOM ROTATIONAL TESTS

By using a sum of sine waves or a computer-generated pseudorandom rotational stimulus, it is theoretically possible to measure the gain and phase of the canal-ocular reflex over a wide frequency range in a much shorter time than is required for multiple discrete sine waves.[44, 68] Frequency analysis of the eye response after saccades have been removed gives the gain and phase at discrete frequencies. Because the sampling time at each frequency is limited, however, this type of test is prone to artifact if the subject is not maximally alert throughout. Furthermore, the techniques used to analyze the data average the response in both directions. Pseudorandom rotational tests have not become popular in clinical laboratories, probably because the readily available impulse test gives a rapid estimate of gain and time constant (in each direction) over a broad frequency range without requiring the complex equipment needed to generate and analyze pseudorandom data.

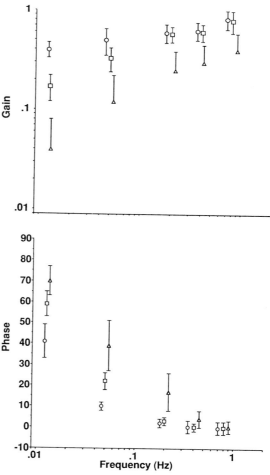

Figure 7–4. Plots of the gain and phase (mean ± 1 standard deviation) of the horizontal vestibulo-ocular reflex as a function frequency in 10 normal subjects (◯), 20 patients with compensated unilateral vestibular lesions (☐) and 22 patients with bilateral peripheral vestibular lesions (△). All subjects were tested with mental alerting in the dark. The unilateral patients had absent caloric response on one side; the bilateral patients had symmetrically decreased response to caloric stimulation.[8] The peak velocities were 0.0125 Hz, 100 deg/sec; 0.05 and 0.2 Hz, 60 deg/sec; 0.4 and 0.8 Hz, 30 deg/sec.

Results in Patients

UNILATERAL PERIPHERAL LESIONS

Patients who suddenly lose vestibular function on one side have asymmetric responses to rotational stimuli because of (1) a dc bias resulting from spontaneous nystagmus and (2) the difference in response to ampullopetal and ampullofugal stimulation of the remaining intact labyrinth.[7, 41] These features are readily seen in the impulsive and sinusoidal data shown in Figures 7–2B and 7–3B. The patient was tested shortly after the acute onset of vertigo due to a right peripheral vestibular lesion (probable viral neurolabyrinthitis). At the time of testing, he exhibited a spontaneous left-beating nystagmus (eyes open in the dark) with an average slow phase velocity of 10 deg/sec. This spontaneous nystagmus added to rotational-induced nystagmus in the same direction and subtracted from that in the opposite direction. The effect of this dc bias and of the asymmetry in response to ampullopetal and ampullofugal stimulation of the intact labyrinth are best illustrated in the plot of eye velocity versus stimulus velocity from sinusoidal rotation (see Fig. 7–3B, right side). The dc bias (the eye velocity at the point of Y-intercept) is equivalent to the average slow phase velocity of the spontaneous nystagmus. The gain (slope) of the response with ampullopetal stimulation of the intact labyrinth is twice that with ampullofugal stimulation.

With compensation, the dc bias gradually disappears and the gain asymmetry between ampullopetal and ampullofugal stimulation decreases but does not disappear.[4, 45] It remains most pronounced after high-intensity stimuli. Figure 7–5 illustrates the results of impulsive rotational testing in a patient with a long-standing compensated left peripheral vestibular lesion (from a slow-growing acoustic neuroma). There is no spontaneous nystagmus, and the induced nystagmus is symmetrical after low intensity stimuli. It is markedly asymmetric after high-intensity stimuli. The 256 deg/sec counterclockwise impulse produced ampullofugal displacement of the cupula in the intact right horizontal semicircular canal, and as expected, the induced nystagmus had a decreased maximum slow component velocity compared with the nystagmus after a clockwise impulse. This asymmetry in response after high-magnitude rotational stimuli (Ewald's second law, Chapter 2) can be used reliably to identify a complete unilateral loss of vestibular function, but unfortunately it cannot be used reliably to identify patients with only partial loss as identified on the bithermal caloric test. Of 25 patients with peripheral vestibular lesions who manifested significant but less than complete unilateral paralysis on bithermal caloric testing, only 10 had significantly ($p < 0.05$) asymmetric responses after large amplitude (256 deg/sec) impulsive rotational stimuli.[12]

Patients with compensated unilateral peripheral vestibular lesions show a characteristic pattern of decreased gain and increased phase lead at low frequencies of sinusoidal stimulation (see Fig. 7–4). These changes appear to be fixed in that they can be observed as long as 10 years after an acute unilateral peripheral vestibular loss.[45, 69] Their functional implications are minimal, however, inasmuch as the visuomotor system can compensate for the loss of vestibular function in the low-frequency range.

BILATERAL PERIPHERAL LESIONS

Rotational stimuli are ideally suited for testing patients with bilateral peripheral vestibular lesions because both labyrinths are stimulated simultaneously and the degree of remaining function is accurately quantified.[5, 42, 69] Because the variance associated with normal rotational responses is less than that associated with caloric responses, diminished function is identified earlier. Furthermore, artifactually decreased caloric responses occasionally occur in patients with angular, narrow external canals or with thickened temporal bones. Inasmuch as the intensity of rotational stimuli is unrelated to these physical features, rotational-induced nystagmus is normal in such patients. Frequently patients with absent response to bithermal caloric stimulation have decreased but recordable rotational-induced nystagmus, particularly at higher frequencies of sinusoidal rotation (see below). The ability to identify remaining vestibular function—even if minimal—is an important advantage of rotational testing, particularly when the physician is contemplating ablative surgery or monitoring the

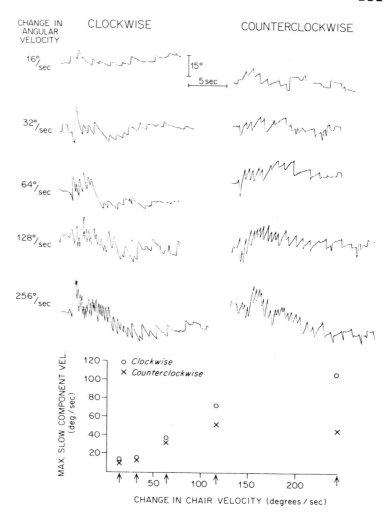

Figure 7–5. ENG recorded responses to a series of step changes in angular velocity (acceleration 140 deg/sec²) in a patient with a left acoustic neuroma. Graph represents maximum slow component velocity for each response determined from computer plots as shown in Figure 7–2. (From Baloh, RW, et al: Cerebellar-pontine angle tumors. Results of quantitative vestibulo-ocular testing. Arch Neurol 33:507, 1976, with permission.)

effects of ototoxic drugs. By using precisely graded rotational stimuli on a serial basis, ototoxic effects are recognized earlier than by using the less-precise caloric stimulus.

Patients with bilateral peripheral vestibular loss show the same pattern of low-frequency gain and phase deficits on sinusoidal testing (only more pronounced) observed in patients with compensated unilateral peripheral vestibular lesions (see Fig. 7–4).[8] Rarely, patients may have no response to rotation at frequencies below 0.05 Hz and yet have normal responses at higher frequencies.[5] These findings have important clinical implications with regard to testing patients with suspected bilateral peripheral vestibular disease.

Given that the results of the bithermal caloric testing reflect the results of low-frequency sinusoidal stimulation, the absense of caloric response does not indicate an absence of vestibular function. In fact, a patient could have absent caloric response yet normal response to rotational testing at high frequencies. On the other hand, early loss of vestibular sensitivity (e.g., secondary to ototoxic drug exposure) could be missed with high-frequency sinusoidal rotational testing alone.

CENTRAL VESTIBULAR LESIONS

As with lesions of the peripheral vestibular structures, lesions of the central vestibulo-ocular reflex pathways can lead to a decrease or an asymmetry in the gain of rotational-induced nystagmus. Lesions involving the nerve root entry zone and vestibular nuclei may produce responses indistinguishable from those produced by peripheral vestibular lesions. The spectrum of abnormalities associated with central lesions, however, is much more diverse than a simple decrease in the slow component velocity. The gain may be increased in some patients with cerebellar lesions.[61] The highly organized pattern of the nystagmus produced in normal subjects may be disorganized, resulting in so-called dysrhythmic nystagmus. If the production of fast components is impaired, the nystagmus waveform is distorted or there may be only a slow tonic deviation of eyes from side to side. Finally, central lesions often interfere with the integration of visual and vestibular signals, producing abnormalities on tests of visual-vestibular interaction (see below).

Sinusoidal rotational stimuli are ideally suited for studying the *pattern of induced nystagmus*. Figure 7–6 illustrates the responses to sinusoidal rotation (eyes open in darkness) in (a) a normal subject, (b) a patient with cerebellar atrophy, (c) a patient with a left pontine lesion (astrocytoma), and (d) a patient with a bilateral lesion of the medial longitudinal fasciculus (MLF). In the normal subject the eyes alternately deviate in the direction of the fast component for each half cycle of induced nystagmus. As discussed in Chapter 3, the eye position in the orbit for initiation of fast components is near the midline. Fast components (saccades) are generated in the paramedian pontine reticular formation, and the cerebellum controls the amplitude of both voluntary and involuntary saccades. In the patient with cerebellar atrophy (Fig. 7–6b), the nystagmus pattern is disorganized with fast components occurring in random fashion, causing marked beat-to-beat variability in amplitude. This type of abnormality has been termed dysrhythmia and is commonly

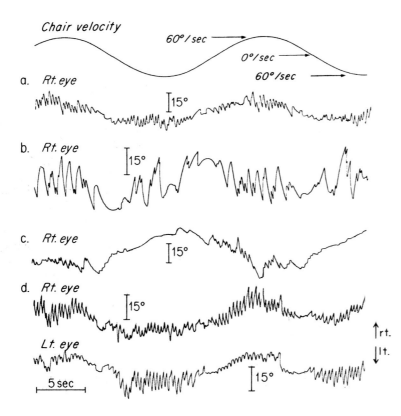

Figure 7–6 ENG recordings of nystagmus response to sinusoidal rotation at 0.05 Hz, peak velocity 60 deg/sec in a normal subject (a) and in patients with cerebellar atrophy (b), left pontine glioma (c) and bilateral MLF lesions caused by multiple sclerosis (d).

found in patients with all varieties of cerebellar lesions. Patients with dysrhythmic vestibular nystagmus also demonstrate dysmetria of voluntary saccades.

The patient with a left pontine lesion (see Fig. 7–6c) could not produce voluntary or involuntary saccades (fast components) to the left, so during the half cycle that normally produced left-beating nystagmus, the eyes tonically deviated to the right. In patients with bilateral pontine lesions, the eyes tonically deviate to the right and left with each half cycle of rotation because of the complete absence of fast components.[3] One might mistakenly interpret this as a decreased or absent vestibular response.

The patient with a bilateral MLF lesion (Fig. 7–6d) demonstrates a dissociation in fast components between the two eyes. When either "paretic" abducting eye is required to make a fast component, the nystagmus beats are rounded because of a decrease in the frequency of action potentials arriving at the medial rectus motor neurons via the damaged MLF. Abducting fast components, however, are normal, because the abducting muscles (abducens nuclei) receive their innervation for fast components directly from the paramedian pontine reticular formation with no involvement of the MLF. Frequently the abducting fast components are actually too large. The oculomotor control centers attempt to overcome the block at the MLF by increasing the innervation sent from the paramedian pontine region to the oculomotor neurons.[14, 15] Because, according to Herring's law, this increased innervation is sent equally to both medial and lateral rectus oculomotor neurons, the difference in amplitude between adducting and abducting fast components is further magnified.

VISUAL-VESTIBULAR INTERACTION

The model introduced in Chapter 3 (Fig. 3–20) identifies two general types of visual-vestibular interaction—one mediated via the "direct" (pursuit) pathway and the other via the indirect (velocity storage) pathway. Inasmuch as the direct pathway

is dominant in humans, clinical tests have focused on pursuit–VOR interaction. In rare patients with selective lesions of the direct pathway it is possible to demonstrate visual-vestibular interaction mediated via the indirect velocity storage pathway (see below).

Methodology

Visual-vestibular interaction is typically tested by rotating the subject either sinusoidally or with a step change in velocity while (1) the surrounding optokinetic drum is stationary (visual-vestibulo-ocular reflex [VisVOR]—a synergistic interaction of the visual and vestibular systems) or (2) the drum and chair are coupled so that they move together (fixation suppression of the vestibulo-ocular reflex [VOR-FIX]—an antagonistic interaction between the visual and vestibular systems).[11] Fixation suppression can also be tested by rotating the subject in the dark with a single fixation light attached to the chair.

Results in Normal Subjects

Typical responses of a normal subject to low-frequency sinusoidal (0.05 Hz) optokinetic (OKN), vestibular (VOR), and visual-vestibular (VisVOR and VOR-FIX) stimulation are shown in Figure 7–7 *(left)*. In each case the peak stimulus velocity is 60 deg/sec. At this low frequency and peak velocity the normal subject has a VisVOR gain of 1 (i.e., the slow phase eye velocity is equal and opposite to the head velocity) and a VOR-FIX gain of 0 (i.e., he is able to completely suppress the VOR with fixation). The mean gain ± standard deviation for similar sinusoidal testing in 20 normal subjects is as follows: $OKN - 0.83 \pm 0.13$; $VOR - 0.50 \pm 0.15$; $Vis\text{-}VOR - 0.99 \pm 0.05$; $VOR\text{-}FIX - 0.03 \pm 0.02$.[11] At high frequencies (>1 Hz) and velocities (>100 deg/sec) the OKN (and pursuit) gain decreases (e.g., see Fig. 6–18). Above 2 Hz, the VisVOR and VOR-FIX gain are approximately the same as the VOR gain (near 1).[43] (For a theoretical discussion see Visual-Vestibular Interaction, Appendix.)

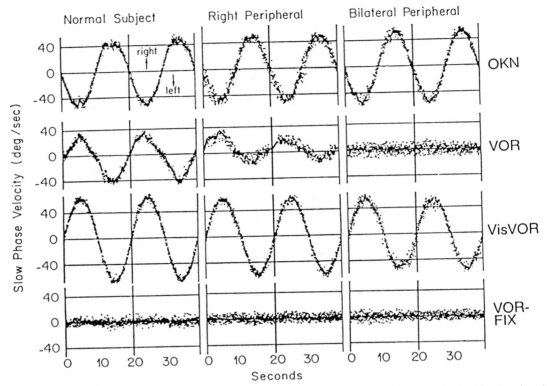

Figure 7–7. Plots of slow phase velocity versus time from a low frequency visual-vestibular test battery (see text for details) in a normal subject *(left)*, a patient who underwent a right labyrinthectomy *(center)*, and a patient with bilateral vestibulopathy secondary to ototoxic drugs *(right)* (0.05 Hz, peak velocity 60 deg/sec). (From Baloh, RW, et al: Quantitative vestibular testing. Otolaryngol Head Neck Surg 92:145, 1984, with permission.)

Results in Patients

Patients with *peripheral* vestibular lesions have decreased and/or asymmetric VOR gain, but visual-vestibular responses are usually normal at low stimulus frequencies and velocities (see Fig. 7–7, *center* and *right*). Even with a complete loss of vestibular function the visuomotor system can provide good ocular stability. At high frequencies and velocities, however, the VisVOR gain decreases if the VOR gain decreases.[43]

Three abnormal patterns of visual-vestibular interaction seen on low-frequency sinusoidal testing in patients with *central* lesions are shown in Figure 7–8.[11] Patients with lesions involving the vestibular nucleus region (e.g., Wallenberg's syndrome) exhibit prominent oculomotor abnormalities (see Infarction of the Brain-

stem and Cerebellum, Chapter 12). With eyes open in the sitting position there is a tonic pulling of the eyes toward the side of the lesion, resulting in spontaneous nystagmus with the fast phase toward the intact side. With eyes closed or with eyes open in darkness the spontaneous nystagmus may change direction. The responses illustrated in Figure 7–8 *(left)* are from a 32-year-old man who had the acute onset of vertigo, nausea, vomiting, dysphagia, and falling to the left. On neurologic examination he exhibited spontaneous nystagmus to the right while fixating, and to the left in the dark. There was also ipsilateral facial hypalgesia, Horner's syndrome, and extremity ataxia, and contralateral extremity hypalgesia. The OKN and VOR responses were asymmetric but in opposite directions, consistent with the changing direction of the patient's spontaneous nys-

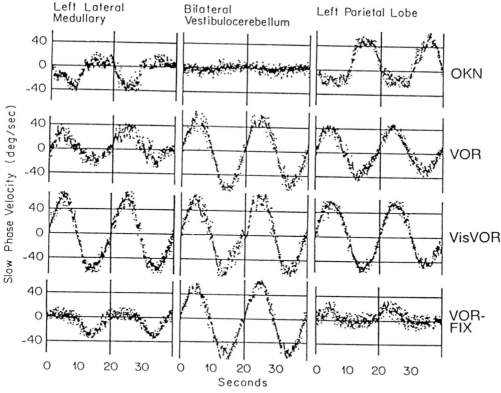

Figure 7–8. Plots of slow phase velocity versus time from a low-frequency visual-vestibular test battery in a patient with infarction of the left lateral medullary region *(left)*, a patient with midline cerebellar atrophy *(center)*, and a patient with a glioma in the deep parietal lobe on the left side *(right)* (0.05 Hz, peak velocity 60 deg/sec). (From Baloh, RW, et al: Quantitative vestibular testing. Otolaryngol Head Neck Surg 92:145, 1984, with permission.)

tagmus from light to dark. Despite the decreased OKN gain, the VisVOR gain was normal in both directions. Fixation suppression of VOR slow phases toward the side of the lesion was impaired. A similar pattern of abnormalities was found in six other patients with infarction in the lateral medulla.[13]

Patients with lesions involving the vestibulocerebellum are unable to modify vestibular responses with vision.[17] This is illustrated by the patient data shown in Figure 7–8 *(center)*, in which the VOR, VisVOR, and VOR-FIX gains are approximately the same (nearly 1) and the OKN gain is markedly decreased in both directions. This patient was a 31-year-old woman who complained only of unsteadiness and oscillopsia. The results of neurologic examination were normal except for spontaneous downbeat nystagmus and

truncal ataxia. Computerized tomography (CT) and magnetic resonance (MR) scanning documented atrophy of the midline cerebellum.

Lesions of the visuomotor pathways from the parieto-occipital cortex to the pons (i.e., those shown in Fig. 3–19) lead to impaired smooth pursuit and optokinetic slow phases toward the side of the lesion.[16] The abnormal visual-ocular control does not impair VOR responses but does alter visual-vestibular interaction. Typical responses to the four sinusoidal rotational test conditions in a patient with a deep parietal lobe lesion are shown in Figure 7–8 *(right)*. This 21-year-old man developed bitemporal headaches and slowly progressive right facial and upper extremity weakness. An angiogram indentified a tumor blush in the left parietal region. A left parietal brain biopsy revealed a grade II astrocytoma. The

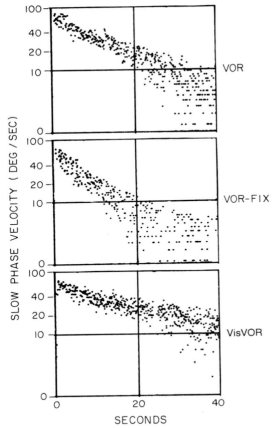

Figure 7–9. VOR, VOR-FIX, and VisVOR responses to step rotational stimuli (0–60 deg/sec, 140 deg/sec^2 acceleration) in a patient with cerebellar atrophy. The log of slow phase eye velocity is plotted against time. For the VOR, the chair was stopped in the dark, for the VOR-FIX the chair was stopped in the light, and for the VisVOR the chair was maintained at a constant velocity in the light with a stationary surround. (From Baloh, RW, et al: Late cortical cerebellar atrophy. Brain 109:159, 1986, with permission.)

OKN gain was normal to the right and markedly decreased to the left. The VOR gain was normal in both directions, but the patient was unable to inhibit VOR slow phases to the right with fixation (i.e., the VOR-FIX gain was increased to the right). The VisVOR gain was slightly asymmetric, with lower gain to the left than to the right.

As noted above in patients with minimal or no sinusoidal VOR, VisVOR, and VOR-FIX responses are almost identical (e.g., Fig. 7–8, *center*). These patients may show evidence of visual-vestibular interaction

with impulse stimuli, however. The patient with cerebellar atrophy whose data are shown in Figure 7–9 had absent pursuit and sinusoidal OKN but exhibited a gradual build-up in OKN after a step onset in drum velocity (see Fig. 6–19). The gain (initial peak eye velocity/peak stimulus velocity) of the impulse responses was the same whether the patient received (1) a VisVOR stimulus (i.e., a step from 0 to 60 deg/sec in the light with a fixed surround), (2) a VOR-FIX stimulus (i.e., stopping the rotating chair in the light with a fixed surround), or (3) a VOR stimulus (i.e., starting or stopping the chair in darkness). However, the rate of decay in slow phase velocity (i.e., the time constant) was prolonged after a VisVOR stimulus and shortened after a VOR-FIX stimulus compared with the VOR stimulus. Thus, one type of visual-vestibular interaction (that mediated via the velocity storage pathway) was preserved in a patient with absent smooth pursuit.

In summary, in addition to tests of the VOR, modern rotational testing includes tests of visual-vestibular interaction. Lesions of the peripheral vestibular system typically impair only the VOR, whereas lesions of the central nervous system (CNS) impair OKN and visual-vestibular interaction. The pattern of abnormal response can help localize lesions within the central pathways.

TESTS OF THE VERTICAL SEMICIRCULAR CANAL AND OTOLITH OCULAR REFLEXES

As suggested above, current rotational tests evaluate only the horizontal semicircular canals. Future tests designed to evaluate other vestibular suborgans (the vertical semicircular canals and otolith organs) will require movements that stimulate these receptors singly or in combination.[38] The determination of which vestibular suborgans are stimulated by a particular movement requires knowledge of three factors: (1) whether the stimulus is an angular or linear acceleration, (2) the orientation of the skull (and thus the labyrinth) with respect to the movement, and (3) the

Table 7–2. VESTIBULAR TESTS AND THE SUBORGANS THEY STIMULATE

Test	Horizontal Canals	Vertical Canals	Otoliths
Conventional rotational chair	+		
Pitch rotation Upright		+	+
Onside		+	
Ocular counterrolling Static			+
Dynamic		+	+
Eccentric rotation	+		+
Off-vertical rotation	+		+
Linear track			+
Parallel swing			+

orientation of the movement with respect to gravity. Table 7–2 lists the tests to be described below and indicates which suborgans they are designed to evaluate.

Pitch Rotation

Rotation of the head in the sagittal plane (e.g., shaking the head yes) stimulates all four vertical semicircular canals. If the pitch stimulus is delivered with the subject seated in the upright position (upright pitch), the head changes orientation with respect to gravity as it tips forward and backward. This change in orientation with respect to gravity stimulates the otolith organs in addition to the vertical semicircular canals. If, however, a subject is seated in a conventional rotational chair with the head tilted toward the shoulder so that one ear is down, the orientation of the subject with respect to gravity does not change during rotation and the otoliths are not activated. This stimulus, called onside pitch, is thus comparable to conventional rotational testing except that the vertical rather than the horizontal semicircular canals are stimulated.

There are major limitations to the clinical use of pitch rotation due to problems with stimulus delivery and measurement of response. Although onside pitch can be delivered with only minor modifications of a conventional rotational chair, upright pitch requires cumbersome and costly equipment. Moreover, the vertical eye movements that are induced by pitch rotation cannot be measured accurately with EOG. Rather, one must use either the magnetic scleral search coil or a video recording system. Preliminary studies in normal animals[26, 62] and humans[6, 10] indicate that there is a difference between the VOR response to pitch in the upright position versus the onside position. The gain was decreased and asymmetries were present in the latter compared with the former. Presumably by positioning a subject so that the rotation occurs in the plane of a vertical canal pair (e.g., the right anterior canal and the left posterior canal), one should be able to identify dynamic asymmetries similiar to those seen in the horizontal VOR after acute and chronic unilateral peripheral vestibular lesions. This has yet to be shown in a clinical study, however.

Ocular Counterrolling

The otolith-ocular reflex produces torsional eye movements during static head tilts. Rotating the head toward the right shoulder causes the eyes to counterrotate to the right (see Characteristics of Eye Movements Induced by Otolith Stimulation, Chapter 3). Such rotation of the head in the coronal plane is called roll, and the counterrotation of the eyes is called ocular counterrolling.[32, 47, 64] Dynamic roll movements also stimulate the vertical semicircular canals because of the angular acceleration of the movement, so when using roll stimulation a distinction should be made between static and dynamic ocular counterrolling.

As with pitch rotation, the clinical use of ocular counterrolling has been hampered by difficulties both in stimulus delivery and in the measurement of response. In order to rotate someone in the coronal plane, the subject must be securely fastened to a cumbersome and costly device. In addition, the amount of torsional eye movement produced by a static tilt in the coronal plane is relatively small. For example, if the head is tilted 45 degrees, the eyes counterroll only about 7 degrees. EOG and infrared reflection techniques are insensitive to this type of movement, so photographic or video recording or the magnetic scleral search coil must be employed.

Unilateral peripheral vestibular lesions produce asymmetries in static ocular counterrolling; roll to the side of the lesion results in less counterrolling than roll away from the side of the lesion.[31, 53] With some types of central lesions one can see a roll rather than a counterroll response (i.e., the eyes rotate in the direction of head tilt).[30, 48] Further research is needed, however, to determine the reliability of this technique for identifying lesions in the clinical vestibular laboratory.

Eccentric Rotation

Eccentric (off-center) rotation is delivered by seating a subject upright in a conventional rotational chair such that the head is away from the axis of rotation as if the head were placed at the end of the arm of a centrifuge. During angular acceleration with the head eccentric the labyrinth is exposed to both rotational and linear (tangential and centrifugal) acceleration, and thus both the otolith organs and the horizontal semicircular canals are stimulated. Once a constant angular velocity is achieved, however, only the otoliths are stimulated. The net linear acceleration delivered to the subject is the vector summation of the linear acceleration produced by the movement itself and the linear acceleration produced by gravity (F_g' in Fig. 1–1c). The advantages of eccentric rotation are that conventional rotational chairs (with minor modifications) and EOG methods can be used for this test.

With sinusoidal angular acceleration the difference between eye movements induced with the head at the center of rotation and those with the head eccentric is the contribution of the otolith organs.[36] Preliminary studies suggest that this might be a useful clinical test of the otolith ocular reflex.[37] An even simpler test of otolith function is to have the subject estimate the subjective vertical (with a vertical light bar) during constant velocity eccentric rotation.[28] Unlike other tests of subjective vestibular sensation, the sensation of

tilt experienced during eccentric rotation appears to be highly reproducible. Patients who have undergone a unilateral vestibular neurectomy experience less of a sensation of tilt when the lesioned ear is outermost.[28] The deficit is maximum in the first postoperative week but persists for at least 24 weeks.

Linear Acceleration on Sleds

Another technique that has been used to study the otolith ocular reflex in the research laboratory is to deliver a pure linear acceleration on a linear track.[24, 54] The device typically consists of a rollercoasterlike sled that runs along a track. As with eccentric rotation, the otolith organs sense the net linear acceleration; that is, the vector summation of the linear acceleration induced by the sled itself and that due to gravity. For the relatively simple case in which the subject is placed on the sled facing the side as if looking out the side window of an automobile moving forward, a consistent horizontal eye movement (including nystagmus) can be recorded with EOG. For other head orientations vertical or torsional eye movements are induced requiring other eye-movement recording techniques such as a magnetic scleral search coil or video system. Use of linear sleds clinically would be severely limited by the expense and size of the equipment.

Parallel Swing

The parallel swing is a simple technique for inducing linear acceleration that may be practical in the clinical laboratory. It consists of a platform suspended from the ceiling by supporting cables at each of its four corners. For small-amplitude displacements almost pure horizontal linear acceleration is experienced by a subject seated on the platform. As with the linear sled, the eye movement response on a parallel swing depends on the orientation of the subject's head relative to the linear acceleration of the swing and gravity. Thus various combinations of horizontal, vertical, and torsional eye movements may be induced. Preliminary studies indicate that horizontal eye movements are reliably induced when normal human subjects are seated in the dark facing the side so that the linear acceleration occurs along the interaural axis (Fig. 7–10A; also see Fig. 3–10).[2] The magnitude of these eye movements is enhanced if the subject imagines a target fixed to the stationary surround. Patients with bilateral peripheral vestibular lesions have diminished or absent responses with or without an imagined fixation target (Fig. 7–10B).[2] So far, parallel swings have been used only at their natural frequency (usually in the range of 0.3 Hz) providing limited information about the dynamic range of the otolith ocular reflex. Spring- or motor-driven devices would allow a more extended evaluation of the reflex.

Off-Vertical Rotation

Off-vertical rotation is performed by seating the subject in a conventional rotational chair and then tilting the entire apparatus, including the chair and subject (see Fig. 3–11).[19, 60] In this way as the subject rotates, the head is continually changing its orientation with respect to gravity. In the extreme case, in which the chair is tipped completely on its side (earth horizontal axis or so-called barbecue rotation), the subject is rotated from supine to lateral to prone to lateral and so on. Once a constant velocity is achieved only the otolith organs are stimulated (inasmuch as the canals respond only to angular acceleration).

A major advantage of this type of otolith test is that a conventional rotatory chair

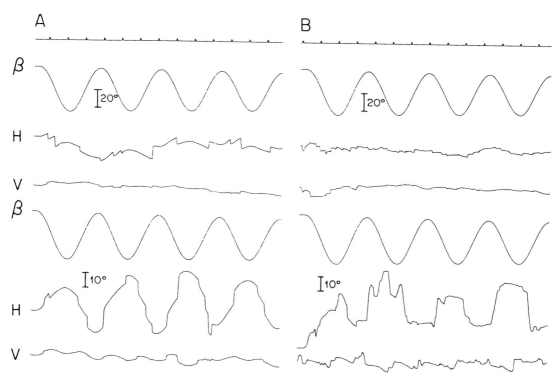

Figure 7–10. Horizontal *(H)* and vertical *(V)* eye movements (recorded with a scleral search coil in the dark) induced on a parallel swing with the subject facing the side (horizontal linear acceleration along the interaural axis) while responding to questions *(upper three traces)* and while imagining an earth-fixed target. *(A)* Normal subject. *(B)* Patient with bilateral Meniere's syndrome and absent response to caloric stimulation. β indicates swing position. Interval between tick marks is 1 second. With mental alerting above both subjects developed horizontal nystagmus (greater in the normal subject). With an imagined target saccades occurred in the same direction as vestibular slow phases. Compared with the normal subject, the patient generated inaccurate and poorly timed saccades. (From Baloh, RW, et al: Eye movements induced on a parallel swing. J Neurophysiol 60:2000, 1988, with permission.)

can be used if the angle of inclination is kept small. Subjects can be placed into or moved from the apparatus easily, and conventional EOG can record the eye movements because they are largely horizontal. A disadvantage is that the stimulus often produces nausea. Off-vertical constant velocity rotation in normal subjects induces two horizontal eye movement components: a bias and a modulation component.[29, 46] In patients with unilateral peripheral vestibular lesions the bias component is diminished when the patient rotates toward the involved ear while the modulation component remains unchanged.[46]

Summary of Vertical Semicircular Canal and Otolith Ocular Testing

The vertical semicircular canal and otolith function tests briefly described above are based on the knowledge that the vertical semicircular canals sense angular acceleration in the sagittal and coronal planes and the otoliths sense linear acceleration in all directions. Each test induces a combination of horizontal, vertical, and torsional eye movements depending on the characteristics of the movement, the orientation of the subject with respect to the movement, and the orientation of the movement with respect to gravity. Future research is needed to determine the potential clinical usefulness of each of these investigational techniques.

VESTIBULO-SPINAL TESTING

Current tests of vestibular function concentrate on the vestibulo-ocular system; the vestibulo-spinal system has been relatively neglected. A major reason for this neglect is that it is difficult to assess the role of the vestibulo-spinal system in isolation of the other sensory systems.

Static-Force Platforms

The simplest method of recording human postural sway employs a so-called force plate. There are several devices of this type, each designed with the basic idea of recording the position of a subject's center of mass during upright stance. In fact, these devices measure the position of the center of force, which is a good estimate of the position of the center of mass if the body is moving slowly. The major limitation of such devices relates to two factors: (1) the nervous system uses a combination of sensory modalities during the maintenance of upright stance, and (2) static-force plates do not yield controlled stimulus-response measures of vestibulo-spinal function and thus must rely on spontaneous movements of the body. This latter consideration is analogous to making assessments of the vestibulo-ocular system by simply monitoring eye position in the absence of vestibular stimulation. The measurement of postural sway might be useful as a screening test for imbalance, but the information it provides is nonspecific and probably not helpful for identifying vestibular lesions.[23, 67]

Moving-Platform Posturography

Moving-force platforms have been designed to overcome the limitations of static-force platforms discussed above by (1) controlling the relative contributions of the visual, somatosensory, and vestibular inputs that are normally used to maintain upright posture; and (2) incorporating stimulus-response measurements. With such a device, one can move the platform upon which the subject stands and simultaneously move the visual surround. By coupling the platform to the sway of the subject it is possible to maintain the angle between the foot and the lower leg at a constant value, thereby reducing a major source of somatosensory input to the postural control system.[52] If the subject simultaneously closes the eyes or if the movement of the visual enclosure is coupled to body sway, the subject is also deprived of visual information about postural sway. In this way the influence of the labyrinth on upright posture via the vestibulo-spinal system can be studied in a more or less isolated fashion.[51] The disadvantage of this technique is that during postural sway many of the suborgans of the vestibular labyrinth are simultaneously stimulated, including the vertical semicircular canals and the otolith organs bilaterally. For this reason, moving-platform studies are incapable of providing an assessment of the individual suborgans of the vestibular labyrinth. In addition, these devices do not assess the subject's strategy in moving other body parts and joints. Not surprisingly, patients with bilateral peripheral vestibular loss perform poorly on these tests when visual and somatosensory signals have been effectively removed.[1, 22] However, preliminary reports that moving-platform posturography can identify sites of lesion or specific vestibular disorders[20, 21] have not been confirmed. More research is required to determine the usefulness of moving-force platforms for assessment of the vestibulo-spinal system.

VESTIBULAR-EVOKED POTENTIALS

The ability to record a human vestibular-evoked potential has obvious merits, inasmuch as it would provide an objective measure of peripheral vestibular function that would be independent of either the oculomotor or postural control systems. Despite the fact that sensory-evoked potentials using auditory, visual, and somatosensory inputs have been developed and are in routine clinical use, short-latency vestibular-evoked potentials have been recorded successfully only in small laboratory animals.[33, 34] The reason for this lack of development is related to the difficulty of delivering a vestibular stimulus that is capable of triggering a coordinated volley of neural activity, a requirement for eliciting a measurable evoked potential. The vestibular equivalent of an auditory click, visual flash, or somatosensory prick is a brief, abrupt high-intensity rotational impulse with an angular acceleration in the range of 7,000 deg/sec^2.

Prior research regarding human vestibular-evoked potentials has focused upon recording long-latency cortical potentials rather than brainstem evoked potentials.[40, 56, 58] The results of these studies are conflicting. It is still unclear whether the recorded potentials are specific for the

vestibular stimulus. Preliminary results from Elidan's group in Israel (personal communication) suggest that it is possible to record brainstem vestibular-evoked responses in normal human subjects. Whether these responses can reliably identify abnormalities of the vestibular labyrinth and vestibular nerve and whether they are safe have yet to be confirmed.

REFERENCES

1. Allum, JHJ and Pfaltz, CR: Visual and vestibular contributions to pitch sway stabilization in the ankle muscles of normals and patients with bilateral peripheral vestibular deficits. Exp Brain Res 58:82, 1985.
2. Baloh, RW, Beykirch, K, Honrubia, V, and Yee, RD: Eye movements induced by linear acceleration on a parallel swing. J Neurophysiol 60:2000, 1988.
3. Baloh, RW, Furman, J, and Yee, RD: Eye movements in patients with absent voluntary horizontal gaze. Ann Neurol 17:283, 1985.
4. Baloh, RW, Honrubia, V, and Konrad, HR: Ewald's second law reevaluated. Acta Otolaryngol 83:475, 1977.
5. Baloh, RW, Honrubia, V, Yee, RD, and Hess, K: Changes in the human vestibulo-ocular reflex after loss of peripheral sensitivity. Ann Neurol 16:222, 1984.
6. Baloh, RW, et al: Vertical visual-vestibular interaction in normal subjects. Exp Brain Res 64:400, 1986.
7. Baloh, RW, Jacobson, KM, Beykirch, K, and Honrubia, V: Horizontal vestibulo-ocular reflex after acute peripheral lesions. Acta Otolaryngol (in press).
8. Baloh, RW, Jacobson, K, Honrubia, V: Idiopathic bilateral vestibulopathy. Neurology 39:272, 1989.
9. Baloh, RW, Langhofer, L, Honrubia, V, and Yee, RD: On-line analysis of eye movements using a digital computer. Aviat Space Environ Med 51:563, 1980.
10. Baloh, RW, et al: The dynamics of vertical eye movements in normal human subjects. Aviat Space Environ Med 54:32, 1983.
11. Baloh, RW, et al: Quantitative vestibular testing. Otolaryngol Head Neck Surg 92:145, 1984.
12. Baloh, RW, Sills, AW, and Honrubia, V: Impulsive and sinusoidal rotatory testing. A comparison with results of caloric testing. Laryngoscope 89:646, 1979.
13. Baloh, RW, Yee, RD, and Honrubia, V: Eye movements in patients with Wallenberg's syndrome. Ann NY Acad Sci 374:600, 1981.
14. Baloh, RW, Yee, RD, and Honrubia, V: Internuclear ophthalmoplegia. I. Saccades and dissociated nystagmus. Arch Neurol 35:484, 1978.
15. Baloh, RW, Yee, RD, and Honrubia, V: Inter-

nuclear ophthalmoplegia. II. Pursuit, optoki-netic nystagmus and the vestibulo-ocular re-flex. Arch Neurol 35:490, 1978.

16. Baloh, RW, Yee, RD, and Honrubia, V: Optoki-netic nystagmus and parietal lobe lesions. Ann Neurol 7:269, 1980.

17. Baloh, RW, Yee, RD, Kimm, J, and Honrubia, V: The vestibulo-ocular reflex in patients with lesions of the vestibulocerebellum. Exp Neu-rol 72:141, 1981.

18. Bárány, R: Physiologie and Pathologie des Bogen-gangsapparates beim Menschen. Deuticke, Vienna, 1907.

19. Benson, AJ: Modification of the response to an-gular accelerations by linear accelerations. In Kornhuber, HH (ed): Handbook of Sensory Physiology; Vestibular System, Vol VI, Part 2. Springer-Verlag, Berlin, 1974, p 281.

20. Black, FO and Nashner, LM: Postural distur-bances in patients with benign paroxysmal positional nystagmus. Ann Otol Rhinol Lar-yngol 93:595, 1984.

21. Black, FO and Nashner, LM: Vestibulospinal con-trol differs in patients with reduced versus distorted vestibular function. Acta Otolaryn-gol 406:110, 1984.

22. Black, FO, Wall, C, III, and Nashner, LM: Effect of visual and support surface references upon postural control in vestibular deficit sub-jects. Acta Otolaryngol 95:199, 1983.

23. Bles, W and De Jong, JMBV: Uni- and bilateral loss of vestibular function. In Bles, W and Brandt, TH (eds): Disorders of Posture and Gait. Elsevier, Amsterdam, 1986, p 127.

24. Buizza, A, Schmid, R, and Droulez, J: Influence of linear acceleration on oculomotor control. In Fuchs, AF and Becker, V (eds): Progress in Oculomotor Research. Elsevier/North-Holland, New York, 1981, p 517.

25. Collewijn, H, Van Der Mark, F, and Jansen, TC: Precise recording of human eye movements. Vision Res 15:447, 1974.

26. Correia, MJ, Perachio, A, and Eden, AR: The monkey vertical vestibulo-ocular response: A frequency domain study. J Neurophysiol 54:532, 1985.

27. Cramer, RL, Dowd, PJ, and Helms, DB: Vestibu-lar responses to oscillations about the yaw axis. Aerospace Med 34:1031, 1963.

28. Dai, MJ, Curthoys, IS, and Halmagyi, M: Effects of unilateral vestibular neurectomy on per-ception of tilt in roll. In Huang, JC, Daunton, NG, Wilson, VJ (eds): Basic and Applied As-pects of Vestibular Function. Hong Kong University Press, 1988, p 234.

29. Denise, P: Rotation d'axe incline par rapport a la gravite. Effets des petits angles et interet clinique. Doctoral thesis. Universite Pierre et Marie Curie, Paris VI Faculte de Medecine Pi-tie, Salpetriere, Dacylosorbonne, 8 rue, Casi-mir-Delavigne, 1986.

30. Diamond, SG, Markham, CH, and Baloh, RW: Ocular counterrolling abnormalities in spasmotic torticollis. Arch Neurol 45:164, 1988.

31. Diamond, SG, Markham, CH, and Furuya, N: Binocular counterrolling during sustained

body tilt in normal humans and in a patient with unilateral vestibular nerve section. Ann Otol 91:225, 1982.

32. Diamond, SG, et al: Binocular counterrolling in humans during dynamic rotation. Acta Oto-laryngol 87:490, 1979.

33. Elidan, J, Langhofer, L, and Honrubia, V: Re-cording of short-latency vestibular evoked potentials induced by acceleration impulses in experimental animals: Current status of the method and its application. EEG Clin Neurophys 68:58, 1987.

34. Elidan, J, Lin, J, and Honrubia, V: Vestibular ototoxicity of gentamicin assessed by the re-cording of short-latency vestibular-evoked re-sponse in cats. Laryngoscope 97:865, 1987.

35. Gonshor, A and Malcolm, R: Effect of changes in illumination level on electro-oculography (EOG). Aerospace Med 42:138, 1971.

36. Gresty, MA and Bronstein, AM: Otolith stimula-tion evokes compensatory reflex eye move-ments of high velocity when linear motion of the head is combined with concurrent angu-lar motion. Neurosci Letters 65:149, 1986.

37. Gresty, MA, Bronstein, AM, and Barratt, H: Eye movement responses to combined linear and angular head movement. Exp Brain Res 65:377, 1987.

38. Gresty, M, et al: Clinical aspects of otolith-oculo-motor relationships. In Keller, EL, Zee, DS (eds): Adaptive Processes in Visual and Ocu-lomotor Systems. Pergamon Press, Oxford, 1986.

39. Hall, RW: Image processing algorithms for eye movement monitoring. Comp Biomed Res 16:563, 1983.

40. Hofferberth, B: Evoked potentials to rotatory stimulation. Acta Otolaryngol (Suppl) 406:134, 1984.

41. Honrubia, V, et al: Vestibulo-ocular reflexes in pe-ripheral labyrinthine lesions. II. Caloric test-ing. Am J Otolaryngol 5:93, 1984.

42. Honrubia, V, et al: Vestibulo-ocular reflexes in pe-ripheral labyrinthine lesions. III. Bilateral dysfunction. Am J Otolaryngol 6:342, 1985.

43. Hydén, D, Istl, YE, and Schwarz, DWF: Human vi-suovestibular interaction as a basis for quan-titative clinical diagnosis. Acta Otolaryngol 94:53, 1982.

44. Hydén, D, Larsby, B, Schwarz, DWF, and Ödk-vist, LM: Quantification of slow compensa-tory eye movements in patients with bilateral vestibular loss. A study with a broad frequen-cy-band rotatory test. Acta Otolaryngol 96:199, 1983.

45. Jenkins, HR, Honrubia, V, Baloh, RW: Evalua-tion of multiple frequency rotatory testing in patients with peripheral labyrinthine weak-ness. Am J Otolaryngol 3:182, 1982.

46. Kamerer, DB, Wall, C, III, and Furman, JMR: Earth horizontal axis rotational responses in patients with unilateral peripheral vestibular deficits (abstr). Bárány Society Meeting, Bo-logna, Italy, 1987.

47. Kirienko, NM, et al: Clinical testing of the oto-liths: A critical assessment of ocular counter-rolling. J Otolaryngol 13:281, 1984.

48. Markham, CH and Diamond, SG: Distinctive counter rolling disruption caused by brain stem compression. In Kunze, K, Zangemeister, WH, Arlt, A (eds): Clinical Problems of Brainstem Disorders. Georg Thieme Verlag, Stuttgart, 1986, p 201.

49. Mathog, RH: Testing of the vestibular system by sinusoidal angular acceleration. Acta Otolaryngol 74:96, 1972.

50. Montandon, A: A new technique for vestibular investigation. Acta Otolaryngol 39:594, 1954.

51. Nashner, LM, Black, FO, and Wall, C, III: Adaptation to altered support and visual conditions during stance: Patients with vestibular deficits. J Neurosci 2:536, 1982.

52. Nashner, LM: A model describing vestibular detection of body sway motion. Acta Otolaryngol 72:429, 1971.

53. Nelson, JR and House, WF: Ocular countertorsion as an indicator of otolith function: Effects of unilateral vestibular lesions. Tr Am Acad Ophthalmol Otolaryngol 75:1313, 1971.

54. Niven, JI, Hixon, WC, and Correia, MJ: Elicitation of horizontal nystagmus by periodic linear acceleration. Acta Otolaryngol 62:429, 1966.

55. Niven, JI, Hinson, C, and Correia, MJ: An experimental approach to the dynamics of the vestibular mechanisms. In Symposium on the Role of the Vestibular Organs in the Exploration of Space. NASA SP-77:43, Pensacola, FL, 1965.

56. Pirodda, E, Ghedini, S, and Zanetti, MA: Investigations into vestibular evoked responses. Acta Otolaryngol 104:77, 1987.

57. Proctor, L, Hansen, D, and Rentea, R: Corneoretinal potential variations. Arch Otolaryngol 106:262, 1980.

58. Salamy, J, Potvin, A, Jones, K, and Landreth, J: Cortical evoked responses to labyrinthine stimulation in man. Psychophysiology 12:55, 1975.

59. Sills, AW, Honrubia, V, and Baloh, RW: Is the adaptation model a valid description of the vestibulo-ocular reflex? Biol Cybernetics 30:209, 1978.

60. Stockwell, CW, Turnipseed, GT, and Guedry, FE: Nystagmus responses during rotation about a tilted axis. NAMRL–1129, Pensacola, FL, 1971.

61. Thurston, SF, Leigh, RR, Abel, LA, and Dell'Osso, LF: Hyperactive vestibulo-ocular reflex in cerebellar degeneration. Neurology 37:53, 1987.

62. Tomko, DL, et al: Gain and phase of cat vertical eye movements generated by sinusoidal pitch rotations with and without head tilt. Aviat Space Environ Med 58:186, 1987.

63. Truong, DM and Feldon, SE: Sources of artifact in infrared recording of eye movement. Invest Ophthal Vis Sci 28:1018, 1987.

64. Uemura, T, et al: Neuro-otological examination. University Park Press, Baltimore, 1977.

65. Van de Calseyde, P, Ampe, W, and Depondt, M: The damped torsion swing test. Quantitative and qualitative aspects of the ENG pattern in normal subjects. Arch Otolaryngol 100:449, 1974.

66. Van Egmond, AAJ, Groen, JJ, and Jongkees, LBW: The turning test with small regulable stimuli. I. Method of examination: cupulometria. J Laryngol Otol 2:63, 1948.

67. Wall, C, III and Black, FO: Postural stability and rotational tests: Their effectiveness for screening dizzy patients. Acta Otolaryngol 95:235, 1983.

68. Wall, C, III, Black, FO, and O'Leary, DP: Clinical use of pseudorandom binary sequence white noise in assessment of the human vestibulo-ocular system. Ann Otol 87:845, 1978.

69. Wolfe, JW, Engelken, EJ, and Olson, JE: Low-frequency harmonic acceleration in the evaluation of patients with peripheral labyrinthine disorders. In Honrubia, V, Brazier, MAB (eds): Nystagmus and Vertigo. Clinical Approaches to the Patient with Dizziness. Academic Press, New York, 1982, p 95.

70. Young, LR and Sheena, D: Eye movement measurement techniques. Am Psychol 30:315, 1975.

Chapter 8

CLINICAL EVALUATION OF HEARING

TYPES OF HEARING DISORDERS

Hearing disorders can be classified as conductive, sensorineural, and central, based on the anatomic site of lesion.[1, 5.]

Conductive

Conductive hearing loss results from lesions involving the external or middle ear. The tympanic membrane and ossicles act as a transformer amplifying airborne sound and efficiently transferring it to the inner ear fluid (see Middle ear, Chapter 2). If this normal pathway is obstructed, transmission may occur across the skin and through the bones of the skull (bone conduction), but at the cost of considerable energy loss.

The most common cause of conductive hearing loss is impacted cerumen in the external auditory canal. This benign condition is often first noticed after bathing or swimming, when water closes the remaining tiny passageway. The most common serious cause of conductive hearing loss is inflammation of the middle ear, otitis media.[13] Either infected (suppurative otitis) or noninfected (serous otitis) fluid accumulates in the middle ear, impairing the conduction of airborne sound. With chronic otomastoiditis the middle ear may be invaded by a cholesteatoma. Otosclerosis produces progressive conductive hearing loss by immobilizing the stapes with new bone growth in front of and below the oval window. Other common causes of conductive hearing loss include large tympanic membrane perforations, trauma, congenital malformations of the external and middle ears, and tumors of the temporal bone.

Sensorineural

Sensorineual hearing loss results from lesions of the cochlea and/or the auditory division of the eighth cranial nerve. The spiral cochlea mechanically analyzes the frequency content of sound. For high-frequency tones only sensory cells in the basal turn are activated, whereas for low-frequency tones maximum stimulation occurs at the apex, even though all or nearly all sensory cells are activated with loud sounds. Therefore, with lesions of the cochlea and its afferent nerve, hearing levels for different frequencies are often unequal, and the timing (phase) relationship between different frequencies may be altered. Patients with sensorineural hearing loss often have difficulty hearing speech that is mixed with background noise and may be annoyed by loud speech.

Distortion of sound is common with sensorineural hearing loss. A pure tone may be heard as noisy, rough, or buzzing, or it may be distorted so that it sounds like a complex mixture of tones. Binaural diplacusis occurs when the two ears are affected unequally so that the same frequency has a different pitch in each ear, i.e., the patient hears different sounds in each ear. Monaural diplacusis occurs when two tones or a tone and noise are heard simultaneously in one ear. With recruitment there is an abnormally rapid growth in the sensation of loudness as the intensity of a sound is increased so that faint or moderate sounds cannot be heard, whereas there is little or no change in the loudness of loud sounds.

The most common cause of acute unilateral sensorineural hearing loss is infection of the inner ear (labyrinthitis). Bacteria can enter the ear directly from the middle ear, or from the cerebrospinal fluid via the cochlear aqueduct, or internal auditory canal. In the former case there is a history of recurrent or chronic otitis media; in the latter case, the patient has bacterial meningitis. Viral labyrinthitis may be part of a systemic viral illness such as measles, mumps, and infectious mononucleosis or an isolated infection of the labyrinth without systemic symptoms. Mumps is a particularly common cause of unilateral hearing loss in school-age children. Other common causes of acute unilateral hearing loss are head trauma and vascular occlusive disease.

Relapsing unilateral sensorineural hearing loss associated with tinnitus, ear fullness, and vertigo is typical of Meniere's syndrome. Ototoxic drugs produce a bilateral subacute hearing loss. Acoustic neuromas (vestibular schwannomas) characteristically produce a slowly progressive unilateral sensorineural hearing loss. The chronic progressive bilateral hearing loss associated with advancing age is called presbycusis. It may include conductive and central dysfunction, but the most consistent effect of aging is on the sensory cells and neurons of the cochlea.[28]

Central Hearing Disorders

Central hearing disorders result from lesions of the central auditory pathways: the cochlear and dorsal olivary nuclear complexes, inferior colliculi, medial geniculate bodies, auditory cortex in the temporal lobes and their interconnecting afferent and efferent fiber tracts. As a rule, patients with central lesions do not have impaired hearing levels for pure tones, and they understand speech if it is clearly spoken in a quiet environment. If the listener's task is made more difficult with the introduction of background or competing messages,

performance deteriorates in patients with central lesions more than in normal subjects. Lesions involving the nerve root entry zone or cochlear nucleus can result in unilateral hearing loss for pure tones (e.g., demyelination or infarction of the lateral pontomedullary region). Because approximately 50 percent of afferent nerve fibers cross central to the cochlear nucleus, this is the most central structure in which a lesion can result in a unilateral hearing loss.

BEDSIDE TESTS OF HEARING

A quick test for hearing loss in the speech range is to observe the response to spoken commands at different intensities (whisper, conversation, shouting). The examiner stands behind the patient to prevent lip reading and occludes and masks the nontest ear by moving a finger back and forth in the patient's external ear canal. Tuning fork tests permit a rough assessment of the hearing level for pure tones of known frequency. The clinician can use his or her own hearing level as a reference standard. The Rinne test compares the patient's hearing by air conduction with that by bone conduction. The fork (preferably 512 Hz) is first held against the mastoid process until the sound fades. It is then placed one inch from the ear. Normal subjects can hear the fork longer by air than by bone conduction. If bone conduction is greater than air conduction, a conductive hearing loss is suggested. The Weber test compares the patient's hearing by bone conduction in the two ears. The fork is placed at the center of the forehead or on a central incisor and the patient is asked where he or she hears the tone. Normal subjects hear it in the center of the head, patients with unilateral conductive loss hear it on the affected side, and patients with unilateral sensorineural loss hear it on the side opposite the loss.

BEHAVIOR AUDIOMETRY

Audiometry typically consists of a battery of tests, the differential results of which provide site-of-lesion information.[20]

It typically begins with pure-tone threshold testing to compare a subject's hearing sensitivity to norms at selected frequencies (the audiogram).

The Audiogram

Pure tones are defined by their frequency and their intensity. In order to quantify the magnitude of hearing loss, normal hearing levels have been established. These levels approximate the intensity of the faintest sounds that can be heard by normal ears. A patient's hearing level (HL) is the difference in decibel (dB) between the faintest pure tone that the patient can hear and the normal reference level given by the standard, where zero dB HL is the sound pressure level (SPL) at which listeners with normal hearing are able to perceive the signal 50 percent of the time. Brief duration tones at selected frequencies are presented by earphones (air conduction) and a vibrator pressed against the mastoid portion of the temporal bone (bone conduction). The results of air and bone conduction testing are plotted on a

graph from which the magnitude of the sensitivity loss (in dB) as a function of frequency is determined (Fig. 8–1).

With a conductive hearing loss, air conduction is impaired while bone conduction remains normal (i.e., an air-bone gap on the audiogram, Fig. 8–1, right ear). Measurement of bone conduction requires careful masking of the nontest ear. Masking involves introducing loud airborne noise into the nontest ear to eliminate cross-hearing via bone conduction. There is less than a 5 dB attenuation between the two ears for a bone conduction receiver placed on any part of the skull.[12] Therefore, a nonhearing ear may appear to have nearly normal hearing via bone conduction if the normal ear is not properly masked. The best masking sound for pure tones is a narrow band of white noise centered about the pure tone being tested.

Lesions producing sensorineural hearing loss impair both air and bone conduction, often with changing pure tone levels at different frequencies. Although the audiogram does not provide specific diagnostic information to identify the site of lesion, certain patterns suggest specific

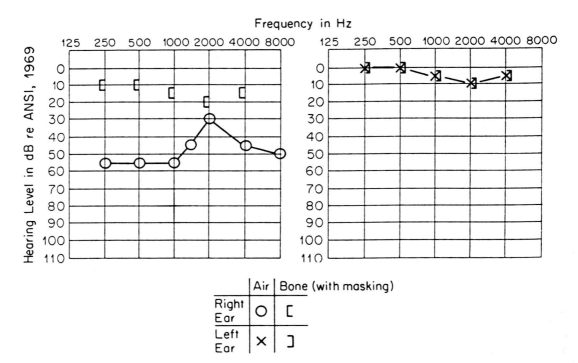

Figure 8–1. Pure tone audiogram: left ear, normal; right ear, conductive hearing loss due to otosclerosis.

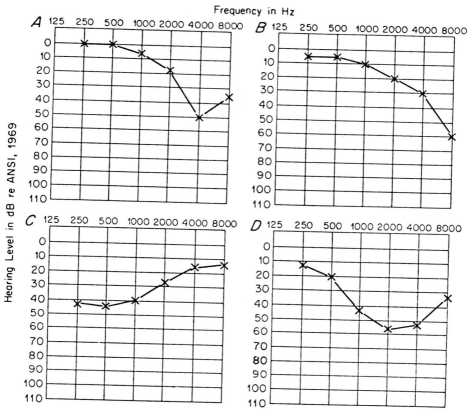

Figure 8–2. Audiograms illustrating four common patterns of sensorineural hearing loss. (*A*) Notched pattern of noise induced hearing loss. (*B*) Downward sloping pattern of presbycusis. (*C*) Low frequency trough of Meniere's syndrome. (*D*) V-pattern of congenital hearing loss.

diagnoses. Typical audiograms seen in patients with four common causes of sensorineural hearing loss are shown in Figure 8–2. None of these patterns is pathognomonic of a given disorder, but they occur often enough to be of diagnostic value.

Speech Recognition Tests

Two categories of tests are used to determine the patient's ability to hear and understand speech: (1) the speech reception threshold and (2) speech discrimination.

The *speech reception threshold* (SRT) is the intensity at which the patient can correctly repeat 50 percent of highly familiar two-syllable words (e.g., airplane, cowboy, sidewalk). The SRT is an estimate of the minimum level of conversation that a person can hear. It provides a check on the va-

lidity of the pure-tone audiogram, inasmuch as it should agree (±5 dB) with an average of the two best pure-tone thresholds in the speech range (500 to 2000 Hz). It is not a test of discrimination, but it does provide information about a patient's ability to recognize and respond to speech. Occasionally, a patient who is profoundly deaf or aphasic cannot repeat words. In such cases a speech detection threshold (SDT) is obtained by having the patient respond to a speech signal. SRT and SDT measurements are particularly useful in young children and infants because they will give an accurate reliable measurement of hearing for speech in just a few minutes.

The *speech discrimination test* is a measure of the patient's ability to understand speech when it is presented at a level that is easily heard. For this test, the patient is usually presented with 50 phonetically balanced monosyllabic words at a comfortable listening level. Each word is presented with a carrier phrase such as "you will say _____" or "say the word _____." The test is scored as a percentage of the correct responses (e.g., 49 out of 50 correct equals 98 percent speech discrimination). In patients with eighth nerve lesions, speech discrimination can be severely reduced even when pure-tone levels are normal or near normal, whereas in patients with cochlear lesions discrimination tends to be proportional to the magnitude of hearing loss.[16]

Evaluation of *rollover* using suprathreshold speech recognition testing can be a sensitive test for retrocochlear lesions. For this test one compares the percentage of words correct for increasing intensities of sound pressure level. In normal subjects, performance increases with increasing intensity, reaching a maximum at about 40 dB HL. In normal subjects performance remains at about the same level with increasing intensity, but there is a drop in performance at higher intensities in patients with retrocochlear lesions. Rollover is quantified as the difference between the percentage of words correct at maximum performance and the lowest score obtained at higher intensities. Differences greater than 20 percent are considered suggestive of retrocochlear involvement.[15]

Loudness Tests

The *alternate binaural loudness balance* (ABLB) test provides a direct measurement of loudness recruitment if the hearing loss is unilateral. A short-duration tone is presented alternately to each ear. The intensity of the tone to one ear is fixed, but the intensity to the other ear is adjusted until the listener perceives the loudness of the two tones to be equal. Recruitment of loudness is present if the patient requires a smaller intensity increase (above threshold in quiet) in the hearing-impaired ear than is required in the better hearing ear to achieve equal loudness between the two ears.

For the *short-increment sensitivity index* (SISI) subjects signal when they detect a change in a steady state tone, on which a

1 dB increment of 200 milliseconds duration is superimposed every 5 seconds. The score is the percentage of correct detections in 20 trials. High scores on the SISI (greater than 70 percent) and recruitment on the ABLB suggest a cochlear loss.[25] These findings do not exclude the possibility of retrocochlear involvement as well, however.

Tone Decay

Tests for tone decay attempt to measure abnormal neural adaptation manifested by a reversible decline in hearing sensitivity in the presence of a sustained tone. A stimulus is presented continuously either near threshold or at suprathreshold levels, and the examiner records the length of time the stimulus is audible to the patient. The suprathreshold test is thought to be more sensitive, inasmuch as high intensities cause greater stress on neural mechanisms. The patient is instructed to signal as long as he or she can hear a sustained tone at 500, 1000, or 2000 Hz, presented at 110 dB SPL for 1 minute, with appropriate contralateral masking. Adaptation or tone decay during this time is considered a positive retrocochlear sign. Rapid tone decay and abnormal findings at multiple frequencies further strengthen the impression of retrocochlear involvement.

Stenger Test

The Stenger test is helpful for determining whether a patient is deliberately exaggerating or feigning a hearing loss. It is based on the psychophysical observation that a tone presented to both ears in the same phase at different intensities above threshold is perceived only in the ear with better hearing. Tones are presented simultaneously to both good and suspect ears. The signals are turned on together and the patient is asked to respond as long as the tone is on. As long as the tone is below the actual threshold in the suspect ear the patient will hear the sound in the other ear and respond. If the tone in the suspect ear is then increased above its true threshold the patient will either fail to respond or show confusion, being unaware of the sound in the good ear and not wanting the examiner to know that he hears the sound in the suspect ear. Although screening tests are usually done at one intensity, a more complete test can be done at multiple intensities or using the same procedure with spondee words. Of course, the Stenger test works only with a unilateral loss, inasmuch as a minimum 20 dB threshold difference is required at the test frequency.[21]

IMPEDANCE AUDIOMETRY

Impedance may be defined as the resistance of a given system to the flow of energy. *Acoustic impedance* refers to the resistance of the middle ear system to the passage of sound. Its reciprocal, *acoustic compliance*, refers to the ease of sound transmission through the middle ear system. In simplified terms, acoustic impedance indicates the stiffness of the middle ear conduction system, whereas acoustic compliance describes the mobility or springiness of the same system. Acoustic impedance measurements are based on the principle that energy that is not absorbed by the ear is reflected.[30] By measuring the difference between the intensity of a sound going into the external auditory canal and that reflected from the tympanic membrane, one can estimate the impedance (or compliance) of the middle ear system.

Acoustic impedance measurements are made by a probe tip hermetically inserted into the ear canal. The probe tip contains three openings: (1) one for air pressure generation and measurement, (2) one for probe tone generation, and (3) one for pickup of sound waves reflected off the tympanic membrane. A schematic drawing of the impedance measurement system is shown in Figure 8–3. With this system the difference between generated and reflected sound is systematically measured at different external ear pressure levels.

Static Impedance Measurements

Static impedance measurements are made when the middle ear system is most compliant; that is, when the air pressure in the canal matches the static pressure in

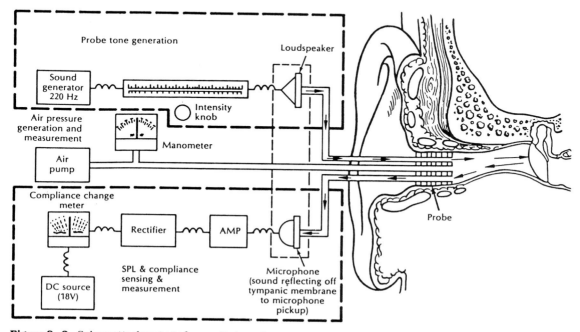

Figure 8–3. Schematic drawing of acoustic impedance measuring system. (See text for details.) (From Goodhill, V: Ear Diseases, Deafness and Dizziness. Harper & Row, Hagerstown, 1979, with permission.)

the middle ear cavity. The normal middle ear and tympanic membrane offer relatively low acoustic impedance, implying that appreciable energy is absorbed and transmitted through the middle ear. If the middle ear contains fluid, or if the tympanic membrane is sclerotic, acoustic impedance is increased and the transmission capability is diminished; that is, the static compliance is decreased. An increase in acoustic impedance can also result from a decrease in flexibility of the ossicular chain, an increase in its mass, or an increase in friction during ossicular movement. An ossicular chain discontinuity causes a decrease in acoustic impedance, because the mass and friction decrease. Unfortunately, acoustic impedance and static compliance measurements rarely provide critical diagnostic information inasmuch as the range of normal values is large and there is overlap in values for different otologic disorders.[19]

Tympanometry

Tympanometry is a method for evaluating changes in acoustic impedance by producing systematic changes in air pressure in the external ear canal. A plot of compliance change versus air pressure (the tympanogram) is made by first introducing a positive pressure into the external canal (usually equivalent to +200 mm of water) and then decreasing the pressure to approximately −200 mm of water (although the negative range can be extended to −600 mm of water). As the pressure is changed, compliance will change if the conduction system is normal. The shape of the normal tympanogram resembles a teepee (Fig. 8−4). The peak of the teepee represents the point of maximum compliance at which the air pressure in the middle ear equals the air pressure in the external auditory canal. Tympanometry can provide useful information about (1) mobility of the tympanic membrane, (2) perforations of the tympanic membrane, (3) pressure within the middle ear, and (4) patency and dynamic function of the eustachian tubes. Artifactual responses can result from inappropriate placement of the probe (against the canal wall or into impacted cerumen) or due to an inadequate seal.

Four characteristic abnormal tympanographic patterns should be recognized (see Fig. 8−4).[19, 22] A *restricted* tympanogram implies normal middle ear pressure and limited compliance relative to normal mobility. It is typically seen in advanced cases of otosclerosis, lateral fixation of the ossicular chain, tympanic membrane fibrosis, and middle ear tympanosclerosis. A *hypermobile* tympanogram indicates a flaccid

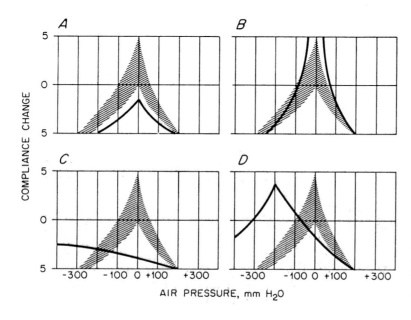

Figure 8−4. Four characteristic abnormal tympanograms. (*A*) Restricted. (*B*) Hypermobile. (*C*) Flat. (*D*) Retracted. *Striped area*, normal range.

tympanic membrane. It occurs with ossicular chain discontinuity and with partial atrophy of the tympanic membrane. A *flat* tympanogram means that there is little or no change in middle ear compliance when ear pressure is varied in the external ear canal. This pattern is more commonly seen with serous otitis media but can also be seen with congenital malformations of the middle ear and occlusion of the external ear canal by cerumen, epithelium, and foreign bodies. Finally, with a *retracted* tympanogram the maximum compliance occurs at negative pressures greater than −100 mm of water. It implies a negative middle ear pressure with a retracted tympanic membrane. This pattern is most commonly seen with poor eustachian tube function.

The Acoustic Reflex

The acoustic reflex refers to contraction of the stapedius muscle in response to a loud sound. It is measured by monitoring the change in acoustic impedance in response to a loud sound introduced into either ear. The stapedius muscle contracts bilaterally, regardless of which ear is stimulated. Contraction of the stapedius muscle produces stiffening of the tympanic membrane and thus an increase in acoustic impedance. This results in an attenuation of sound transmitted to the cochlea by about 10 dB. In a normal subject the acoustic reflex will be observed when a pure-tone signal is presented between 70 and 100 dB above hearing level (median value 82 dB), and when a white noise stimulus is presented at 65 dB above hearing level.[14]

The stimulus sound can be presented to either the contralateral ear or to the ear with the recording probe tip. In the former case, one tests the contralateral eighth nerve, brainstem crossover pathways, and the ipsilateral seventh nerve and middle ear system. In the latter case, one tests the ipsilateral eighth nerve, ipsilateral brainstem connections, and the ipsilateral seventh nerve and middle ear system. By systematically presenting the stimulus sound to each ear and recording with the probe tip in each ear, the location of a lesion within the reflex pathway can be isolated. The results of acoustic reflex testing in patients with four different common unilateral lesions are summarized in Table 8–1.

Patients with conductive hearing loss often have an absent acoustic reflex because the lesion prevents a change in compliance with stapedius muscle contraction. An air-bone gap as small as 5 dB may obscure the acoustic reflex.[17] The acoustic reflex is particularly useful for identifying the site of lesion for different types of sensorineural hearing loss. With cochlear lesions the acoustic reflex often can be demonstrated at a sensation level less than 60 dB above the auditory pure-tone threshold. This is another form of abnormal loudness growth or recruitment. A cochlear hearing loss must be severe before the acoustic reflex is lost. An absent reflex is rarely associated with a cochlear hearing loss less than 50 dB, and only when the hearing loss exceeds 85 dB is the reflex absent in 50 percent of patients.[18] By contrast, patients with eighth nerve lesions often have either

Table 8–1. PATTERN OF ACOUSTIC REFLEX MEASUREMENTS WITH UNILATERAL LESIONS

| | Stimulus Presented: | C* | I | C | I |
	Reflex Measured:	I†	C	C	I
Type of Lesion					
Conductive (>30 dB HL)		−	−	+	−
Cochlear (<85 dB HL)		+	+	+	+
VIII nerve		+	−	+	−
VII nerve		−	+	+	−

*Contralateral to lesion.
†Ipsilateral to lesion.
+ = reflex present.
− = reflex absent.

normal hearing or only mildly impaired hearing (less than 20 dB), yet they have an abnormal acoustic reflex. The reflex may be absent, exhibit an elevated threshold, or exhibit abnormal decay. Reflex decay is present if the amplitude decreases to one half of its original size within 10 seconds of tonal stimulation. The acoustic reflex is abnormal in approximately 80 percent of patients with surgically documented acoustic neuromas.[29]

AUDITORY-EVOKED RESPONSES

The advent of averaging computers has made it possible to collect and analyze a variety of evoked electrical potentials from the auditory system.[9] Repetitive sounds are delivered to the external ear and an "averaged" series of specific brain wave potentials are recorded with disk electrodes for up to 500 milliseconds after signal onset. The latencies (re: signal onset) of each of the potentials are used as the most reliable means by which generator sources for the potentials are identified. Electrical events in the cochlea (so-called electrocochleography) can best be monitored by an electrode inside the external canal or from a transtympanic electrode on the cochlear promontory.[27, 31] A series of waves in the first 5 milliseconds after the stimulus reflects the cochlear microphonics and the compound cochlear action potential (Fig. 8–5).[32] Other evoked potentials from the auditory nerve and central nervous system (CNS) can be recorded with differential scalp electrodes. One electrode is placed at the vertex (the positive electrode) and another on the earlobe or mastoid (the negative electrode) ipsilateral to the acoustic stimulation. A third electrode (contralateral mastoid or earlobe) serves as the ground. Acoustic signals are presented via earphones, or bone vibrator and responses are amplified, filtered, and averaged. The early (0 to 10 millisecond) evoked responses reflect the far field representation of electrical events generated at points from the periphery (eighth nerve action potential) to the level of the brainstem. The five to seven waves in the first 10 milliseconds are referred to as the brainstem-evoked response. The

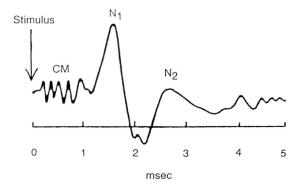

Figure 8–5. Electrical responses of the cochlea. An electrode near the round window records the cochlear microphonic potential (*CM*) and a compound action potential (N_1 and N_2). (Adapted from Sohmer, H and Feinmesser, M: Electrocochleography in clinical audiological diagnosis. Arch Oto-Rhino-Laryngol [Berl] 1974, 206:91.)

middle latency responses (12 to 50 milliseconds) have received less systematic study but probably reflect electrical activity in the upper brainstem and in the primary and nearby secondary auditory projection areas. The late evoked responses (50 to 300 milliseconds) reflect cortical electrical activity.

Electrocochleography

Up to the present, this technique has been most useful for identifying cochlear responses in infants or in very young children who are unable to cooperate with behavioral testing.[12, 27] A rough estimate of the cochlear response at multiple frequencies and intensities can be obtained. Of course, the presence of these responses does not indicate that the subject actually "hears" but rather documents that electrical activity is being generated within the cochlea. The presence of cochlear microphonics and summating potentials (see Fig. 8–5) in the absence of a compound action potential suggests a denervated cochlea. Electrocochleography is useful in conjunction with brainstem auditory-evoked responses in adults when one is attempting to identify whether a hearing loss is cochlear or retrocochlear. The presence of a normal electrocochleogram in a patient with an absent brainstem auditory-evoked response suggests a retrocochlear lesion. Absence of both can occur with either cochlear or retrocochlear lesions.

Brainstem Auditory-Evoked Response (BAER)

As noted above, the BAER reflects the far field representation of electrical events occurring in the eighth nerve and brainstem. It is highly reproducible in a given subject, and the latency of the various waves shows little variation among normal subjects. With rare exceptions the BAER is not affected by inattention to the stimulus, alterations in the level of consciousness, or drugs. For this reason it can be used to test the integrity of the peripheral and brainstem auditory pathways in patients who cannot cooperate with subjective auditory testing (e.g., infants, comatose patients).

GENERATING POTENTIALS

A schematic drawing of a BAER and the neural centers that are thought to generate each component of the response is shown in Figure 8–6. Wave I (average latency 1.9 milliseconds) results from activation of the eighth nerve terminals within the cochlea, whereas the remainder of the waves are generated by the retrocochlear part of the eighth nerve and the brainstem auditory nuclei and pathways.[23, 33, 35] Although a useful working tool, this schematic electroanatomic correlation is an oversimplification. Clearly, each vertex positive and vertex negative potential after wave I reflects simultaneous activity in multiple brainstem loci. The more caudal generators— such as the eighth nerve, cochlear nuclei, and superior olivary complex—contribute to the response beyond waves II and III. By the time waves VI and VII appear, the summation of potentials

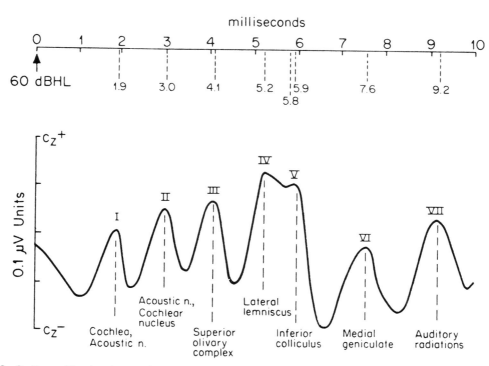

Figure 8–6. Normal brain stem auditory evoked response evoked by clicks of 60 dB HL (60 dB above normal hearing threshold) at a rate of 10 per second. Normal mean latencies for waves I through VII are shown on the time scale (the intermediate latency, 5.8 ms, between waves IV and V is the mean peak latency of a fused wave IV/V when present). The neural centers thought to be responsible for generating each wave are shown at the bottom. (Adapted from Stockard, JJ, Stockard, JE, Sharbrough, FW: Detection and localization of occult lesions with brain stem auditory responses. Mayo Clinic Proc 1977, 52:761.)

from the different neural centers is so complex that the concept of single principle contributors to individual waves no longer applies.

TEST METHODOLOGY

The standard stimulus for eliciting a BAER is a click caused by a very short (less than 1 millisecond) pulse. This signal produces a spectrally diffused acoustic stimulus, with most of the energy concentrated in the high frequencies (around 2000 Hz with most of the commercially available speakers). The absolute latency of the BAER waves is dependent on the intensity of the click stimulus. The BAERs to unfiltered clicks presented at various intensity levels from a normal subject are shown in Figure 8–7. Wave V is most robust, often being identifiable at only 10 dB above hearing level. At 60 dB above hearing level all waves are identifiable. Such latency-intensity functions provide a basis for estimating the degree of hearing loss in patients who cannot cooperate with standard pure-tone behavioral testing.[6, 8] On the other hand, because of this latency-intensity relationship BAERs must be interpreted with caution in patients with severe conductive or cochlear hearing loss (particularly if it involves high frequencies).

RESULTS IN PATIENTS

In practice, only waves I, III, and V are used to define response abnormalities.

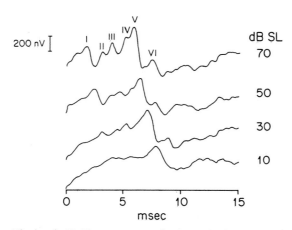

Figure 8–7. Brain stem auditory evoked responses in a normal subject induced by clicks at varying intensity levels (10 to 70 dB SL, sensation level).

Waves II, IV, VI, and VII are sufficiently variable in the normal population to preclude their routine use in defining response abnormalities on the basis of a single recording. Often waves IV and V fuse into a single complex, which is designated as wave IV/V. Because wave I disappears before wave IV/V with decreasing stimulus intensity (e.g., see Fig. 8–7), the absence of wave IV/V in the presence of wave I indicates a retrocochlear lesion. The absence of all waves, on the other hand, often reflects a peripheral lesion (conductive or cochlear) or a technical problem.[4, 35] If peak I occurs at normal latency, then prolongation of the I–III or I–IV/V interval indicates a lesion of the eighth nerve or brainstem.

In clinical neurotology BAERs have been most useful for (1) evaluation of the cause and reversibility of coma, (2) the diagnosis of multiple sclerosis (MS), and (3) the detection and localization of lesions involving the eighth nerve, particularly those in the cerebellopontine angle.[34] Because BAERs are relatively resistant to metabolic insults they can help differentiate between metabolic and structural causes of brainstem dysfunction. The presence of an intact BAER in a patient with global brainstem dysfunction on neurologic examination suggests the possibility of a metabolic, reversible cause of coma. On the other hand, the absence of waves III and/or V in the presence of wave I suggests widespread structural damage of the brainstem and implies a poor prognosis.[10, 11] The complete absence of a BAER may have a similar poor prognosis but requires more cautious interpretation, inasmuch as there may be other explanations for the lack of response (technical or otologic problems).

In patients suspected of having MS who present with lesions outside of the brainstem (e.g., optic nerve or spinal cord), an abnormal BAER supports the likely diagnosis.[26, 34] Obviously, if the initial lesion involves the brainstem, the finding of an abnormal BAER provides little additional information. Stockard and associates[34] studied the BAERs of 135 patients with possible MS who presented with clinical evidence of a single non-brainstem CNS lesion. Eighty-four had unilateral optic neuritis, and 51 had an acute or subacute thoracic or lumbar myelopathy with normal myelograms. The patients developed their symptoms and were tested between ages 21 and 46 years. They were predominantly women (91 females/44 males), and none had audiometric abnormalities or subjective auditory complaints. Of these patients, 31 (23 percent) had BAER abnormalities; of these, 15 (48 percent) developed clinically definite MS within 1 to 3 years. Of the 104 patients with normal BAERs, 13 (12 percent) developed definite MS over the same period of follow-up. Therefore, a patient with a single, non-brainstem CNS lesion who had an abnormal BAER was four times more likely to develop clinically definite MS than a similar patient with a normal BAER. It is important to note, however, that a normal initial BAER had no predictive value with regard to the subsequent development of MS.

BAERs have been particularly useful for the early detection of acoustic neuromas. Abnormal BAERs occur in approximately 95 percent of surgically proven cases.[3, 24, 34] Furthermore, an abnormal BAER can be found in the presence of normal or nearly normal pure-tone hearing. The most common abnormality overall is absence of all waves beyond wave I. The next most common is absence of all waves including wave I (helpful only if electrocochleography shows normal cochlear responses). When both waves I and III are present, the most common abnormality is prolongation of the I–III interwave interval (Fig. 8–8). Large cerebellopontine (CP) angle tumors compressing the brainstem often lead to abnormalities in the contralateral BAER. Prolongation of the III–V interwave interval in the face of a normal I–III wave interval is the most common finding.

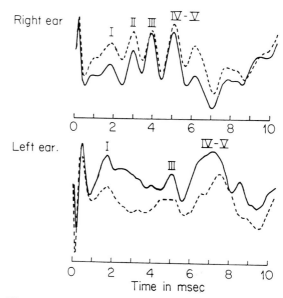

Figure 8–8. Brain stem auditory evoked responses in a patient with a left acoustic neuroma. *Dashed lines* indicate repeat test. Wave I occurs at normal latency on both sides, but the I–III and I–V intervals are prolonged on the left side.

CENTRAL AUDITORY SPEECH TESTS

Patients with lesions of the central auditory pathways usually have normal pure-tone hearing levels. Routine speech tests are also usually normal because speech contains a great deal of redundancy. Within the central auditory pathways, redundancy is enhanced by the multiple crossings and interactions. One of the few diagnostically useful central audiologic findings is the reduced ability of patients with temporal lobe lesions to discriminate speech in the ear contralateral to the lesion when the task is complicated by distorting the speech.[2] Apparently, by making the speech less redundant, heavier demands are placed on the integrating, synthesizing function of the auditory cortex.

There are several varieties of central auditory speech tests currently in use, each involving methods of presenting distorted speech. Portions of the frequency spectrum of speech can be filtered, the speech can be time compressed, it can be presented at very low intensties, and the speech can be interrupted at irregular intervals. Dichotic stimulation involves presenting two different messages to each ear.[7] Both monosyllabic and spondee words can be used. As with distorted speech tests, when a temporal lobe lesion exists, the ear contralateral to the lesion performs poorer than the ear ipsilateral to the lesion.

SUMMARY OF AUDITORY TEST RESULTS

Hearing loss for pure tones is typically divided into conductive and sensorineural;

Table 8–2. SUMMARY OF AUDITORY TEST RESULTS WITH LESIONS AT DIFFERENT LOCATIONS

| Test | Conductive | Sensorineural | | Central |
		Cochlea	Nerve	
Speech discrimination	N	Relatively preserved	Abnormal early, rollover	N
Tympanometry	Abn: restricted, hypermobile, flat	N	N	N
Stapedius reflex	Absent	N	Absent or decay	N
BAER	N	N	Absent, delayed I–III, I–V	Delayed III–V
Special tests	—	Loudness recruitment	Tone decay	Dichotic listening, alternating speech, filtered speech

N = Normal.

central lesions rarely produce such hearing loss (Table 8–2). Conductive and sensorineural loss can usually be differentiated with an audiogram based on the finding of an air-bone gap with the former and a characteristic frequency intensity profile with the latter. The causes of a conductive hearing loss can be differentiated with tympanometry. There are several test results that help distinguish between a cochlear and retrocochlear sensorineural hearing loss. Speech discrimination is relatively preserved with a cochlear loss, whereas it is impaired early and there may be a roll-over at higher intensities with a sensorineural loss. Loudness recruitment is commonly seen with a cochlear loss, whereas tone decay is a common feature of a sensorineural loss. Abnormalities of the stapedius reflex and brainstem auditory-evoked response provide an objective differentiation between cochlear and retrocochlear lesions. These measurements remain normal unless there is profound cochlear hearing loss, but they are usually abnormal with only mild to moderate hearing loss due to nerve damage. Central hearing disorders may show abnormalities of the late waves of the BAER or of cortical-evoked responses or in discriminating speech when the task is complicated by distorting the content of the speech.

REFERENCES

1. Beagley, HA (ed): Audiology and Audiologic Medicine. Oxford University Press, New York, 1981.
2. Berlin, C, Lowe-Bell, S, Janetta, P, and Kline, D:
   Central auditory deficits after temporal lobectomy. Arch Otolaryngol 96:4, 1972.
3. Clemis, JD and McGee, T: Brain stem electric response audiometry in the differential diagnosis of acoustic tumors. Laryngoscope 89:31, 1979.
4. Coats, AC: Human auditory nerve action potentials and brain stem evoked responses. Arch Otolaryngol 104:799, 1978.
5. Davis, H and Silverman, SR (eds): Hearing and Deafness, ed. 4. Holt, Rinehart, and Winston, New York, 1978.
6. Davis, H: Principles of electric response audiometry. Ann Otol Rhinol Laryngol (Suppl) 28:1, 1976.
7. Denes, G and Cariezel, F: Dichotic listening in crossed aphasia. Arch Neurol 38:182, 1981.
8. Don, M, Eggermont, JJ, and Brachmann, DE: Reconstruction of the audiogram using brain stem responses and high-pass noise masking. Ann Otol Rhinol Laryngol (Suppl 57) 88:1, 1979.
9. Galambos, R: Electrophysiological measurement of human auditory function. In Eagles, EL (ed): Human Communication and Its Disorders, Vol 3. Raven Press, New York, 1975.
10. Goldie, WD, Chiappa, KH, Young, RR, and Brooks, EB: Brain stem auditory and short somatosensory evoked responses in brain death. Neurology 31:248, 1981.
11. Hall, JW, Mackey-Hargadine, JR, and Kim, EE: Auditory brain stem response in determination of brain death. Arch Otolaryngol 111:613, 1985.
12. Heffernan, HP, Simons, MR, and Goodhill, V: Audiologic assessment, functional hearing loss and objective audiometry. In Goodhill, V (ed): Ear Diseases, Deafness and Dizziness. Harper & Row, Hagerstown, MD, 1979.
13. Jaffee, BF (ed): Hearing Loss in Children. University Park Press, Baltimore, 1977.
14. Jepson, O: Middle ear muscle reflexes in man. In Jerger, J (ed): Modern Developments in Audiology. Academic Press, New York, 1963.
15. Jerger, J and Hayes, D: Diagnostic speech audiometry. Arch Otolaryngol 103:216, 1977.
16. Jerger, J and Jerger, S: Diagnostic significance

of PB word functions. Arch Otolaryngol 93:573, 1971.

17. Jerger, J, et al: Studies in impedance audiometry. III. Middle ear disorders. Arch Otolaryngol 99:165, 1974.

18. Jerger, J, Jerger, S, and Maulden, L: Studies in impedance audiometry. I. Normal and S-N ears. Arch Otolaryngol 96:513, 1972.

19. Jerger, J: Clinical experience with impedance audiometry. Arch Otolaryngol 92:311, 1970.

20. Katz, J (ed): Handbook of Clinical Audiology, ed 2. Williams & Wilkins, Baltimore, 1977.

21. Kintsler, DP, Phelan, JG, and Lavender, RB: Efficiency of the Stenger and speech Stenger tests in functional hearing loss, Audiology 11:187, 1972.

22. Liden, G, Pederson, JL, and Bjorkman, G: Tympanometry. Arch Otolaryngol 92:248, 1970.

23. Møller, AR, Janetta, PJ, and Møller, MB: Neural generators of brain stem evoked potentials. Results from human intracranial recordings. Ann Otol Rhinol Laryngol 90:591, 1981.

24. Musiek, FE, Josey, AF, and Glasscock, ME: Auditory brain stem response in patients with acoustic neuromas. Wave presence and absence. Arch Otolaryngol 112:186, 1986.

25. Owens, E: Differential intensity discrimination. In Rintelman, WF (ed): Hearing Assessment. University Park Press, Baltimore, 1979.

26. Paludetti, G, et al: Auditory brain stem responses (ABR) in multiple sclerosis. Scand Audiol 14:27, 1985.

27. Portmann, M: Electrocochleography. J Laryngol 91:665, 1977.

28. Schuknecht, HL: Pathology of the Ear. Harvard University Press, Cambridge, MA, 1974.

29. Sheehy, JL and Inzer, BE: Acoustic reflex test in neurotologic diagnosis. Arch Otolaryngol 102:647, 1976.

30. Simons, MR: Acoustic impedance tests. In Goodhill, V (ed): Ear Diseases, Deafness and Dizziness. Harper & Row, Hagerstown, MD, 1979.

31. Sohmer, H and Feinmesser, M: Cochlear action potentials recorded from the external ear in man. Ann Otol Rhinol Laryngol 76:427, 1967.

32. Sohmer, H and Feinmesser, M: Electrocochleography in clinical audiological diagnosis. Arch Oto-Rhino-Laryngol (Berlin) 206:91, 1974.

33. Starr, A and Hamilton, AE: Correlation between confirmed sites of neurological lesions and abnormalities of far-field auditory brain stem responses. Electroencephalography Clin Neurophysiol 41:595, 1976.

34. Stockard, JJ, Stockard, JE, and Sharbrough, FW: Brain stem auditory evoked potentials in Neurology: Methodology, interpretation, and clinical application. In Aminoff, MJ (ed): Electrodiagnosis in Clinical Neurology. Churchill Livingstone, New York, 1986; p 467.

35. Stockard, JJ, Stockard, JE, and Sharbrough, FW: Detection and localization of occult lesions with brain stem auditory responses. Mayo Clinic Proc 52:761, 1977.

ذ

Part III

DIAGNOSIS AND MANAGEMENT OF COMMON NEUROTOLOGIC DISORDERS

Chapter 9

INFECTIOUS DISORDERS

OTITIS MEDIA

Inflammation of the middle ear (otitis media) is a common cause of conductive hearing loss, particularly in children. Either infected (suppurative otitis) or noninfected (serous otitis) fluid accumulates in the middle ear, impairing conduction of airborne sound. Because the air cavity of the middle ear is in direct communication with the mastoid air cells, infection can spread throughout the pneumatized parts of the temporal bone. Typical patterns of progression of middle ear infections are summarized in Figure 9–1.

Pathophysiology

The middle ear is involved with most viral upper respiratory tract infections. The nasal, paranasal, and pharyngeal mucositis spreads to involve the eustachian tube and middle ear mucosa, producing a tubotympanitis. As noted in Chapter 1, the mucosa of the pharyngeal end of the eu-

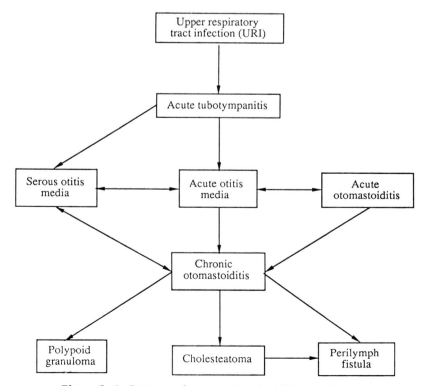

Figure 9–1. Patterns of progression of middle ear infections.

stachian tube is continuous with the mucociliary system of the middle ear. This tubotympanitis is usually transitory and subsides without sequela. In a small percentage of cases, however, a secondary bacterial suprainfection occurs. Eighty percent of children between the ages of 1 and 6 years have at least one bout of acute otitis media.[7] It is the most common disease treated with antibiotics in the United States. The symptoms typically include unilateral otalgia, fever, and hearing loss. The peak incidence occurs during the first year of life, reaching an incidence rate of almost 50 percent and then gradually decreasing to an incidence rate less than 10 percent beyond age 8. With acute otitis media the tympanic membrane initially appears hyperemic and then bulges outward due to the accumulation of purulent exudate within the middle ear. Often spontaneous perforation occurs, allowing the purulent effusion to drain into the external ear. With prompt antibiotic therapy the effusion is rapidly cleared of inflammatory cells, but a serous or mucinous effusion can persist for months.

Serous otitis media often follows acute otitis media although in about a third of cases there is no previous history of acute infection.[42] Fever and constitutional symptoms are typically absent. Unlike acute bacterial otitis media, serous otitis media reaches its peak incidence between ages 5 and 7. Abnormalities in eustachian tube function have long been implicated in the pathogenesis of serous otitis media. It has been suggested that mechanical or functional obstruction of the eustachian tube leads to absorption of gas within the middle ear and a resultant transudation of serous fluid into the middle ear cleft. This theory is supported by the common observation that eustachian tube blockage leads to accumulation of serous fluid in the middle ear. However, other factors, including allergy and chronic infection, probably also play a role.[7, 42]

Diagnosis and Management

The diagnosis of acute otitis media rests on finding the characteristic changes in the tympanic membrane in a patient complaining of acute otalgia and hearing loss. The most common organisms associated with acute otitis media are *Streptococcus pneumoniae* and *Hemophilus influenza*.[27] Once the clinical diagnosis is made, empiric therapy with either ampicillin or amoxicillin is initiated.[4] If the infection fails to resolve within a few days, a myringotomy can be performed to obtain material for culture, and a second antibiotic is started (typically cefaclor to cover the ampicillin-resistant strains of *H. influenza*). The antibiotics are then adjusted based on the results of culture.

Serous otitis media is more difficult to diagnose because constitutional symptoms are usually absent and changes in the tympanic membrane are more subtle. The normal translucent appearance of the tympanic membrane is lost, and the membrane may be retracted and the middle ear, atelectatic. Impaired mobility of the tympanic membrane during pneumatic otoscopy is the most useful diagnostic sign with this disorder. Tympanometry can complement the otoscopic examination, often showing a flat tympanogram (see Fig. 8–4). Decongestants and antihistamines have long been used for the prevention and treatment of serous otitis media although a recent placebo-controlled double-blind study did not support their efficacy.[6] Some physicians recommend an initial course of antibiotics, such as amoxicillin or trimethoprim/sulfamethoxazole, even though many cases are not associated with infection. If the serous effusion persists beyond 2 to 3 months, a myringotomy with insertion of a ventilating tube is recommended.[7, 42]

CHRONIC OTOMASTOIDITIS

Pathophysiology

Chronic otomastoiditis results from an untreated or nonresponsive acute otomastoiditis or serous otitis media.[5, 7] Pathology is characterized by thickened edematous mucosa with obliteration of the mastoid air cell lumen, perivascular fibrosis, and osteitis. Chronic obstruction of the mastoid antrum leads to irreversible changes in the mucosa and bone of the mastoid. *Polypoid granulomas* composed of hyperplastic mucosa may fill the mastoid antrum, extend into the middle ear, and extrude through a tympanic membrane perforation into the external auditory canal. Keratinized squamous epithelium *(cholesteatoma)* can invade the middle ear and other pneumatized areas of the temporal bone through the typanic membrane. The term cholesteatoma is a misnomer because it neither contains cholesterol nor is a neoplasm. Cholesteatomas usually develop in the epitympanic space after penetrating a perforation in the pars flaccida region of the tympanic membrane (see Fig. 5–1). From here they extend posteriorly into the antrum, into the central mastoid tract, or inferiorly into the middle ear to erode the ossicles and bony labyrinth, producing a mixed conductive sensorineural hearing loss and vertigo. The mechanism by which a cholesteatoma erodes bone is not entirely clear, but it is not a simple pressure necrosis. Ultrastructural studies in humans and experimental studies in animals suggest that the bone resorption is caused primarily by activation of multinucleated osteoclasts on the bone.[8] Ultimately, a cholesteatoma may erode through the temporal bone into the intracranial cavity, producing central nervous system (CNS) symptoms and signs.

Cholesteatomas are prone to recurrent infection, because they contain keratin debris enclosed in a tissue space. The bacteria seen with chronic cholesteatomas are different from those seen with acute otitic infections, with the most common aerobe being *Pseudomonas aeruginosa* and the most common anaerobe being bacteroides.[33] When acutely infected, cholesteatomas can rapidly cause bone destruction. With chronic otomastoiditis and cholesteatoma formation a *fistula* may develop in the bony labyrinth, producing an artificial communication between the perilymph and the middle ear.[29] The fistula can be caused by either progressive rarefying osteitis or erosion by the cholesteatoma. Patients with a perilymph fistula experience incapacitating episodes of vertigo when they sneeze or cough because the sudden

change of pressure in the middle ear is transmitted directly to the inner ear.

Diagnosis

Patients with chronic otomastoiditis typically present with painless purulent otorrhea. Otoscopic examination of the tympanic membrane may reveal evidence of a perforation, particularly in the pars flaccida region, and a cholesteatoma or granuloma may be visible in the epitympanic region of the middle ear. The otoscopic appearance of a cholesteatoma can be quite variable. The typical attic retraction cholesteatoma appears as a "pearly tumor" in the posterior superior portion of the tympanic membrane. In other cases, a cholesteatoma develops at the margin of a perforation and migrates into the middle ear. Cholesteatomas sometimes appear behind or within an intact tympanic membrane (so-called primary cholesteatomas). Rarely, a cholesteatoma is not seen otoscopically but is discovered at the time of mastoid surgery. A perilymph fistula can be identified on examination by transiently changing the pressure in the external canal using a pneumatic bulb attached to the otoscope (see Fistula test, Chapter 5). With a positive fistula test the patient develops vertigo and nystagmus lasting 10 to 20 seconds. The nystagmus can be in either direction but usually is in the same direction with both positive and negative pressure. Computerized tomography (CT) scanning of the temporal bone may reveal a nonpneumatized or poorly pneumatized mastoid, haziness of air spaces, or bony erosion from a cholesteatoma or osteitis. (Fig. 9–2). One can also identify erosion of the bony wall of the horizontal semicircular canal or the facial canal.

Management

Initial management is directed at medical treatment of the chronic infection.[29, 33] Chronic otomastoiditis that is unresponsive to medical management requires surgical eradication of all diseased tissue. A complete transcortical mastoidectomy is

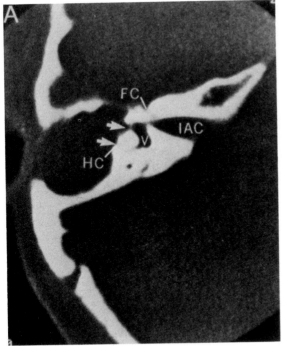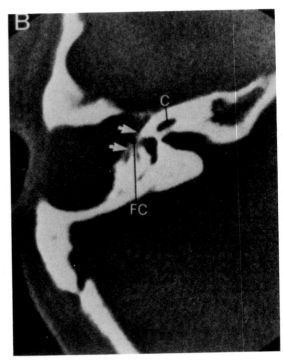

Figure 9—2. CT scan of the temporal bone in a patient with a cholesteatoma eroding the wall of the horizontal semicircular canal *(A)* and the facial canal *(B)*. *Arrows* point toward area of bony erosion. *FC*, facial canal; *HC*, horizontal semicircular canal; *V*, vestibule; *IAC*, internal auditory canal.

performed with attention to establishing good communication from the mastoid into the middle ear space. A bony fistula requires microsurgical removal of the lesion and closure with either perichondrium or fascia.

BACTERIAL LABYRINTHITIS

Pathophysiology

Labyrinthitis refers to an inflammatory process of the labyrinth. The inflammation may involve primarily the bony or membranous labyrinth, but for symptoms to occur the membranous labyrinth and its contents must be involved. Bacterial infections initially affect the otic capsule from which they extend into the perilymphatic space and ultimately involve the membranous labyrinth. By contrast, viral infections initially affect the membranous labyrinth, presumably by hematogenous spread. There are two types of labyrinthitis

associated with acute and chronic bacterial infections of the temporal bone: (1) serous or toxic labyrinthitis, in which bacterial toxins or chemical products invade the inner ear; and (2) suppurative labyrinthitis, in which bacteria invade the inner ear.[45] The former often leads to only subtle symptoms such as an insidious high-frequency sensorineural hearing loss, whereas the latter typically leads to a profound combined auditory and vestibular loss with little or no recovery.

Serous labyrinthitis is probably the single most common complication of acute or chronic middle ear infections. With acute otitis media small molecules such as bacterial toxins and enzymes rapidly diffuse through the round window into the scala tympani. Acute and chronic inflammatory cells also infiltrate the round window, and a fine serofibrinous precipitate forms just medial to the round window membrane. The toxins and/or inflammatory cells may penetrate the basilar membrane and invade the endolymph at the basal turn of the cochlea. Such changes could explain the high incidence of high-frequency sensorineural hearing loss in patients with chronic otitis media.[36] A more rapid onset of serous labyrinthitis results in a more complete sensorineural hearing loss along with vestibular symptoms including episodic vertigo and unsteadiness.

Acute suppurative labyrinthitis has become relatively rare since the introduction of antibiotics, but it produces a clinical syndrome that should be easily recognized. Symptoms include the sudden onset of severe vertigo, nausea, vomiting, and unilateral hearing loss. The infection originates either in the middle ear or in the cerebrospinal fluid (CSF). When the labyrinthitis is a direct complication from middle ear disease it is more likely to occur from chronic otitis media and mastoiditis than from acute middle ear infection. The most common port of entry of bacteria into the inner ear, however, is from the spinal fluid in patients with meningitis (which may or may not be a complication of middle ear infection).[33] Patients with bacterial meningitis develop labyrinthitis when bacteria enter the perilymphatic space by way of the cochlear aqueduct or internal auditory canal. Meningogenic bacterial labyrinthitis is usually bilateral, whereas direct invasion from a chronic otitic infection is almost always unilateral. The most common route for a direct bacterial invasion of the labyrinth is via a horizontal semicircular canal fistula from a cholesteatoma. Endolymphatic hydrops can be a sequela of both serous and suppurative labyrinthitis.[45]

Diagnosis

The diagnosis of labyrinthitis in association with acute or chronic ear infections is based on finding the characteristic symptoms and signs of inner ear dysfunction. As noted above, serous labyrinthitis most commonly produces a slowly progressive insidious high-frequency sensorineural hearing loss, which may be discovered only with audiometric testing. Suppurative labyrinthitis produces a much more fulminant course, with both auditory and vestibular loss. Intermediate clinical pictures are not uncommon, however, and it may

be impossible to differentiate between a toxic and suppurative labyrinthitis on the basis of the symptoms alone. Bacterial labyrinthitis should be considered in any patient with acute or chronic ear infection who develops progressive auditory and vestibular symptoms. A positive fistula test suggests that the source of inner ear infection is a fistula in the horizontal semicircular canal.

Management

Management of labyrinthitis is directed at the associated infection of the middle ear, mastoid, and, if present, meninges. Any patient with acute or chronic bacterial ear disease associated with sudden or rapidly progressive inner ear symptoms should be hospitalized and treated with local cleansing and topical antibiotic solutions to the affected ear as well as parenteral antibiotics capable of penetrating the blood-brain barrier.[33] Surgical intervention to eradicate the middle ear and mastoid infection is usually required after a few days of antibiotic treatment. If the labyrinthitis is secondary to a primary meningitis, it is best treated by treating the underlying meningitis. If the labyrinthitis and meningitis are secondary to chronic ear infection, a labyrinthectomy might be indicated if the meningitis fails to respond to adequate medical treatment. A resistant or recurrent meningitis may result from unrecognized posterior fossa epidural abscesses with dural perforation or from congenital direct communications with the CSF.

PETROSITIS

Pathophysiology

Infections involving the perilabyrinthine bone may extend into the apical regions of the petrous bone, producing petrositis. Although only about 30 percent of petrous bones are pneumatized into the petrous apex, when infection does spread into this region management can be difficult because drainage is more restricted and the proximity of the apical air cells to diploic spaces predisposes to osteomyelitis.[33] Because of these problems petrositis is commonly associated with both bacterial labyrinthitis and with intracranial extension of the infection.

Diagnosis

The main symptom of an indolent infection in the petrous bone is a deep boring pain. With infection in the perilabyrinthine region, pain is often referred to the occipital, parietal, or temporal regions. Infection confined to the petrous apex is referred to the deep retro-orbital area. In 1904, Gradenigo described a classic triad associated with lesions of the petrous apex: (1) deep retro-orbital pain, (2) paralysis of the ipsilateral lateral rectus muscle from involvement of the abducens nerve as it crosses the petrous bone, and (3) otitic infection with purulent discharge from the ear.[16] The syndrome may be associated with vertigo and hearing loss, either from a concomitant bacterial labyrinthitis or from involvement of the eighth nerve in its bony canal. Radiologic evidence for infection of the petrous apex can be difficult to establish even with high-resolution CT scanning, so one must be alert to this diagnosis in patients with the typical clinical presentation.

Management

Management is usually a combined medical-surgical approach. After appropriate antibiotic therapy, the mucosal and bone infection must be removed. Surgically one usually begins with a radical mastoidectomy and dissection along the cell tracts to the petrous bone. If infection persists in the petrous apex—even though the middle ear may have responded—a middle fossa approach to exenterate the pneumatized spaces of the temporal bone may be necessary.[20]

INTRACRANIAL EXTENSION OF EAR INFECTIONS

Background

Extension of infection from the temporal bone into the cranial cavity demands rapid

Table 9–1. CNS COMPLICATIONS OF 100 EAR INFECTIONS IN ONE HOSPITAL OVER A 20-YEAR PERIOD

Meningitis	76
Brain abscess	6
Subdural effusion	5
Lateral sinus thrombosis	5
Otitic hydrocephalus	5
Subdural empyema	3
	100

Adapted from Gower and McGuirt.[15]

diagnosis and effective therapy to prevent permanent neurologic sequelae or death. Complications can result directly from either acute otitis media and mastoiditis or with chronic otomastoiditis and bone destruction. In a patient with an otitic infection who is febrile and continues to complain of severe ear and mastoid pain or headache despite appropriate antibiotic therapy, intracranial extension of the infection should be considered. Localized neurologic signs frequently do not develop until late in the disease process, and the diagnosis should be considered before focal signs develop.

Although the incidence of morbidity and mortality with CNS complications of ear infections has markedly decreased since the antibiotic era, these disorders have not disappeared. Gower and McGuirt[15] recently reviewed 100 cases with intracranial complications from otitic infections seen in a single hospital over a 20-year period. They found that even though the incidence of these complications has declined since the antibiotic era, their natural history remains the same and the resulting mortality is still alarmingly high. Of the complications (Table 9–1), 73 resulted from acute otitis media, and 46 occured in infants 2 years of age or younger.

Routes of Spread

Infection within the temporal bone can reach the intracranial space via three routes: (1) direct extension, (2) hematogenous spread, and (3) thrombophlebitis. Extracranial subperiosteal abscesses, intracranial extradural abscesses, and sigmoid sinus thrombophlebitis almost always result from a direct extension of the temporal bone infection. Subdural and brain abscesses may also result from direct extension along the soft tissue planes through the petromastoid canal to the posterior fossa or along the petrosquamous suture line to the middle fossa. There is a rich network of veins in and around the temporal bone, and these veins directly communicate with extracranial, intracranial, and cranial diploic veins. Thrombophlebitis of any of these veins may spread to the others, resulting in osteomyelitis of the calvaria or brain abscess at some distance from the temporal bone. Meningitis, particularly in young children, typically results from hematogenous dissemination. The frequent association between acute otitis media, pneumonia, and meningitis is probably due to the fact that all three diseases result from a systemic bacterial infection that has entered via the upper respiratory tract. Chronic bacterial otomastoiditis produces meningitis by direct extension through bone and dura or through the inner ear via a labyrinthine fistula produced by a cholesteatoma.

Meningitis

Meningitis secondary to ear disease is primarily a disease of infants with acute otitis media. Of the 76 patients with meningitis reported by Gower and McGuirt (Table 9–1),[15] 56 were less than 10 years of age. As a general rule, the bacteria causing the meningitis are similar to those causing the acute ear infection. With chronic ear infections and cholesteatoma, however, multiple microorganisms may be involved in the meningitis. Recurrent meningitis associated with middle ear infections suggests a CSF fistula with *S. pneumoniae* being the most common organism responsible.[33]

Epidural Abscess

Probably the most common intracranial complication of chronic otitic infections is extradural abscess, a collection of purulent fluid between the dura mater and bone of the middle or posterior fossa.[45] The dura mater is usually an effective barrier, and the infection remains localized outside the nervous system. Extradural abscesses are frequently asymptomatic and are discovered incidentally during mastoidectomies for acute or chronic disease.[22] Extradural abscesses in the middle fossa may become large and compress the temporal lobe, whereas abscesses in the posterior fossa remain small because of the tight attachments of the dura. The initial symptoms of fever, severe headache, and vomiting without focal neurologic signs can create a diagnostic and therapeutic dilemma.

Lateral Sinus Thrombophlebitis

Of the three dural sinuses intimately connected with the temporal bone, the lateral sinus is most commonly affected by acute or chronic temporal bone infection. Inflammation in the extradural space adjacent to the lateral sinus causes a local phlebitis and formation of a mural thrombus. The thrombus enlarges within the lumen of the vessel and may occlude it or become infected. A bland or infected thrombus may propagate in either direction and become organized. When infected, septic emboli are released into the bloodstream, causing septicemia and its systemic manifestations (i.e., fever, chills). When the cerebral veins are involved, the patient may develop focal or generalized seizures.[11]

Brain Abscess

As noted earlier, brain abscesses associated with ear infections predominantly originate from venous thrombophlebitis rather than direct extension through the dura mater.[21] The temporal lobe is most commonly involved followed by the cerebellum. Both aerobic and anaerobic organisms are found in pure or mixed cultures within brain abscesses. Multiple organisms are found in more than half of the cases.[17] Surprisingly, although *H. influenza* and *Pseudomonas* species are common organisms with ear infections, they are rare with brain abscesses.

Neurologic signs associated with temporal lobe abscess are often subtle, particularly if the patient has received inadequate antibiotic therapy.[19] An upper quadrant hemianopia can result from involvement of the optic radiations on either side, and when the abscess is in the dominant hemisphere, speech may be abnormal. Usually some weakness of the contralateral face and arm occurs, but gross paralysis is rare. The signs of a cerebellar abscess are usually more prominent. The patient complains of severe neck stiffness and holds the head rigid in a tilted position. Neurologic examination reveals ataxia, dysrhythmia, and dysmetria of the ipsilateral extremities, and the gait is markedly ataxic—if the patient is able to walk at all. Asymmetric gaze-evoked nystagmus is usually present with larger amplitude directed toward the side of the abscess. As the disease progresses, the speech be-

comes thick and slurred and swallowing difficulty develops.

Otitic Hydrocephalus

In 1931, Symonds[51] coined the term otitic hydrocephalus to describe the syndrome of increased intracranial pressure without evidence of meningitis or brain abscess in patients with chronic ear infections (i.e., pseudotumor cerebri). Symonds later hypothesized that the brain edema resulted from thrombosis of the superior sagittal sinus, leading to impared CSF resorption. This is primarily a diagnosis by exclusion, and a clear pathophysiology has

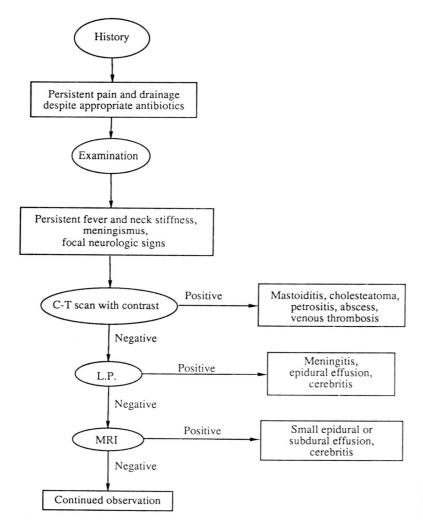

Figure 9–3. Algorithm for the diagnosis of intracranial complications of ear infections. *CT*, computerized tomography; *MRI*, magnetic resonance imaging; *LP*, lumbar puncture.

yet to be identified with modern neuro-imaging techniques.

Diagnosis

An intracranial complication of an otitic infection should be considered in any patient with a known ear infection who continues to complain of severe pain and headache despite appropriate antibiotic therapy (Fig. 9–3). The presence of fever, neck rigidity, and a positive Kernig's or Brudzinski's sign support the initial impression. As noted above, focal neurologic signs develop late in the course, even with localized brain abscesses, so one must have a high degree of suspicion based on the clinical presentation. After a detailed history and a careful physical examination, a CT scan with infusion is the initial diagnostic test. The CT scan will identify bone erosion, collections of pus within the intracranial cavity, and thrombosis of the venous sinuses.[26, 52] It can miss small collections of extradural or subdural pus and early stages of brain abscess formation, however, which might be identified with magnetic resonance (MR) scanning. If a mass lesion has been ruled out, a lumbar puncture is performed for analysis of the CSF. The characteristic profile of bacterial meningitis (pleocytosis, decreased glucose, and increased protein) is readily identified. More subtle changes (monocytic pleocytosis and mildly increased protein) can be seen with collections of pus in the epidural spaces or with brain abscess. The finding of increased intracranial pressure without a structural lesion suggests the possibility of a sagittal sinus thrombosis. The venous phase of cerebral angiography can sometimes identify a sinus thrombophlebitis that was not recognized with CT scanning.

Management

Treatment of the intracranial complications secondary to ear infections is directed along two lines: (1) eradication of the infection with appropriate antibiotics and (2) establishing adequate drainage and excision of infected tissue when neces-sary.[33] Complications due to acute otitis media are usually effectively controlled by a myringotomy and adequate parenteral antibiotics. Complications associated with bone destruction from chronic otitis media and mastoiditis usually require some type of mastoidectomy along with parenteral antibiotics. As a general rule, when there is a collection of pus within the intracranial cavity, treatment is directed first to reduce intracranial pressure—usually by evacuating the empyema. Appropriate management of meningitis consists of first identifying the offending organism, beginning appropriate intravenous antibiotics, and periodic monitoring of the progress by lumbar puncture.

MALIGNANT EXTERNAL OTITIS

Pathophysiology

Otitis externa, usually a benign disorder, produces a debilitating disease called malignant external otitis in elderly diabetic patients.[49] It typically begins with a nonspecific infection of the external canal resulting in complaints of pain, drainage, and fullness of the ear. The pain becomes severe and continuous as the infection spreads to contiguous soft tissues and adjacent bony structures. The invading organism is almost always *P. aeruginosa*. The organism invades the junction of the cartilaginous and osseous portions of the external auditory canal and spreads to the temporo-occipital bones. The most common neurologic sequela is involvement of the facial nerve in the fallopian canal or at the stylomastoid foramen. Occasionally multiple cranial nerves are compressed extradurally, and in rare cases, the infection spreads across the dura to produce a purulent meningitis.

Diagnosis

Diagnosis rests on finding the characteristic granulation tissue in the external canal along with a positive culture for *P. aeruginosa*. CT scan of the temporal bone may reveal (1) a soft tissue mass in the external canal, (2) clouding of the mastoid air cells, (3) sequestra of the bony canal, (4) erosion of bony structures at the base of the skull, and (5) soft tissue masses within the parapharynx and nasopharynx.[14] Radionuclide scanning is useful for determining the duration of therapy (see below).[30]

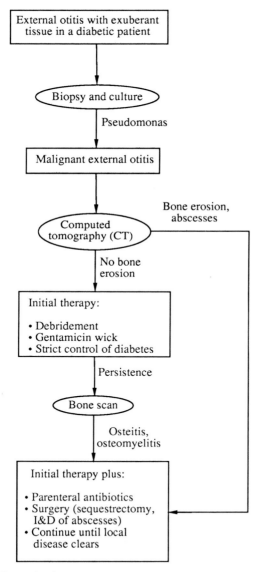

Figure 9—4. Algorithm for the management of malignant external otitis. (Adapted from Smith and Lucente.[49])

Management

An algorithm for the management of malignant external otitis is given in Figure 9—4.[49] Initial local treatment consists of removal of all accumulated debris and granulation tissue from the external canal and instillation of a gentamicin wick (gentamicin sulfate drops on 1/2-inch gauze packing) in the external canal. This, along with strict control of the underlying diabetes, can be sufficient in some patients with early stages of disease. In patients with more advanced disease including bony erosion or in those who fail to respond promptly to this initial therapy, a bone scan is indicated to assess the possibility of osteitis or osteomyelitis. If positive, the patient should undergo a 6-week course of parenteral antibiotic therapy in conjunction with local cleansing and debridement as required. Antibiotic therapy for *Pseudomonas* usually requires an aminoglycoside such as gentamicin, tobramycin, or amikacin. Penicillin derivatives such as carbenicillin, ticarcillin, and piperacillin may also be effective and can be used in combination with an aminoglycoside.

VIRAL NEUROLABYRINTHITIS

Pathophysiology

Viral neurolabyrinthitis may be part of a systemic viral illness such as measles, mumps, and infectious mononucleosis, or it may be an isolated infection of the labyrinth and/or eighth nerve without systemic involvement. In the latter case, the infecting agent is rarely identified, but substantial pathologic evidence exists that the sudden onset of hearing loss and/or vertigo can be caused by an isolated viral infection of the inner ear.[44]

Of the thousands of infants born deaf every year, about 20 percent are thought to be the result of congenital viral infections.[37] More than 4000 persons are stricken each year with "sudden deafness"—a unilateral, infrequently bilateral, sensorineural hearing loss of acute onset, presumed to be of viral origin in most cases.[54] A like number of individuals are stricken with the acute onset of intense vertigo (so-called vestibular neuronitis or neuritis) unaccompanied by any neurologic or audiologic symptoms and also presumed to be of viral origin.[44, 46] Despite this strong suspicion of a viral origin for these common neurotologic disorders, proof of a viral pathophysiology in a given case is difficult to obtain. Routine otologic examination is usually unremarkable, and CT scanning of the temporal bone reveals only a normal-appearing bony labyrinth; it provides no information about the state of the membranous labyrinth. The membranous labyrinth can often be visualized with MR scanning, but the resolution is too poor to identify even the grossest pathology. Serologic studies can demonstrate that a virus infected the patient but do not prove that the infectious agent caused the inner ear damage. Furthermore, isolation of an infectious agent from the nasopharynx or other tissue other than the membranous labyrinth does not prove a causal relationship between the virus and the inner ear disease. Although a few viruses have been cultured directly from perilymph samples in infected ears, this is not a practical method for routine diagnosis of viral infections of the inner ear.[10]

Epidemiologic evidence supports a viral cause in most patients with either sudden deafness or acute prolonged vertigo. A large percentage of such patients report an upper respiratory tract illness within 1 to 2 weeks prior to the onset of symptoms. Both syndromes occur in epidemics, may affect several members of the same family, and erupt more commonly in the spring and early summer.[12, 18, 31] A list of the viruses that have been clinically associated with cases of deafness and/or vertigo is given in Table 9–2.[10] In most cases, however, proof that these viruses caused the symptoms is circumstantial.

The most convincing evidence for a viral cause of these isolated auditory and vestibular syndromes comes from the temporal bone studies of Schuknecht and his colleagues[44, 46, 47] in Boston. These and other investigators have reported pathologic evidence for isolated viral involvement of the cochlea and auditory nerve in patients with sudden deafness and of the vestibular

Table 9–2. VIRUSES THAT HAVE BEEN CLINICALLY ASSOCIATED WITH HEARING LOSS AND/OR VERTIGO

Cytomegalovirus	Hepatitis
Rubella	Adenovirus
Mumps	Influenza
Rubeola	Parainfluenza
Varicella-zoster	Poliomyelitis
Herpes simplex	Coxsackie
Epstein-Barr	Lymphocytic choriomeningitis
Variola	Yellow fever

Adapted from Davis and Johnsson.[10]

end-organs and vestibular nerve in patients with isolated sudden vertigo. The atrophy of the nerves and end-organs was identical to that associated with well-documented viral disorders (such as mumps or measles). In all of these cases the vasculature was intact; there was no evidence for a vascular cause for the sudden deafness or vertigo. These pathologic studies are supported by experimental studies in animals where it has been shown that several viruses will selectively infect the labyrinth and/or eighth nerve.[10, 35]

Clinical Features

Viral neurolabyrinthitis can present with sudden deafness (usually unilateral, although rarely, bilateral), acute vertigo (with associated autonomic symptoms), or with some combination of auditory and vestibular symptoms. Although the term "sudden deafness" is commonly used, the hearing loss due to viral infection usually comes on over several hours and may even extend over several days.[47] As noted above, the loss is often profound and may be permanent, although it reverses at least partially in most cases. It returns to normal in more than 50 percent of patients (with or without treatment).[28] Tinnitus and fullness in the involved ear are common.

Vestibular neurolabyrinthitis (vestibular neuronitis, vestibular neuritis) is typically manifested by the gradual onset of vertigo, nausea, and vomiting over several hours.[9, 13, 46] The symptoms usually reach a peak within 24 hours and then gradually resolve over several weeks. During the first day there is severe truncal unsteadiness and imbalance and the patient has difficulty focusing because of the spontaneous nystagmus. Most patients have a benign course with complete recovery within 3 months. There are important exceptions to this rule, however. Occasionally patients,—particularly the elderly—will have intractable dizziness that persists for years. Twenty to 30 percent of patients will have at least one recurrent bout of vertigo (usually less severe than the initial episode).[9] This may represent reactivation of a latent virus, inasmuch as it is often associated with systemic viral illness. A small percentage of these patients will have multiple recurrent episodes of vertigo leading to a profound bilateral vestibulopathy (so-called bilateral sequential vestibular neuritis).[48] The episodic vertigo is eventually replaced by persistent dysequilibrium and oscillopsia.

Diagnosis

The diagnosis of viral neurolabyrinthitis rests on finding the characteristic clinical profile along with laboratory evidence of peripheral auditory and/or vestibular dys-

function in the absence of neurologic symptoms and signs. When the hearing loss is partial, it tends to be most prominent in the high frequencies—consistent with neuropathologic studies demonstrating the greatest degree of damage in the basilar turn of the cochlea.[39] BAER studies are usually normal, consistent with a cochlear site of pathology. When the vestibular system is involved, the caloric responses are decreased and/or absent on the side of the lesion. Recently it has been shown that patients with vestibular neurolabyrinthitis often have hearing loss in the ultrahigh-frequency range, suggesting that the auditory end-organ may be involved to a minor degree even though clinically silent.[3, 40] Similarly, vestibular abnormalities have been identified on electronystagmography (ENG) in patients with "sudden hearing loss" but without associated vestibular symptoms.[53]

Viral neurolabyrinthitis must be differentiated from other forms of labyrinthitis (bacterial and syphilitic) and from acute labyrinthine ischemia and from perilymph fistula (Table 9–3). As noted earlier, bacterial labyrinthitis is typically associated with acute and chronic otomastoiditis, which should be easily identified on exami-

Table 9–3. DIFFERENTIAL DIAGNOSIS OF ACUTE PERIPHERAL VESTIBULOPATHY

	History	Examination	Laboratory
Viral neurolaby-rinthitis	Developing over hours, resolving over days, prior flulike illness	Normal except for signs of acute unilateral vestibular loss	ENG: Caloric hypoexcitability Audio: may show ultrahigh-frequency loss
Bacterial labyrin-thitis	Abrupt onset, associated hearing loss, prior ear infections	Signs of otitis media or meningitis	ENG: Absent caloric response Audio: Profound sensorineural loss CSF: Pleocytosis
Syphilitic labyri-nthitus	Recurrent episodes, associated tinnitus and hearing loss, prior congenital or acquired syphilis	May be stigmata of congenital syphilis, rarely associated signs of neurosyphilis	ENG: Caloric hypoexcitability Audio: Low-frequency loss Serology: positive FTA-ABS CSF: Usually normal
Labyrinthine ischemia	Abrupt onset, usually associated neurologic symptoms, prior vascular disease	May be signs of brainstem or cerebellar infarction	ENG: Absent caloric response Audio: Profound sensorineural loss Neuroimaging: May show brain infarction
Perilymph fistula	Abrupt onset associated with head trauma, barotrauma, or sudden strain during heavy lifting, coughing, or sneezing; chronic otomastoiditis with cholesteatoma	Positive fistula test, may be chronic otitis with tympanic membrane perforation	ENG: Caloric hypoexcitability Audio: Usually sensorineural loss CT of temporal bone may show erosion from cholesteatoma

nation of the ear and with CT of the temporal bone. Suppurative labyrinthitis invariably results in a fulminate profound loss of both auditory and vestibular function, usually with only minimal recovery. Serous labyrinthitis may produce only a high-frequency sensorineural hearing loss if the toxic products remain confined to the basilar region of the cochlea. Syphilitic labyrinthitis might initially be confused with viral neurolabyrinthitis, but the former leads to recurrent episodes of vertigo and hearing loss, usually progressing to severe bilateral dysfunction over a period of months. Unlike the gradual onset of symptoms over hours with viral neurolabyrinthitis, infarction of the labyrinth results in a sudden profound loss of auditory and vestibular function—often in a setting of prior episodes of transient ischemia within the vertebrobasilar system (see Chapter 12). Without major risk factors and without a prior history of occlusive vascular disease, there would be little reason to suspect a vascular cause for isolated auditory or vestibular symptoms in a patient under the age of 50. In older patients, ischemic vascular disease involving the labyrinth is more common, but in our experience it is still much less common than viral neurolabyrinthitis as a cause of isolated auditory and vestibular symptoms.

Like viral neurolabyrinthitis, perilymph fistulae can present with hearing loss, vertigo, or a combination of auditory and vestibular symptoms. With the latter, however, the onset is usually abrupt, and there is nearly always a precipitating event such as head trauma, barotrauma, or a sudden strain during heavy lifting, coughing, or sneezing. Perilymph fistulae are particularly common in patients who have undergone stapedectomy for otosclerosis. Fluctuating symptoms (particularly if induced by coughing or sneezing) and/or a positive fistula test are indications for exploratory surgery (see Chapter 14).

Management

The management of patients who present with isolated episodes of auditory and/or vestibular loss is controversial because the pathophysiology is often uncertain. As suggested above, unless there is convincing evidence to suspect a vascular or nonviral infectious cause, the patient should be managed as a presumed viral neurolabyrinthitis, that is, symptomatic treatment with antivertiginous medications when vertigo is a prominent symptom (see Table 11–1). Although steroids have been recommended for their anti-inflammatory effect,[1] there have been no controlled studies to assess the risk–benefit ratio for these drugs. Numerous so-called vasodilating regimens have been proposed, but they would have little effect on the presumed viral pathophysiology. Although about a third of patients with vestibular neurolabyrinthitis are left with a permanent loss of vestibular function (as documented by serial caloric examinations), the CNS is able to adapt to the vestibular loss, and residual symptoms are usually minimal once the compensation has occured. Vestibular exercises (see Table 11–2) should be started immediately after the acute nausea and vomiting subside, and they should be continued until dizziness and imbalance are minimal.[2] Although antiviral agents such as cytosine arabinase and acyclovir have been used for treating systemic viral illnesses in children, it is unclear whether the hearing loss that is often associated with disorders such as cytomegalovirus and rubella infections is altered by such treatment. There have been no reports on the efficacy of antiviral agents in adults with presumed viral neurolabyrinthitis.

HERPES ZOSTER OTICUS

Pathophysiology

A clear example of a viral syndrome involving the eighth nerve is *herpes zoster oticus* (also known as the Ramsay Hunt syndrome).[41] Presumably, the zoster virus remains dormant in the ganglia associated with the seventh and eighth nerves and is reactivated during a period of lowered immunity. The patient initially develops a deep burning pain in the ear followed a few days later by vesicular eruption in the external auditory canal and concha. At some time after the onset of pain, either before or after the vesicular eruption, the patient may develop hearing loss, vertigo, and facial weakness. These symptoms may occur singly or collectively. A small percentage of patients with idiopathic facial palsy (Bell's palsy) have a rise in complement fixation antibodies to zoster antigen.[38] The pathologic findings in patients with *H. zoster oticus* consist of perivascular, perineural, and intraneural round cell infiltration in the seventh nerve and in both divisions of the eighth nerve.[55]

Diagnosis and Management

The diagnosis rests on finding the characteristic cutaneous eruptions about the auricle and external ear canal. *H. zoster* can be cultured from these vesicles in the early stages. Although the herpetic external otitis is self-limiting, the seventh and eighth nerve damage is often profound and nonreversible. During the acute stages, warm moist compresses applied locally can provide symptomatic relief, although often systemic analgesics are required. The role of corticosteroids and antiviral drugs such as acyclovir is yet to be established with regard to whether they alter the outcome of the seventh and eighth nerve damage.

SYPHILITIC INFECTIONS OF THE EAR

Syphilitic infections remain an important cause of vertigo and hearing loss despite the general availability and use of penicillin. Involvement of the eighth nerve and/or labyrinth can be an early or late manifestation of both congenital and acquired syphilis. Morrison[32] calculated that the prevalence of congenital syphilis in England in 1972 was approximately 1 in 700, or 0.14 percent. About one in three patients with congenital syphilis develop otologic manifestations. Although the number of new cases of congenital syphilis progressively declined from 1930 to 1968, the incidence of new cases appears to have stabilized since 1968. After a long period of decline, new cases of acquired syphilis are again on the increase, so one might well expect an increased incidence of otologic manifestations in the future.

Pathophysiology

Syphilitic infections produce auditory and vestibular symptoms by two different pathophysiologic mechanisms: (1) meningitis with involvement of the eighth nerve, and (2) osteitis of the temporal bone with associated labyrinthitis.[25, 43] The former typically occurs as an early manifestation of acquired syphilis, whereas the latter occurs as a late manifestation of both congenital and acquired syphilis. With early congenital syphilis there may be a lymphocytic infiltration of both the membranous labyrinth and eighth nerve, leading to profound bilateral deafness. Spirochetes have been demonstrated in temporal bones obtained at autopsy in such patients. With early acquired syphilis the predominant pathologic finding is basilar meningitis affecting the eighth nerve, particularly the auditory branch. The hearing loss typically occurs with the rash and lymphadenopathy of secondary syphilis.[43] It is usually abrupt in onset, tends to be bilateral, and is rapidly progressive. Vestibular symptoms are often absent. Patients demonstrate symptoms and signs of meningitis including headache, stiff neck, cranial nerve palsies, and optic neuritis.

Both congenital and acquired syphilitic infections produce temporal bone osteitis and labyrinthitis as a late manifestation. The congenital variety is approximately three times as common as the acquired variety.[32] The time of onset of congenital syphilitic labyrinthitis is anywhere from the first to seventh decades, with the peak incidence in the fourth and fifth decades, whereas acquired syphilitic labyrinthitis rarely occurs before the fourth decade and has a peak incidence in the fifth and sixth decades. The congenital variety is often associated with other stigmata of congenital syphilis, such as interstitial keratitis, Hutchinson's teeth, saddle nose, frontal bossing, and rhagades. Of these associated signs, interstitial keratitis is by far the most common, occurring in approximately 90 percent of patients.[32] Pathologic changes in the labyrinth are similar in the congenital and acquired variety, consisting of inflammatory infiltration of the membranous labyrinth and osteitis of all three layers of the otic capsule.[25, 45] A combination of hydrops of the membranous labyrinth and atrophy of the cochlear and vestibular end-organs resembles the pathologic findings in idiopathic Meniere's syndrome.

The natural history of syphilitic labyrinthitis is a slow relentless progression to profound or total bilateral loss of vestibular and auditory function.[32, 50] This progression is marked by episodes of sudden deafness and vertigo and fluctuation in the magnitude of hearing loss and tinnitus.

Diagnosis

Infants with congenital syphilis exhibit a profound bilateral sensorineural hearing loss along with extensive damage to multiple organs (Table 9–4). The hearing loss associated with early acquired syphilis may be the only manifestation of a basilar meningitis, or it may be associated with headaches, stiff neck, and multiple neurologic findings. The rash of secondary syphilis may precede or accompany the onset of hearing loss. CSF examination is invariably abnormal with a pleocytosis and elevated protein.[43] The CSF VDRL may or may not be positive.

The diagnosis of syphilitic labyrinthitis as a late manifestation of either congenital or acquired syphilis is based on the finding of a positive serum fluorescent treponemal antibody absorption (FTA-ABS) test in a patient with the typical clinical history of fluctuating hearing loss and vertigo (see Table 9–4).[23] The serum VDRL is positive in only about 75 percent of cases, making it an unreliable test for syphilitic labyrinthitis.[32] As noted above, patients with congenital syphilitic labyrinthitis often have associated stigmata of congenital syphilis, whereas patients with the acquired variety may have other clinical symptoms and signs of tertiary syphilis. The CSF examination is usually normal in both the congenital and acquired varieties of syphilitic labyrinthitis.

Management

Penicillin is the treatment of choice for the otologic manifestations of syphilis, although the optimal regimen for each variety remains uncertain. Because CSF infection accompanies the early manifestations of both congenital and acquired syphilis,

Table 9–4. DIFFERENTIAL FEATURES OF DIFFERENT OTOLOGIC MANIFESTATIONS OF SYPHILIS

	Early		Late	
	Congenital	*Acquired*	*Congenital*	*Acquired*
Patho-physiology	Inflammation of membranous labyrinth and eighth nerve	Meningitis with involvement of eighth nerve	Temporal bone osteitis and petrositis with secondary degeneration of membranous labyrinth leading to endolymphatic hydrops	
Hearing loss	Congenital deafness	Abrupt onset, bilateral, progressive	Begins unilateral, fluctuating, progresses to bilateral over months; associated tinnitus and ear pressure	
Vertigo	No	Infrequent	Episodic (hours) with fluctuating hearing loss	
Age of peak incidence	At birth	20–30 years	30–50 years	40–60 years
Associated features	Infection involving multiple organs	Rash of secondary syphilis	Interstitial keratitis, other stigmata of congenital syphilis	Other features of tertiary syphilis
CSF	Usually abnormal (pleocytosis, elevated protein, VDRL ±)		Usually normal	
Treatment	IV aqueous penicillin, 20 million U/day ×2 weeks		IM benzathine penicillin, 2.4 million U, weekly ×3 months; prednisone 30–60 mg QOD, 3–6 months, slow tapering	

high-dose intravenous penicillin seems appropriate. Prognosis following treatment is poor in the early congenital form, but it is excellent in the early acquired variety. Complete recovery of both hearing and vestibular function usually occurs with the latter.[43]

For the late manifestations of both congenital and acquired syphilitic labyrinthitis the combination of steroids and penicillin appears to be superior to penicillin alone.[32, 50] Numerous penicillin regimens have been used, with the most popular being benzathine penicillin (2.4 million units) given weekly for 6 weeks to 3 months. Along with the penicillin, prednisone, beginning at a dose of 60 mg per day on an alternate day regimen, is given for 3 months, followed by a slow tapering. If symptoms recur during the tapering, a more long-term maintenance dose of prednisone may be required. The majority of patients can be expected to stabilize or improve on this therapeutic regimen.[50]

TUBERCULOSIS AND MYCOTIC INFECTIONS OF THE EAR

Tuberculous Mastoiditis

Although less common than in the past, tuberculous mastoiditis accompanies both pulmonary and nonpulmonary infections—presumably due to hematogenous spread. In contrast to bacterial infections, tuberculosis of the temporal bone runs an indolent course and usually produces little pain.[24] The main finding on examination is a foul-smelling otorrhea which, when cultured, shows nonspecific mixed organisms. It may mimic chronic otomastoiditis with cholesteatoma formation because there is often tympanic membrane perforation and prominent granulomatous tissue. CT scan of the temporal bone shows an irregular punched-out lesion resembling a cholesteatoma. Diagnosis rests on culturing tuberculosis from the otorrhea or by histologic examination of the mastoid granulomatous tissue. Management consists of antituberculous drugs and surgical eradication of the lesion.

Mycotic Mastoiditis

Primary mycotic infections such as actinomycosis and coccidioidomycosis can occur in the temporal bone. Their manifestations are comparable to those of tuberculosis. Although the mucorales group of fungi are usually of low virulence, mucormycosis of the mastoid bone can lead to a life-threatening illness in patients who are chronically ill (particularly with diabetes or malignancy) or are receiving chemotherapy or broad-spectrum antibiotic therapy.[34] The organism enters the sinuses from the nose and penetrates the muscular wall of arteries, inciting thrombosis and infarction of tissue. The infection may then spread to the petrous apices, the middle and inner ears, and into the intracranial cavity. Thrombosis of the major cerebral arteries often develops despite therapy with amphotericin.

Basilar Meningitis

Tuberculosis, cryptococcosis, and coccidioidomycosis produce basilar meningitis with involvement of multiple cranial nerves, including the eighth nerve. The clinical picture is that of an insidious febrile illness associated with progressive bilateral sensorineural hearing loss. The diagnosis rests on finding the characteristic CSF profile of lymphocytic pleocytosis, elevated protein, and decreased glucose. Often, there are associated systemic symptoms and signs, including multiple pulmonary lesions. *Mycobacterium tuberculosis* may be seen on acid-fast smears and cultured from the CSF. The diagnosis of fungal meningitis relies on identifying the appropriate antigen in the CSF.

REFERENCES

1. Adour, KK, Sprague, MA, and Hilsinger, RL: Vestibular vertigo. A form of polyneuritis. JAMA 246:1564, 1981.
2. Baloh, RW: The dizzy patient. Symptomatic treatment of vertigo. Postgrad Med 73:317, 1983.
3. Bergenius, J and Borg, E: Audio-vestibular findings in patients with vestibular neuronitis. Acta Otolaryngol 906:389, 1983.
4. Bluestone, CD: Otitis media in children: To treat or not to treat. N Engl J Med 306:1399, 1982.
5. Bluestone, CD and Klein, JO: Otitis media with

effusion, atelectasis and eustachian tube dysfunction. In Bluestone, CD and Stool, SE (eds): Pediatric Otolaryngology, Vol I. WB Saunders, Philadelphia, 1983.

6. Cantekin, EI, et al: Lack of efficacy of a decongestant-antihistamine combination for otitis media with effusion ("secretory" ototis media) in children: Results of a double-blind randomized trial. N Engl J Med 308:297, 1983.

7. Chole, RA: Acute and chronic infection of the temporal bone including otitis media with effusion. In Cummings, CW, Fredrickson, JM, Harker, LA, Krause, CJ, and Schuller, DE (eds): Otolaryngology—Head and Neck Surgery. CV Mosby, St Louis, 1986, p 2963.

8. Chole, RA: Cellular and subcellular events of bone resorption in human and experimental cholesteatoma: The role of osteoclasts. Laryngoscope 94:76, 1984.

9. Coats, AC: Vestibular neuronitis. Acta Otolaryngol 251 (Suppl): 1, 1969.

10. Davis, LE and Johnsson, LG: Viral infections of the inner ear: Clinical, virologic and pathologic studies in humans and animals. Am J Otolaryngol 4:347, 1983.

11. Dawes, J: Complications of infections of the middle ear. In Scott-Brown, W, Ballantyne, J, and Groves, J (eds): Diseases of the Ear, Nose, and Throat. London, Butterworth, 1965.

12. Dishoeck, H Van and Bierman, T: Sudden perceptive deafness and viral infection (report of first one hundred patients). Ann Otol Rhinol Laryngol 66:963, 1957.

13. Dix, M and Hallpike, C: The pathology, symptomatology and diagnosis of certain common disorders of the vestibular systems. Ann Otol Rhinol Laryngol 61:987, 1952.

14. Gold, S, et al: Radiographic findings in progressive necrotizing "malignant" external otitis. Laryngoscope 94:363, 1984.

15. Gower, D and McGuirt, WF: Intracranial complications of acute and chronic infectious ear disease: A problem still with us. Laryngoscope 93:1028, 1983.

16. Gradenigo, G: Sulla leptomeningite circoscritta e sulla paralisi dell' abducente di origine otitica. G Accad Med Torino 10:59, 1904.

17. Harrison, MJG: The clinical presentation of intracranial abscesses. QJ Med 204:461, 1982.

18. Hart, C: Vestibular paralysis of sudden onset and probable viral etiology. Ann Otol Rhinol Laryngol 74:33, 1965.

19. Heineman, HS, Braude, AI, and Osterholm, JL: Intracranial suppurative disease. Early presumptive diagnosis and successful treatment without surgery. JAMA 218:1542, 1971.

20. Hendershot, EL and Wood, JW: The middle fossa approach in the treatment of petrosites. Arch Otolaryngol 98:426, 1973.

21. Hirsch, JF, et al: Brain abscess in childhood. Childs Brain 10:251, 1983.

22. Holt, GR and Gates, GA: Masked mastoiditis. Laryngoscope 93:1034, 1983.

23. Hughes, GB and Rutherford, I: Predictive value of serologic tests for syphilis in otology. Ann Otol Rhinol Laryngol 95:250, 1986.

24. Jeanes, A and Friedmann, I: Tuberculosis of the middle ear. Tubercle, The Journal of the British Tuberculosis Association 41:109, 1960.

25. Karmody, C and Schuknecht, H: Deafness in congenital syphilis. Arch Otolaryngol 83:18, 1966.

26. Kaufman, DM and Leeds, NE: Computed tomography (CT) in the diagnosis of intracranial abscesses. Brain abscess, subdural empyema, and epidural empyema. Neurology 27:1069, 1977.

27. Klein, JO: Microbiology of otitis media. Ann Otol Rhinol Laryngol 89:98, 1980.

28. Laird, N and Wilson, WR: Predicting recovery from idiopathic sudden hearing loss. Am J Otolaryngol 4:161, 1983.

29. McCabe, BF: The incidence, site, treatment and fate of labyrinthine fistulae. Clin Otolaryngol 3:329, 1978.

30. McShane, D, Chapnik, JS, Noyek, AM, and Vellend, H: Malignant external otitis. J Otolaryngol (Can) 15:2, 1986.

31. Merifield, D: Self-limited idiopathic vertigo (epidemic vertigo). Arch Otolaryngol 81:355, 1965.

32. Morrison, AW: Late syphilis. In Management of Sensorineural Deafness. Boston, Butterworth, 1975.

33. Neely, JG: Complications of temporal bone infection. In Cummings, CW, Fredrickson, JM, Harker, LA, Krause, CJ, and Schuller, DE (eds): Otolaryngology—Head and Neck Surgery. CV Mosby, St Louis, 1986, p 2988.

34. New England Journal of Medicine: Case records of the Massachusetts General Hospital. N Engl J Med 279:1220, 1968.

35. Nomura, Y, Kurata, T, and Saito, K: Sudden deafness: Human temporal bone studies and an animal model. In Nomura, Y (ed): Hearing Loss and Dizziness. Igaku-Shoin, Tokyo, 1985, p 58.

36. Paparella, MM, Goycoolea, MV, and Meyerhoff, WL: Inner ear pathology and otitis media: A review. Ann Otol Rhinol Laryngol 89:249, 1980.

37. Pappas, DG: Hearing impairments and vestibular abnormalities among children with subclinical cytomegalovirus. Ann Otol Rhinol Laryngol 92:552, 1983.

38. Peitersen, E and Anderson, P: Spontaneous course of 220 peripheral nontraumatic facial palsies. Acta Otolaryngol (Suppl 224):296, 1967.

39. Portmann, M, Dauman, R, and Aran, JM: Audiometric and electrophysiological correlations in sudden deafness. Acta Otolaryngol 99: 363, 1985.

40. Rahko, T and Karma, P: New clinical finding in vestibular neuritis: High frequency audiometry hearing loss in the affected ear. Laryngoscope 96:198, 1986.

41. Robillard, RB, Hilsinger, RL, and Adour, KK: Ramsay Hunt facial paralysis: Clinical analysis of 185 patients. Otolaryngol Head Neck Surg 95:292, 1986.

42. Sade, J: Secretory Otitis Media and Its Sequela. Churchill Livingstone, New York, 1979.

43. Saltiel, P, Melmed, CA, and Portnoy, D: Sensorineural deafness in early acquired syphilis. Can J Neurol Sci 10:114, 1983.

44. Schuknecht, HF: Neurolabyrinthitis. Viral infections of the peripheral auditory and vestibular systems. In Nomura, Y (ed): Hearing Loss and Dizziness. Igaku-Shoin, Tokyo, 1985, p 1.

45. Schuknecht, HF: Pathology of the Ear. Harvard University Press, Cambridge, MA, 1974.

46. Schuknecht, HF and Kitamura, K: Vestibular neuritis. Ann Otol Rhinol Laryngol 90 (Suppl):1, 1981.

47. Schuknecht, HF, Kimura, RR, and Nanfal, PM: The pathology of idiopathic sensorineural hearing loss. Arch Otorhinolaryngol 243:1, 1986.

48. Schuknecht, HF and Witt, RL: Acute bilateral sequential vestibular neuritis. Am J Otolaryngol 6:255, 1985.

49. Smith, PG and Lucente, FE: External ear: Infections. In Cummings, CW, Fredrickson, JM, Harker, LA, Krause, CJ, and Schuller, DE (eds): Otolaryngology—Head and Neck Surgery. CV Mosby, St Louis, 1986, p 2899.

50. Steckelberg, JM and McDonald, TJ: Otologic involvement in late syphilis. Laryngoscope 94:753, 1984.

51. Symonds, CP: Otitic hydrocephalus. Brain 54:55, 1931.

52. Venezio, FR, Naiclich, TP, and Shulman, ST: Complications of mastoiditis with special emphasis on venous sinus thrombosis. J Pediatr 101:509, 1982.

53. Wilson, WR, Laird, N, and Kavesh, DA: Electronystagmographic findings in idiopathic sudden hearing loss. Am J Otolaryngol 3:279, 1982.

54. Wilson, WR, et al: Viral and epidemiologic studies of idiopathic sudden hearing loss. Otolaryngol Head Neck Surg 91:653, 1983.

55. Zajtchuk, J, Matz, G, and Lindsay, J: Temporal bone pathology in herpes oticus. Ann Otol Rhinol Laryngol 81:331, 1972.

Chapter 10

BENIGN POSITIONAL VERTIGO

Benign positional vertigo is the single most common cause of vertigo seen in our neurotology clinic. It is not a disease but, rather, a syndrome that can be the sequela of several different inner ear diseases; in about half the cases no cause can be found.[1] Patients with benign positional vertigo develop brief episodes of vertigo (usually lasting less than 30 seconds) with position change—typically when turning over in bed, getting in and out of bed, bending over and straightening up, and extending the neck to look up. So-called top shelf vertigo, in which a patient experiences an episode of vertigo while reaching for something on a high shelf is nearly always due to benign positional vertigo. The syndrome is important to recognize because, in the vast majority of patients, the symptoms will spontaneously remit and extensive diagnostic procedures are not warranted. As will be discussed below, the diagnosis is based on finding the characteristic paroxysmal positional nystagmus with rapid positional testing.

In a review of 240 cases of benign positional vertigo we did not identify a single case in which an episode of positional vertigo lasted longer than 1 minute.[1] Often, after a flurry of episodes, however, patients complained of more prolonged nonspecific dizziness (lightheaded, swimming sensation) and nausea that lasted for hours to days. Typically, bouts of benign positional vertigo were intermixed with variable periods of remission. The mean age of onset was 54 years, with a range of 11 to 84 years. At the time of examination, one third of the patients reported durations longer than 10 years. The spectrum of the clinical course is illustrated by two patients: (1) a 43-year-old man, who de-veloped a flurry of episodes of benign positional vertigo lasting 1 week without recurrence in more than 10 years of follow-up, (2) a 67-year-old woman who experienced recurrent bouts of benign positional vertigo for 21 years, the longest period of remission being 1 year.

In slightly more than one half of the cases (122 of 240), a likely cause was determined (Table 10–1). The two largest diagnostic categories were post-traumatic and post-viral neurolabyrinthitis. Patients with the former had the onset of positional vertigo within 3 days of well-documented head trauma. Although many others reported a prior history of head trauma months to years before the onset of positional vertigo, they were not included in this group (i.e., they were included in the idiopathic group). Patients in the viral neurolabyrinthitis group reported a prior episode of acute vertigo gradually resolving over 1 to 2 weeks. In 25 out of 37 there was an associated sudden hearing loss that also improved as the vertigo subsided, although most patients were left with a re-

Table 10–1. DIAGNOSES IN 240 PATIENTS WITH BENIGN PAROXYSMAL POSITIONAL VERTIGO[1]

Idiopathic	118
Post-traumatic	43
Viral neurolabyrinthitis	37
Miscellaneous	(42)
Basilar vertebral insufficiency	11
Meniere's disease	5
Postsurgery (general)	5
Postsurgery (ear)	5
Ototoxicity	4
Luetic labyrinthitis	2
Chronic otomastoiditis	2
Other	8

sidual unilateral sensorineural hearing loss. Episodes of benign positional vertigo began as soon as 1 week and as long as 8 years after the acute attack. Most patients reported a cold or flulike illness within 2 weeks of the acute vertiginous episode. Eleven patients reported typical symptoms of vertebrobasilar insufficiency (in addition to vertigo) prior to the onset of benign positional vertigo. In these cases, the benign positional vertigo resulted from prior ischemic damage to the labyrinth (see Chapter 12). It is important to recognize that episodes of positional vertigo in such patients do not indicate recurrent vascular insufficiency.

Females outnumbered males by a ratio of 1.6 to 1 combining all diagnostic categories. This ratio was approximately 2 to 1, if one considers only the idiopathic and miscellaneous groups. Others have reported an even higher female-to-male preponderance with idiopathic benign positional vertigo.[8] The age of onset peaked in the sixth decade in the idiopathic group, in the fourth and fifth decades in the postviral group, and was evenly distributed over the second to sixth decade in the posttraumatic group.

PATHOPHYSIOLOGY

The pathophysiology of benign positional vertigo is not entirely understood, although an abnormality of the posterior semicircular canal is strongly implicated. Bárány[3] initially suggested that benign positional vertigo was caused by a lesion of the otolith organs, inasmuch as it was induced by a change in head position relative to gravity. Dix and Halpike[5] supported this notion by finding unilateral degeneration of the utricular macula at necropsy in a typical case of benign positional vertigo. More recently, Schuknecht[9, 10] proposed that benign positional vertigo resulted from a lesion of the posterior semicircular canal. He found basophilic deposits on the cupulae of the posterior canals in two patients who manifested benign positional vertigo prior to death from unrelated disease; the deposits were present only on the side that was undermost when benign positional vertigo was induced (Figure 10–1).

Schuknecht proposed that otoconia from a degenerating utricular macula settles on the cupula of the posterior canal, causing it to become heavier than the surrounding endolymph. When the patient moves from the sitting to the head-hanging position (standard positioning maneuver), the posterior canal moves from the inferior to a superior position, and utriculofugal displacement of the cupula occurs. The latency before nystagmus onset reflects the period of time required for the otoconial mass to be displaced, and the fatigability is caused by disbursement of particles in the endolymph.

The two most convincing pieces of clinical evidence supporting a posterior semicircular canal origin for benign positional vertigo are (1) the positional nystagmus is in the plane of the posterior canal[2, 7] and (2) sectioning of the ampullary nerve from the posterior canal stops benign positional vertigo.[6] Schuknecht's cupulolithiasis theory[9] could explain the varied etiologies of benign positional vertigo, inasmuch as any type of damage to the inner ear (trauma, infection, ischemia) could lead to dislodging of the calcium carbonate crystals from the otolith and deposition on the cupula of the posterior semicircular canal. The idiopathic variety could result from degeneration of the otolithic membrane with aging. Also, many of the patients in the idiopathic category may have had inner ear damage from subclinical infection or minor head trauma that was forgotten.

DIAGNOSIS

The diagnosis of benign positional vertigo rests on finding the characteristic fatigable paroxysmal positional nystagmus in a patient with a typical history of positional vertigo. The nystagmus is torsional, consistent with the known anatomic connections between the posterior semicircular canal of the undermost ear and the eye muscles. (See Fig. 3–5c and Paroxysmal Positional Nystagmus, Chapter 5). It is readily seen on visual inspection and can be recorded with electronystagmography (ENG).[2] It is important to keep in mind, however, that ENG does not record torsional eye movements and that the major

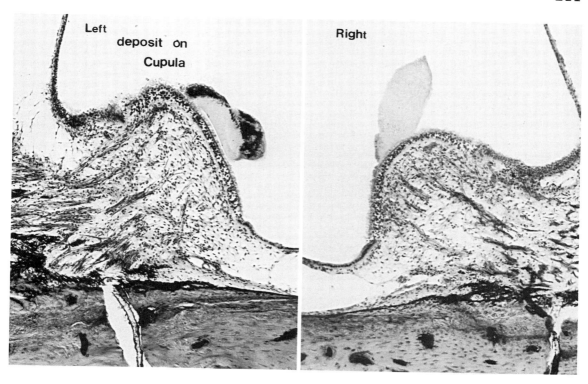

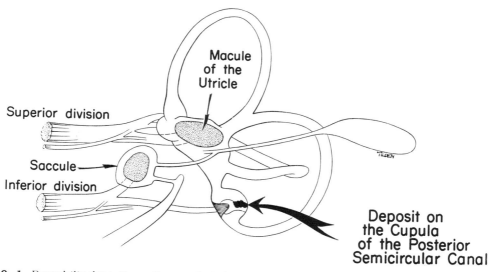

Figure 10–1. Basophilic deposits on the cupula in benign positional vertigo. *(Top)* Histopathological section through the cristae of the posterior semicircular canals of a patient who exhibited typical benign paroxysmal positional vertigo and nystagmus in the head-hanging left position prior to death from unrelated causes. Attached to the cupula of the left posterior canal is a granular, basophilic staining deposit. *(Bottom)* Drawing illustrating relationship between the macule of the utricle and the ampulla of the posterior semicircular canal when the head is erect. (From Schuknecht,[11] with permission.)

linear component of the nystagmus is vertical (see Fig. 6–9). If vertical eye movements are not recorded as part of the ENG examination, the nystagmus might be missed. The nystagmus fatigues (decreases with repeated positioning) in more than 90 percent of patients, but there are occasional patients with otherwise typical positional vertigo and nystagmus who do not show fatigue with repeated positioning.[1] The presence of positional nystagmus correlates with the clinical symptoms. Unless the patient is tested during a period in which he or she is having acute episodes of vertigo, positional nystagmus will not be observed. In the study mentioned above, many patients who had typical paroxysmal positional nystagmus on the initial examination did not have it on repeat examination weeks to months later.

In addition to finding the characteristic paroxysmal positional nystagmus on ENG, patients with benign positional vertigo may also exhibit a static positional nystagmus in one or both lateral positions and either a vestibular paresis or directional preponderance to caloric stimulation.[1] In most patients with caloric hypoexcitability, the decreased response is on the side that was undermost when positional nystagmus was induced. Presumably, such patients have involvement of both the horizontal and posterior semicircular canals on the same side.

MANAGEMENT

Once the diagnosis is made, a simple explanation of the nature of the disorder and its favorable prognosis can help relieve the patient's anxiety. Because of the dramatic nature of these episodes of vertigo, many patients believe they have a life-threatening disorder such as a tumor or stroke and they are reassured to learn that they have a benign inner ear disorder. It is important to be aware, however, that although it is a benign disorder the course is often protracted. In the study mentioned earlier,[1] one third of the patients reported episodes occurring for more than a year, and seven reported episodes dating back more than 10 years. The episodes of positional vertigo occurred in flurries, and nearly all patients

had at least one exacerbation after an initial remission. The likelihood of a recurrence should be explained to patients so that they are not unduly frightened if it occurs.

Positional exercises can accelerate remissions in most cases of benign positional vertigo.[4] The patient is instructed to sit on the edge of a bed and then rapidly assume the lateral position to induce positional vertigo. After the vertigo subsides, the patient returns to the upright position, usually experiencing a lesser episode of vertigo (Fig. 10–2). These positional changes are repeated in each session until the vertigo fatigues, and the sessions are repeated three times a day until the vertigo no longer occurs. In our experience patients who show the most prominent fatigue on the standard diagnostic positional test will derive the most benefit from positional exercises. It has been hypothesized that these positional maneuvers work by dislodging the calcium carbonate material from the cupula of the posterior semicircular canal.[4] Central adaptation is another possible explanation for their benefit. Antivertiginous medications such as meclizine or phenergan (25 mg each) can be used for symptomatic treatment of the vertigo during an acute exacerbation while the patient is performing positional exercises. These medications are useful for suppressing the nausea and nonspecific dizziness between acute episodes but have only minimal effect on the severe abrupt episodes. They do not seem to interfere with the beneficial effects of the exercises.

For those rare patients with prolonged intractable benign positional vertigo unresponsive to conventional therapy, a surgical procedure whereby the ampullary nerve is sectioned from the posterior semicircular canal crista may be considered. This operation, known as a singular neurectomy, has been effective in relieving benign positional vertigo in more than 90 percent of patients.[6] The main complication is a sensorineural hearing loss occurring in about 8 percent of patients. Transection of the vestibular nerve through a middle cranial fossa approach is another procedure that can relieve the positional vertigo while preserving hearing, but it is associated with greater potential risks than the singular neurectomy operation.

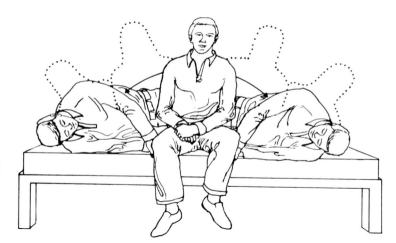

Figure 10–2. Positioning exercises for treatment of benign paroxysmal positional vertigo. (Adapted from Brandt, T and Daroff, RB: Physical therapy for benign paroxysmal positional vertigo. Arch Otolaryngol 106:484, 1980.)

REFERENCES

1. Baloh, RW, Honrubia, V, and Jacobson, K: Benign positional vertigo. Clinical and oculographic features in 240 cases. Neurology 37:371, 1987.
2. Baloh, RW, Sakala, SM, and Honrubia, V: Benign paroxysmal positional nystagmus. Am J Otolaryngol 1:1, 1979.
3. Bárány, R: Diagnose von Krankheitserschernungen in bereiche des otolithenapparates. Acta Otolaryngol 2:434, 1921.
4. Brandt, T and Daroff, RB: Physical therapy for benign paroxysmal positional vertigo. Arch Otolaryngol 106:484, 1980.
5. Dix, M and Hallpike, C: The pathology, symptomatology and diagnosis of certain common disorders of the vestibular systems. Ann Otol Rhinol Laryngol 61:987, 1952.
6. Gacek, RR: Further observations on posterior ampullary nerve transection for positional vertigo. Ann Otol Rhinol Laryngol 87:300, 1978.
7. Harbert, F: Benign paroxysmal positional nystagmus. Arch Ophthalmol 84:298, 1970.
8. Katsarkas, A and Kirkham, TH: Paroxysmal positional vertigo: A study of 255 cases. J Otolaryngol 7:320, 1978.
9. Schuknecht, H: Cupulolithiasis. Arch Otolaryngol 90:765, 1969.
10. Schuknecht, H and Ruby, R: Cupulolithiasis. Adv Otorhinolaryngol 20:434, 1973.
11. Schuknecht, HF: Pathology of the Ear. Harvard University Press, Cambridge, MA, 1974.

Chapter 11

ENDOLYMPHATIC HYDROPS (MENIERE'S SYNDROME)

CLINICAL FEATURES

Meniere's syndrome is characterized by fluctuating hearing loss and tinnitus, episodic vertigo, and a sensation of fullness or pressure in the ear. The clinical syndrome was first described by Prosper Meniere in 1861,[3] but Hallpike and Cairns[11] made the first clinical pathologic correlation with hydrops of the labyrinth. Subsequently numerous pathologic studies have been reported, and the findings of endolymphatic hydrops are remarkably consistent in patients with the syndrome originally described by Meniere.

Typically, the patient with Meniere's syndrome develops a sensation of fullness and pressure along with decreased hearing and tinnitus in one ear. Vertigo rapidly follows, reaching a maximum intensity within minutes and then slowly subsides over the next several hours. The patient is usually left with a sense of unsteadiness and dizziness for days after the acute vertiginous episode. In the early stages the hearing loss is completely reversible but in later stages a residual hearing loss remains. Tinnitus may persist between episodes but usually increases in intensity immediately before or during the acute episode. It is typically described as a roaring sound (the sound of the ocean or a hollow seashell sound). After vomiting the patient prefers to lie in bed without eating until the acute symptoms pass. Such episodes occur at irregular intervals for years, with periods of remission unpredictably intermixed.[9] Eventually, severe permanent hearing loss develops and the episodic nature sponta-neously disappears ("burnt-out phase"). In about one third of patients bilateral involvement will eventually occur.[11, 28]

Variations from this classic picture occur, particularly in the early stages of the disease process, but the diagnosis remains uncertain unless the combination of fluctuating hearing loss and vertigo occur. Rarely, isolated episodes of vertigo or hearing loss will precede the characteristic combination of symptoms by months or even years. Although so-called "vestibular Meniere's" and "cochlear Meniere's" have been proposed as variations of the classic syndrome, clinical-pathologic correlation of isolated vestibular and auditory disorders with selective endolymphatic hydrops of the vestibular and auditory labyrinth is lacking. Some patients with well-documented Meniere's syndrome experience abrupt episodes of falling to the ground without loss of consciousness or associated neurologic symptoms. These episodes have been called otolithic catastrophies by Tumarkin[26] because of his suspicion that they represented acute stimulation of the otoliths from the hydrops. Patients often report feeling as though they were pushed to the ground by some external force. These episodes can be confused with drop attacks seen with vertebrobasilar insufficiency and may suggest an inaccurate diagnosis in a patient with otherwise typical symptoms and signs of Meniere's syndrome.

So-called delayed endolymphatic hydrops develops in an ear that has been damaged years before usually by a viral or bacterial infection.[16, 20] With this disorder, the patient reports a long history of hearing loss since early childhood followed many years later by typical symptoms and signs of endolymphatic hydrops. If the hearing loss is profound, as it often is, the episodic vertigo will not be accompanied by fluctuating hearing levels and tinnitus. Pathologic studies in such patients suggest that delayed endolymphatic hydrops results from damage to the resorptive mechanism of the inner ear from the initial insult; it eventually leads to an imbalance between secretion and resorption of endolymph. Delayed endolymphatic hydrops can be unilateral or bilateral, depending on the extent of damage at the time of the original insult.

PATHOPHYSIOLOGY

As indicated above, the principal pathologic finding in patients with Meniere's syndrome is an increase in the volume of endolymph associated with distension of the entire endolymphatic system (Fig. 11–1).[17] The membranous labyrinth progressively dilates until the saccular wall makes

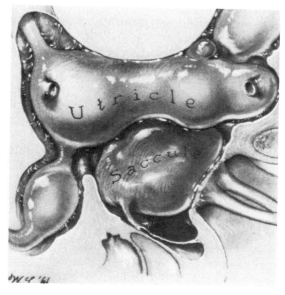

Figure 11–1. Dilated membranous labyrinth in Meniere's syndrome. The drawing was made from a three-dimensional model developed from serial sections of the ear of a patient with Meniere's syndrome. (From Schuknecht,[21] with permission.)

contact with the stapes footplate and the cochlear duct occupies the entire vestibular scala. The cochlear and vestibular end-organs and nerves show minimal pathologic changes. Membranous labyrinth herniations and ruptures are common, the latter frequently involving Reissner's membrane and the walls of the sacculus, utriculus, and ampullae. Occasionally, a rupture is followed by complete collapse of the membranous labyrinth.

Although the pathologic changes in Meniere's syndrome have been well described, the mechanism for its fluctuating symptoms and signs are still not completely understood. The leading theory is that the episodes of hearing loss and vertigo are caused by ruptures in the membranes separating endolymph from perilymph, producing a sudden increase in potassium concentration in the latter. If the perilymph space of animals is infused with a potassium solution, the bioelectric activity of the labyrinthine receptors is inhibited.[23] When the artificial infusate is stopped, potassium is slowly cleared from the perilymph, and labyrinthine function returns to normal in 2 to 3 hours (the typical duration of a Meniere's attack). Another possible explanation for fluctuating symptoms with Meniere's syndrome is mechanical deformation of the end-organ, which is reversible as the endolymphatic pressure decreases.[2] The dramatic sudden falling attacks initially described by Tumarkin are likely due to sudden deformation or displacement of one of the otolith organs.

ETIOLOGY

Several diseases are known to produce Meniere's syndrome but in the majority of cases the cause is unknown. Bacterial, viral, and syphilitic labyrinthitis all can lead to endolymphatic hydrops and typical symptoms and signs of Meniere's syndrome. The hydrops results from damage to fluid-resorptive mechanisms due to inflammation and scarring of the endolymphatic duct and sac. Multiple etiologic possibilities have been proposed for idiopathic Meniere's syndrome including allergy, endocrine disturbance, infection, sympathetic vasomotor disturbances, and even psychosomatic factors.[21] Patients with idiopathic Meniere's syndrome frequently have a positive family history (in some reports as high as 50 percent), suggesting genetic predisposing factors.[5, 6] Developmental hypoplasia of the endolymphatic duct and sac may be a unifying concept. The similarity in pathologic findings between so-called delayed endolymphatic hydrops and idiopathic Meniere's syndrome has suggested a possible common viral etiology. A subclinical viral infection could damage the resorptive mechanism of the inner ear, leading to an eventual decompensation in the balance between secretion and resorption of endolymph.[19]

Endolymphatic hydrops can be reliably produced in animals by either blocking the endolymphatic duct or destroying the endolymphatic sac.[4, 14] Although the extent of the hydrops in the cochlear and vestibular labyrinths is similar to that seen with Meniere's syndrome, the characteristic ruptures in the membranous wall allowing an intermixing of endolymph and perilymph are rarely seen with the animal model. Several drug and surgical treatment protocols have been tried with the experimental animal model of hydrops, but so far none has been effective in reliably controlling or preventing the disorder.[13]

DIAGNOSIS

The key to the diagnosis of Meniere's syndrome is to document fluctuating hearing levels in a patient with the characteristic clinical history.[1] A shift of more than 10 dB at two different frequencies is pathognomonic. In the early stages, the sensorineural hearing loss is usually greater in the lower frequencies (see Fig. 8–2C). Speech discrimination is relatively preserved, and recruitment often occurs consistent with a cochlear site of dysfunction. Brainstem auditory-evoked response (BAER) and stapedius reflex measurements are normal. Electronystagmography (ENG) examination may reveal a peripheral spontaneous nystagmus and either a vestibular paresis or directional preponderance on caloric testing. During an acute attack of Meniere's disease the nystagmus may be directed toward the involved ear,

suggesting an excitatory rather than a destructive effect. However, this "wrong-direction nystagmus" may be a reversal phenomena due to central compensation, because episodes that have been monitored from the onset begin with nystagmus in the correct direction (i.e., fast component toward the good ear).[15] Radiologic studies of the temporal bones in patients with idiopathic Meniere's syndrome often show narrowing of the endolymphatic duct or decreased pneumatization of the temporal bone.[27] However, these features are also seen in normal subjects and therefore are of limited value in the diagnosis of Meniere's syndrome.

MANAGEMENT

Because the cause of Meniere's syndrome is usually unknown, treatment is empiric. Medical management consists of symptomatic treatment of the acute spells (Table 11–1) and long-term prophylaxis with salt restriction and diuretics.[7, 12] Phenergan, 25 to 50 mg, orally or via suppository, is usually effective for relieving the acute vertigo, nausea, and vomiting. It should be taken as soon as possible, preferably during the prodrome if there are reliable warning symptoms. Antiemetics such as proclorperazine (Compazine) are sometimes useful if nausea and vomiting are severe. The mechanism by which a low-salt diet decreases the frequency and severity of attacks with Meniere's syndrome is unclear, but there is extensive empiric evidence for its efficacy. In some patients the results are dramatic. We have seen patients who had had severe disabling episodes on a weekly basis have prolonged remissions (years) on a low-salt diet. Other patients show little or no improvement, possibly reflecting the multifactorial pathogenesis of Meniere's syndrome. We recommend salt restriction in the range of 1 to 2 grams per day, with a minimum therapeutic trial of 2 to 3 months. If a good response is obtained, then the level of salt intake can be gradually increased while symptoms and signs are carefully monitored. Fluid and food intake should be regularly distributed throughout the day, and binges (particularly foods with high sugar

Table 11–1. DOSAGE AND EFFECTS OF COMMONLY USED
ANTIVERTIGINOUS MEDICATIONS

Class	Drug	Dosage	Sedation	Anti-emetic Actions	Dryness of Mucous Membranes	Extra-pyramidal Symptoms
Anticholinergic	Scopolamine	0.6 mg orally q4–6h or 0.5 mg transdermally q3d	+	+	+ + +	—
Monoaminergic	Amphetamine	5 or 10 mg orally q4–6h	—	+	+	+
	Ephedrine	25 mg orally q4–6h	—	+	+	—
Antihistamine	Meclizine (Antivert)	25 mg orally q4–6h	+	+	+	—
	Dimenhydrinate (Dramamine)	50 mg orally or intra-muscularly q4–6h or 100-mg suppository q8h	+	+	+	—
	Promethazine (Phenergan)	25 or 50 mg orally, in-tramuscularly, or as suppository q4–6h	+ +	+ +	+	—
Phenothiazine	Prochlorperazine (Compazine)	5 or 10 mg orally or in-tramuscularly q6h or 25 mg suppository q12h	+	+ + +	+	+ + +
Benzodiazepine	Diazepam (Valium)	5 or 10 mg orally, intra-muscularly, or intra-venously q4–6h	+ + +	+	—	—

and/or salt content) should be avoided. Occasionally, patients will notice that certain foods (e.g., alcohol, coffee, chocolate) may precipitate attacks. Diuretics (acetazolamide, 250 mg two times a day or hydrochlorothiazide, 50 mg two times a day) provide additional benefit in some patients, although, in our experience, they cannot replace a salt-restriction diet. Recently it has been shown that acetazolamide decreases the osmotic pressure of the inner ear in experimental endolymphatic hydrops in guinea pigs.[22]

Two different types of surgery have been used for treating Meniere's syndrome: endolymphatic shunts and destructive procedures. Although shunts are logical, based on the presumed pathophysiology of Meniere's syndrome, several factors limit the probability of achieving a functional shunt with this disorder.[18] The most popular shunt procedure at the present time drains the endolymphatic sac to the mastoid cavity. A major conceptual problem with this procedure is that pathologic studies of temporal bones in patients with Meniere's syndrome usually show evidence of blockage of the endolymphatic pathways proximal to the endolymphatic sac. Furthermore, Schuknecht[18] pointed out that any drain device that is implanted in the endolymphatic sac will almost certainly become rapidly encapsulated in fibrous tissue. Revision operations and temporal bone studies in patients who have had shunts implanted have shown fibrous encapsulation of shunt devices. Not surprisingly there are conflicting reports regarding the clinical efficacy of these surgical shunt procedures.[25]

The rationale for ablative surgery in treatment of Meniere's syndrome is that the nervous system is better able to compensate for complete loss of vestibular function than for partial loss, that is, fluctuating in degree. Ablative procedures are most effective in patients with unilateral involvement who have no functional hearing on the damaged side. Obviously, ablative surgery should not be considered if the abnormal side is not well defined or if the nature of the underlying disorder is not absolutely clear. Severe vertigo is expected during the immediate postoperative period, but most patients who follow a structured vestibular exercise program can return to normal activity within 1 to 3 months (Table 11–2).[8, 24] Ablative surgical procedures generally should be avoided in elderly patients because the elderly have great difficulty adjusting to the vestibular imbalance.

The two main types of destructive surgery are labyrinthectomy and vestibular nerve section.[10] Labyrinthectomy is useful only when there is no functional hearing on the damaged side. The purpose of a labyrinthectomy is to remove the neural epithelium of the vestibular end-organ. Transoval window or transround window exenteration are simple procedures that may be effective, but parts of the neural epithelium are often left behind which may lead to return of episodic vertigo. For total removal of the vestibular neural epithelium a translabyrinthine labyrinthectomy is required. In this procedure, the surgeon first performs a simple mastoidectomy to outline the three semicircular canals. Next, the canals are opened, their neuroepithelium is removed, and the dissection is carried into the vestibule where the remaining neuroepithelium is identified and removed. The procedure can be extended

at this point to include sectioning of the superior and inferior divisions of the vestibular nerve in the internal auditory canal. Major complications are infrequent with this procedure, inasmuch as hearing is not a factor, the subarachnoid space is not violated, and the facial nerve is usually not exposed in areas where it is not covered by a thick sheath.

Vestibular neurectomy has the advantage of preserving hearing in patients with salvageable residual cochlear function, but the risks of complication are greater than with labyrinthectomy. Initially, the neurosurgical suboccipital approach to the cerebellopontine angle was used for intracranial sectioning of the vestibular nerve. Inasmuch as this procedure involves considerable risk to the patient, its use in treating episodic vertigo is probably unwarranted. More recently, a retrolabyrinth approach to the vestibular nerve has been developed, offering the possibility of hearing conservation where salvageable residual cochlear function exists. Major complications of this procedure include trauma to the facial and/or cochlear nerves.

Table 11–2. VESTIBULAR EXERCISES

A. In bed
    Eye movements at first slow, then quick
    Gazing up and down
    Gazing from side to side
    Focusing on finger moving from 30 to 10 cm
       away from face
B. Sitting
    Head movements as above
    Shoulder shrugging and circling
    Bending forward and picking up objects from
       ground
C. Standing
    Eye and head movements, shoulder shrugging
       and circling as above
    Changing from sitting to standing position
       with eyes open and closed
    Throwing small ball from hand to hand (above
       eye level)
    Throwing ball from hand to hand under knee
    Changing from sitting to standing position,
       turning around in between
D. Moving about
    Walking across room with eyes open and then
       closed
    Walking up and down slope with eyes open and
       then closed
    Performing any game involving stooping and
       stretching and aiming

REFERENCES

1. Alford, B: Meniere's disease: Criteria for diagnosis and evaluation of therapy for reporting. Report of Subcommittee on Equilibrium and Measurement. Trans Am Acad Ophthalmol Otolaryngol 76:1462, 1972.
2. Altman, F and Zechner, G: The pathology and pathogenesis of endolymphatic hydrops. New investigations. Arch Klin Exper Ohr-Nas-Kehlkheilk 192:1, 1968.
3. Atkinson, M: Meniere's original papers: Reprinted with an English translation together with commentaries and biographical sketch. Acta Otolaryngol (Suppl 162):14, 1961.
4. Beal, D: Effect of endolymphatic sac ablation in the rabbit and cat. Acta Otolaryngol 66:333, 1968.
5. Bernstein, J: Occurrence of episodic vertigo and hearing loss in families. Ann Otol Rhinol Laryngol 74:1011, 1965.
6. Birgerson, L, Gustavson, K-H, and Stahle, J: Familial Meniere's disease. Acta Otolaryngol 412(Suppl):71, 1984.
7. Boles, R, Rice, DH, Hybels, R, and Work, WP: Conservative management of Meniere's disease: Furstenberg regimen revisited. Ann Otol Rhinol Laryngol 84:513, 1975.
8. Brandt, TH: Episodic vertigo. In Rake, RE (ed): Conn's Current Therapy. WB Saunders, Philadelphia, 1985, p 741.

9. Eggermont, JJ and Schmidt, PH: Meniere's disease: A long-term follow-up study of hearing loss. Ann Otol Rhinol Laryngol 94:1, 1985.
10. Glasscock, ME, Davis, ME, Hughes, GB, and Jackson, CG: Labyrinthectomy versus middle fossa vestibular nerve section in Meniere's disease. Ann Otol Rhinol Laryngol 89:318, 1980.
11. Hallpike, C and Cairns, H: Observations on the pathology of Meniere's syndrome. J Laryngol 53:625, 1938.
12. Jackson, CG, et al: Medical management of Meniere's disease. Ann Otol 90:142, 1981.
13. Kimura, RS: Surgical and drug intervention in experimentally induced endolymphatic hydrops. In Nomura, Y (ed): Hearing Loss and Dizziness. Tokyo, Igaku-Shoin, 1985, p 16.
14. Kimura, RS: Experimental blockage of the endolymphatic duct and sac and its effect on the inner ear of the guinea pig: A study on endolymphatic hydrops. Ann Otol Rhinol Laryngol 76:664, 1967.
15. McClure, JA, Copp, JC, and Lycett, P: Recovery nystagmus in Meniere's disease. Laryngoscope 91:1727, 1981.
16. Nadol, JB, Weiss, AD, and Parker, SW: Vertigo of delayed onset after sudden deafness. Ann Otol 84:841, 1975.
17. Paparella, MM: Pathology of Meniere's disease. Ann Otol Rhinol Laryngol 93(Suppl 112):31, 1984.
18. Schuknecht, HF: Endolymphatic hydrops: Can it be controlled? Ann Otol Rhinol Laryngol 95:36, 1986.
19. Schuknecht, HF: Neurolabyrinthitis. Viral infections of the peripheral auditory and vestibular systems. In Nomura, Y (ed): Hearing Loss and Dizziness. Tokyo, Igaku-Shoin, 1985, p. 1.
20. Schuknecht, HF: Delayed endolymphatic hydrops. Ann Otol 87:743, 1978.
21. Schuknecht, HF: Pathology of the Ear. Harvard University Press, Cambridge, MA, 1974.
22. Shinkawa, H and Kimura, RS: Effect of diuretics on endolymphatic hydrops. Acta Otolaryngol 101:43, 1986.
23. Silverstein, H: The effects of perfusing the perilymphatic space with artificial endolymph. Ann Otol Rhinol Laryngol 79:754, 1970.
24. Takemori, S, Ida, M, and Umezu, H: Vestibular training after sudden loss of vestibular functions. ORL 47:76, 1985.
25. Thomsen, J, Brettan, P, Tos, M, and Johnsen, NJ: Placebo effect of surgery for Meniere's disease. Arch Otolaryngol 107:271, 1981.
26. Tumarkin, I: Otolithic catastrophe; a new syndrome. Br Med J 2:175, 1936.
27. Valvassori, GE and Dobben, GD: Multidirectional and computerized tomography of the vestibular aqueduct in Meniere's disease. Ann Otol Rhinol Laryngol 93:547, 1984.
28. Wladislavosky-Waserman, P, Facer, GW, Mokri, B, and Kurland, LT: Meniere's Disease: A 30-year epidemiologic and clinical study in Rochester, MN, 1951–1980. Laryngoscope 94:1098, 1984.

Chapter 12

VASCULAR DISORDERS

VERTEBROBASILAR INSUFFICIENCY (VBI)

Pathophysiology

As discussed in Chapter 2, the vascular supply to the labyrinth, eighth nerve, and brainstem arises from a common source: the vertebrobasilar circulation. The vestibular system is subject to two general categories of vascular ischemia: (1) hypoperfusion in the vertebrobasilar system, in which case multiple areas (both peripheral and central) become simultaneously ischemic, or (2) hypoperfusion in the distribution of a single smaller feeding vessel, in which case there is a circumscribed area of ischemia. In the former case the site of origin of hypoperfusion can be anywhere from the heart and major vessels in the chest and neck to the basilar artery, whereas in the latter case an occlusion is usually situated near the origin or, less frequently, in the smaller feeding vessel itself. These two categories of ischemia are not mutually exclusive, however; a patient with small vessel disease may be as asymptomatic because of collateral circulation, but an added hypoperfusion in the vertebrobasilar system can lead to focal ischemia and/or infarction.

The cause of VBI is usually atherosclerosis of the subclavian, vertebral, and basilar arteries.[13, 19, 41] Other less common causes of arterial occlusion include dissection, arteritis, emboli, polycythemia, thromboangitis obliterans, and hypercoagulation syndromes. In rare cases occlusion or stenosis of the subclavian or innominate arteries just proximal to the origin of the vertebral artery results in the so-called subclavian steal syndrome. In this syndrome VBI results from siphoning of blood down the vertebral artery from the basilar system to supply the upper extremity. Occasionally, episodes of VBI are precipitated by postural hypotension, Stokes-Adams attacks, or mechanical compression from cervical spondylosis. Regarding the latter, cervical spondylosis is extremely common in the elderly, but documented cases of mechanical compression of the vertebral arteries by neck turning or extension are rare.

Clinical Features

VBI is a common cause of vertigo in patients over the age of 50.[21, 55] Whether the vertigo originates from ischemia of the labyrinth, brainstem, or both structures is not always clear. It is abrupt in onset, usually lasts several minutes, and is frequently associated with nausea and vomiting. In a series of 65 patients with VBI reported by Williams and Wilson,[55] vertigo was the initial symptom in 48 percent. Invariably, the vertigo is associated with symptoms resulting from ischemia in the remaining territory supplied by the posterior circulation (those listed in Table 12–1). These symptoms occur in episodes either in combination with the vertigo or in isolation. Vertigo may be an isolated initial symptom of VBI or may occur in isolation intermixed with more typical episodes of VBI,[25] but long-standing (>6 months) recurrent episodes of vertigo without other symptoms should suggest a disorder other than VBI.[21]

Diagnosis

The diagnosis of VBI rests on finding the characteristic combination of symptoms

Table 12–1. INITIAL SYMPTOMS OF VERTEBROBASILAR INSUFFICIENCY IN 65 PATIENTS[55]

Symptom	Number	Percentage
Vertigo	32	48
Visual hallucinations	7	10
Drop attacks or weakness	7	10
Visceral sensations	5	8
Visual field defects	4	6
Diplopia	3	5
Headaches	2	3
Other	5	8

listed in Table 12–1, typically occurring in episodes lasting minutes. One can usually find multiple risk factors for atherosclerotic vascular disease, and often there is a prior history of myocardial infarction or occlusive peripheral vascular disease. Between episodes, the neurologic examination is usually normal, although there may be residual signs of prior brainstem and/or cerebellar infarction. Both peripheral and central signs can occur on electronystagmography (ENG) testing, with the most common finding being a unilateral vestibular paresis to caloric stimulation (present in approximately 25 percent of patients).[25] The latter presumably results from ischemic damage to the vestibular labyrinth. Computerized tomography (CT) and magnetic resonance (MR) scans of the brain are normal unless there was prior infarction. Angiography is unlikely to lead to definitive surgical treatment inasmuch as the occlusions are usually intracranial.[21] Furthermore, angiographic findings often do not correlate with clinical symptoms and signs.

Management

Knowledge of the natural history of VBI is critical in assessing any treatment regimen.[12] Although some patients with VBI go on to develop infarction, the great majority do not. Furthermore, patients with episodes of vertigo of typical vascular onset and duration, with or without associated symptoms, may have the most benign course of all the VBI syndromes.[25] More worrisome are patients who present with

episodes of quadraparesis, perioral numbness, bilateral blindness, or loss of consciousness. These latter symptoms are prodroma of basilar artery thrombosis; they require more aggressive investigation (including angiography).

Treatment of VBI usually consists of controlling risk factors (diabetes, hypertension, hyperlipidemia) and using antiplatelet drugs (aspirin 330 mg/day).[34] Anticoagulation is reserved for patients with frequent incapacitating episodes or in patients with symptoms and signs suggesting a stroke in evolution, particularly basilar artery thrombosis. In these instances heparin is used, with an intravenous (IV) bolus of 5000 units followed by a continuous infusion of 1000 units per hour. The dose is titrated to keep the partial thromboplastin time at approximately 2.5 times control. After 3 to 4 days warfarin is begun with an oral dose of 15 mg. The daily dose is then adjusted (5 to 15 mg) until the prothrombin time is approximately twice the control value. Heparin is then discontinued. In some patients, symptoms and signs will recur as heparin is discontinued, and the heparin must then be restarted and more gradually tapered.

Although surgical reconstruction and revascularization procedures have been performed successfully in the vertebrobasilar system, their specific indications have yet to be defined.[34] Controlled studies with modern angiographic and surgical techniques are needed to assess the risk/benefit ratio.

LABYRINTHINE ISCHEMIA AND INFARCTION

The internal auditory artery arises from the anterior inferior cerebellar artery in approximately 85 percent of individuals and from the basilar or vertebral arteries in the other 15 percent.[47] After supplying all of the eighth nerve, the internal auditory artery (about 200 microns in diameter) divides into two main branches to supply the auditory and vestibular labyrinth (see Fig. 2–8). Occlusion of the internal auditory artery leads to a sudden, profound loss of both auditory and vestibular function. Hearing loss is usually permanent, and a vestibular imbalance remains, although symptoms gradually improve with central compensation. Pathologic studies in such patients reveal widespread necrosis of inner ear tissues with subsequent proliferation of fibrous tissue and new bone formation.[47] Most documented cases have been seen in association with ischemia in the distribution of the anterior inferior cerebellar artery accompanied by infarction of the dorsal lateral pontomedullary region and the inferolateral cerebellum. Not infrequently, infarction of the labyrinth is preceded by typical episodes of VBI, in some cases isolated episodes of vertigo.[25] The diagnosis should be considered in any patient with the sudden onset of unilateral deafness and vertigo, particularly if there is a prior history of transient ischemic attack (TIA), stroke, or known atherosclerotic vascular disease.

Cochlea

The role of vascular occlusion in the production of sudden unilateral deafness is controversial.[43] There is little reason to suspect that unilateral deafness in a young, healthy individual is caused by vascular disease. As already suggested, most of these cases are probably due to viral infections. However, the sudden onset of deafness without associated vertigo or brainstem signs in a patient with known vascular disease or hypercoagulation syndrome should suggest the possibility of ischemia within the distribution of the common cochlear artery or one of its branches. Sudden deafness (reversible or permanent) has been reported in patients with fat emboli,[31] thromboangitis obliterans,[33] and macroglobulinemia.[45] Atherosclerotic disease is also associated with sudden deafness, but pathologic confirmation of the site of vascular occlusion is often lacking. Examination of the cochlea at necropsy in such patients reveals loss of the organ of corti, and degenerative changes in the stria vascularis, spiral ligament, and distal cochlear nerve fibers (findings similar to those seen in animals who have had their internal auditory artery occluded).[47]

Vestibular Labyrinth

Ischemia confined to the anterior vestibular artery distribution can result in transient episodes of vertigo (lasting minutes) or a prolonged attack (lasting days) due to infarction of the vestibular labyrinth.[25] The former are often associated with hyperviscosity syndromes such as polycythemia, macroglobulinemia, and sickle cell anemia.[2] The clinical picture of infarction is that of a sudden onset of vertigo without hearing loss or brainstem symptoms. After recovering from the acute manifestations, patients may develop episodes of paroxysmal positional vertigo months to years later. Schuknecht[46] postulated that this positional vertigo resulted from ischemic necrosis of the utricular macula, causing a release of octoconia that settle on the intact cupula of the posterior semicircular canal (see Chapter 10). Lindsay and Hemenway[38] reported seven cases of this syndrome—with examination of the temporal bone in one case. All were elderly patients with atherosclerotic vascular disease. The lesion consisted of degeneration of part of Scarpa's ganglion and the nerves to the utriculus and the anterior and horizontal semicircular canals, with a mass of convoluted vessels in the internal auditory canal—indicating a vascular occlusion as the cause.

Diagnosis

The diagnosis of ischemia or infarction of the labyrinth rests on finding the characteristic clinical picture of a sudden onset of hearing loss and/or vertigo in a patient with known cerebral vascular disease (manifested by prior TIA or stroke) or in a patient with risk factors for vascular occlusions (such as vasculitis, hypercoagulation, or hyperviscosity). The common occurrence of transient isolated episodes of vertigo preceding the onset of typical episodes of VBI or infarction (particularly in the distribution of the anterior inferior cerebellar artery) indicates that the vestibular labyrinth is selectively vulnerable to ischemia within the vertebrobasilar system.[25] As with other TIAs, patients with transient ischemia of the labyrinth have normal diagnostic studies between episodes. With infarction of the labyrinth, hearing loss is profound, and auditory-evoked (cochlear and brainstem) and caloric responses are absent.

Management

Management of labyrinthine infarction is primarily symptomatic. Antivertiginous medications (meclizine 25 mg, phenergan 25 mg) can help relieve the acute vertigo and nausea. Vestibular exercises (see Table 11–2) should be started as soon as the patient is able to cooperate.[56] Patients with recurring symptoms of VBI are treated with antiplatelet drugs and anticoagulation as discussed above. Reduction in blood viscosity is indicated in patients with hyperviscosity syndromes.[2]

INFARCTION OF THE BRAINSTEM AND CEREBELLUM

Lateral Medullary Infarction (Wallenberg's Syndrome)

The zone of infarction producing the lateral medullary syndrome consists of a wedge of the dorsal lateral medulla just posterior to the olive (Fig. 12–1). Although the syndrome is commonly known as that of the posterior inferior cerebellar artery, Fisher and coworkers[22] demonstrated that it usually results from occlusion of the ipsilateral vertebral artery, and only rarely from occlusion of the posterior inferior cerebellar artery. Major symptoms include vertigo, nausea, vomiting, intractable hiccuping, ipsilateral facial pain, diplopia, dysphagia, and dysphonia.

On examination, any or all of the follow-

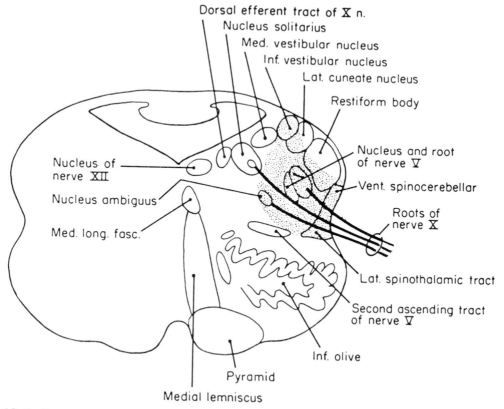

Figure 12–1. Cross-section of the medulla illustrating the zone of infarction with Wallenberg's syndrome (*stippled area*).

ing abnormalities may be found: (1) ipsilateral Horner syndrome from involvement of the preganglionic sympathetic fibers originating in the hypothalamus; (2) ipsilateral loss of pain and temperature sensation on the face due to involvement of the nucleus and descending tract of the fifth nerve; (3) ipsilateral paralysis of the palate, pharynx, and larynx from involvement of the nucleus ambiguous and the exiting fibers of the ninth and tenth nerves; (4) ipsilateral facial and lateral rectus weakness from involvement of the sixth and seventh nerves; (5) ipsilateral dysmetria, dysrhythmia, and dysdiadochokinesia from involvement of the cerebellum; and (6) contralateral loss of pain and temperature sensation on the body from involvement of the crossed spinothalamic fibers. Hearing loss does not occur because the lesion is caudal to the cochlear nerve entry zone and cochlear nuclei.

Patients with Wallenberg's syndrome suffer a prominent motor disturbance that causes their body and extremities to deviate toward the side of the lesion as if being pulled by a strong external force.[9] This so-called lateropulsion also affects the oculomotor system, causing excessively large voluntary and involuntary saccades directed toward the side of the lesion while saccades away from the lesion side are abnormally small.[4, 35] Patients also may exhibit a transient ocular tilt reaction (ipsilateral head tilt, skew deviation, and ocular torsion) that is associated with a deviation of the subjective visual vertical in the direction of the head tilt (see Chapter 5). Even with their head fixed in the true vertical, they perceive it as tilted opposite to the direction of the tilt reaction.

Lateral Pontomedullary Infarction

Ischemia in the distribution of the anterior inferior cerebellar artery usually results in infarction of the dorsolateral pontomedullary region and the inferior lateral cerebellum.[1] As noted above, because the labyrinthine artery arises from the anterior inferior cerebellar artery, in approximately 85 percent of cases infarction of the membranous labyrinth is a common accompaniment. Severe vertigo, nausea, and vomiting may be the initial and most prominent symptoms. Other associated symptoms include unilateral hearing loss, tinnitus, facial paralysis, and cerebellar asynergy. In addition to the signs of ipsilateral hearing loss, facial weakness, and cerebellar dysfunction, the examination discloses ipsilateral loss of pain and temperature sensation on the face from involvement of the trigeminal nucleus and tract and contralateral decreased pain and temperature sensation on the body from involvement of the crossed spinothalamic tract.

Cerebellar Infarction

Frequently, occlusion of the vertebral artery, the posterior inferior cerebellar artery, or the anterior inferior cerebellar artery results in infarction confined to the cerebellum without accompanying brainstem involvement.[17, 52] The initial symptoms are severe vertigo, vomiting, and ataxia, and because typical lateral brainstem signs are not present, a mistaken diagnosis of an acute peripheral labyrinthine disorder might be made.[29] The key differential point is the finding on examination of prominent cerebellar signs, including asymmetric gaze-evoked nystagmus (larger amplitude directed toward the side of the lesion). After a latent interval of 24 to 96 hours some patients develop progressive brainstem dysfunction due to compression by a swollen cerebellum. A relentless progression to quadriplegia, coma, and death follows unless the compression is surgically relieved.[52]

Diagnosis

The diagnosis of the lateral medullary and lateral pontomedullary syndromes, when complete, are readily apparent based on the characteristic combination of symptoms and signs listed above. Partial syndromes are more common than complete syndromes, however; presumably collateral circulation supports the border zones between the distribution of these and other brainstem arteries. Isolated cerebel-

lar infarction is the most difficult to identify, although careful neurologic examination should demonstrate ataxia beyond
that which could be seen with a peripheral
vestibular lesion. ENG typically identifies
central signs (spontaneous central nystagmus, gaze-evoked nystagmus, asymmetric
pursuit, and impaired fixation suppression of vestibular nystagmus), although a
vestibular paresis to caloric stimulation is
not uncommon (indicating ischemic damage to the labyrinth and/or eighth nerve).
Modern neuroimaging techniques are
most useful for differentiating cerebellar
infarction from more benign peripheral
causes of vertigo. CT scans are usually normal in the acute phase, but cerebellar infarction becomes apparent within a few
days.[29] With high-resolution MR scanning
both the brainstem and cerebellar infarction can be identified (Fig. 12–2).[10] An-

giography is unlikely to lead to definitive
therapy unless one suspects a vascular
malformation or dissecting aneurysm.

Management

As with other completed strokes, management of brainstem and/or cerebellar infarction is symptomatic. The clinical
course is typically that of an acute onset
followed by gradual incomplete recovery.
Vertigo may persist for months because of
damage to central structures important for
compensation.[30] Many patients complain
of disabling oscillopsia due to spontaneous
nystagmus and damaged central vestibular and cerebellar pathways. Antivertiginous medications are less effective for controlling vertigo than with peripheral
vestibular lesions, and vestibular exercises

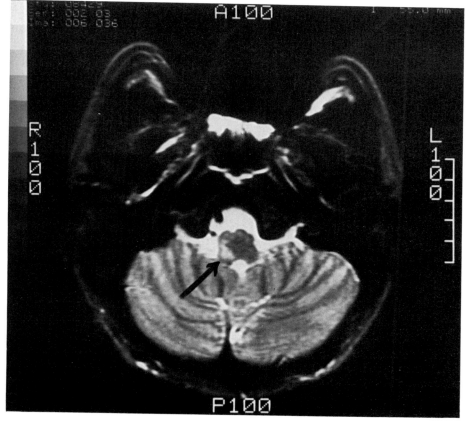

Figure 12–2. MR scan of the posterior fossa (T$_2$ weighted, transverse section) demonstrating infarction of the
right lateral medulla *(arrow).*

are often of little use. As noted above, patients with cerebellar infarction must be watched carefully for evidence of brainstem dysfunction from compression by a swollen cerebellum.

INTRALABYRINTHINE HEMORRHAGE

Spontaneous hemorrhage into the inner ear typically occurs in patients with an underlying bleeding diathesis.[47] Leukemia is the most common cause. Such patients experience the sudden onset of unilateral deafness and severe vertigo. Pathologic examination of the inner ear reveals hemorrhage into the perilymphatic space with smaller focal hemorrhages in the endolymphatic space. The vestibular and cochlear end organs, although morphologically intact are rendered nonfunctional, apparently from altered fluid chemistry. A similar condition may follow from a blow to the head without the occurrence of a bony fracture (so called labyrinthine concussion).

Diagnosis and Management

Diagnosis of intralabyrinthine hemorrhage is based on finding a sudden auditory and vestibular loss in a patient with an underlying bleeding diathesis (particularly leukemia) or in a patient who has received a blow to the head. Hearing loss and vestibular loss (documented with audiometric and ENG tests) are profound and usually permanent. Management consists of symptomatic treatment of the vertigo (see Table 11–1) and correcting the underlying bleeding diathesis when possible.

HEMORRHAGE INTO THE BRAINSTEM AND CEREBELLUM

Spontaneous intraparenchymal hemorrhage into the brainstem or cerebellum produces a dramatic clinical syndrome frequently progressing to loss of consciousness and death.[15] The cause of hemorrhage is hypertensive vascular disease in

approximately two thirds of patients. Anticoagulation therapy, cryptic arteriovenous malformations, and bleeding diathesis are also important etiologic factors whether alone or in combination with hypertension.

Vertigo may be an initial symptom with brainstem hemorrhage, but it is never an isolated symptom and is usually only fleeting as the patient rapidly plunges into coma. Hemorrhage into the pons typically results in a rapid onset of coma, flaccid quadriplegia, loss of horizontal eye movements, pinpoint reactive pupils, and ocular bobbing.[36] Hemorrhage into the medulla is associated with rapid cardiorespiratory failure and death.

Because of its potential reversibility, cerebellar hemorrhage deserves particular emphasis. The initial symptoms of acute cerebellar hemorrhage are vertigo, nausea, vomiting, headache, and inability to stand or walk.[23, 42] As with cerebellar infarction, these symptoms might be confused with an acute peripheral vestibular lesion. Unlike the latter, however, examination in the initial period usually reveals nuchal rigidity, prominent cerebellar signs, ipsilateral facial paralysis, and ipsilateral gaze paralysis. Pupils are often small bilaterally but reactive. Approximately 50 percent of patients lose consciousness within 24 hours of the initial symptoms, and 75 percent become comatose within 1 week of onset.[11] The condition is often fatal unless surgical decompression is performed. Midline cerebellar hemorrhage is particularly difficult to diagnose because it produces bilateral signs and generally runs a more fulminant course than a lateralized hemorrhage. Such patients have profound ataxia, usually being unable to stand—a finding never associated with benign peripheral vestibular lesions.

Diagnosis and Management

The diagnosis of hemorrhage into the brainstem and cerebellum has been revolutionized with the introduction of CT and MR scanning. CT is usually superior to MR for identifying intraparenchymal blood (Fig. 12–3). Any patient who presents with the acute onset of vertigo and who exhibits

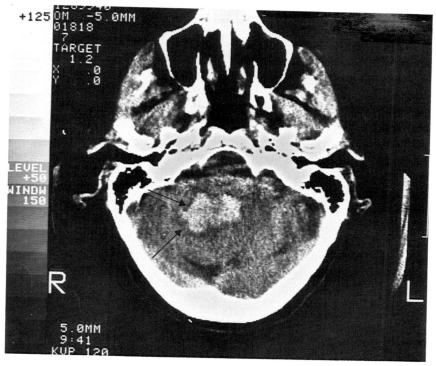

Figure 12–3. CT scan showing a cerebellar hemorrhage *(arrows).*

prominent ataxia, either of the trunk and/or extremities, should have a CT scan of the brain. If the CT is negative, an MR scan may still show evidence of cerebellar infarction.[10]

As indicated above, hemorrhage into the cerebellum is often fatal unless surgical decompression is performed. The earlier the syndrome is recognized, the more likely the surgery will be successful. Once the patient is comatose, almost none survive.[11] Small hemorrhages into the brainstem and cerebellum may spontaneously resolve.

MIGRAINE

Migraine is a syndrome characterized by periodic headaches along with many other symptoms, including dizziness and vertigo. It is nearly always familial and occurs in complex patterns and settings.[24] Migraine is estimated to affect nearly 25 percent of women and 15 percent of men.[53] Approximately 20 percent of adults with migraine indicate that their headaches be-

gan before the age of 10 years.[48] In the prepubertal periods boys with migraine outnumber girls by nearly two to one, but at puberty migraine decreases in boys and increases in girls so that a 2.5 to 1 female preponderance is established by adulthood. Although migraine usually begins before the age of 40, it is such a common disorder that a substantial number of adults become affected later in life.

Vertigo is a common symptom with migraine. It can occur with the headaches or in separate isolated episodes, and it can predate the onset of headache. Kayan and Hood[32] compared the incidence of nonspecific dizziness (a giddy sensation) and vertigo (an illusion of rotation) in 200 patients with migraine and 116 patients with tension headache. The headache sufferers were taken in sequence as they presented to a large outpatient headache clinic. Although the incidence of nonspecific dizziness was about the same in the migraine and tension headache groups (28 percent and 22 percent, respectively), the migraine patients had a much higher incidence of vertigo than the tension headache patients

(27 percent compared with 8 percent, difference significant at p<0.001). In 10 of the migraine patients the vertigo was severe enough that the patient sought help for this symptom independent of the headache.

Classifications of migraine vary, but most include classic migraine, common migraine, posterior fossa migraine, and migraine equivalents. It should be emphasized, however, that the patterns of symptomatology change over time and patients often move from one category to another.

Classic Migraine

A classic migraine headache begins with an aura and continues with a severe throbbing, usually unilateral headache. The aura symptoms slowly progress over several minutes, last 15 to 60 minutes, and then gradually abate. In about 25 percent of patients, however, onset is abrupt. The headache begins as the aura diminishes, usually reaching its peak in about an hour and gradually subsiding over the next 4 to 8 hours. Nausea and vomiting typically accompany the onset of head pain.

The migraine aura consists of transient neurologic dysfunction, usually visual disturbances, but may include prominent vertigo or somatosensory symptoms. Both positive and negative visual phenomena occur. The latter include complete blindness, hemianopsia or quadrantanopsia, tunnel vision, altitudinal defects, monocular blindness, or one or more scotomata. Positive phenomena are more common and may consist of stars, sparkling lights, unformed flashes of light (photopsia), geometric patterns, or a jagged sparkling zigzag (teichopsia or fortification spectra). Although usually black and white, the visual phenomena can be in color. The positive and negative visual phenomena are combined in the so-called scintillating scotoma. Patients describe a hole in their vision with a sparkling border. The scotoma will begin in one hemifield but gradually enlarge and move across to involve the other hemifield with the leading edge being a zigzag of sparkling lights.[39]

The second most common symptom of a migraine aura is somatosensory—a numbness, tingling, or both that may affect the hands, lower face, or half of the body.[39] Rarely dysarthria, aphasia, hemiparesis, or unilateral incoordination are seen. Vertigo occurs during the aura in up to one third of patients.[48] When focal neurologic symptoms such as hemianopsia or unilateral paresthesias occur in an aura, they usually occur on the side opposite that of the headache. Only about 12 percent of patients with migraine regularly experience classic attacks, but approximately two thirds have occasional classic attacks with common migraine or migraine equivalents at other times.[6]

Common Migraine

Common migraine can best be described as a "sick headache." Vague prodromal symptoms precede it, but aura phenomena are absent. The headache, unilateral or bilateral, builds slowly in intensity and may go on for several days. Nausea, vomiting, diarrhea, chills, and prostration often accompany the headache. Nonspecific dizziness is a common complaint, and patients frequently report visual blurring and a sense of unsteadiness during the entire headache period. Vertigo can occur before, during, or entirely separate from the episodes of headache.[32]

Posterior Fossa Migraine

Bickerstaff[8] described a type of migraine similar to the classic variety in that it consisted of an aura followed by a headache but different in that the aura consisted of posterior fossa symptoms such as vertigo, ataxia, dysarthria, and tinnitus along with visual phenomena consistent with ischemia in the distribution of the posterior cerebral arteries. Motor and sensory symptoms, such as circumoral or extremity paresthesias, weakness, and drop attacks are occasionally seen as well. When vertigo occurs it usually has an abrupt onset and lasts 5 to 60 minutes.[27] The headache following the aura is usually unilateral occipital or frontal, but it can occur anywhere, especially in children.

Bickerstaff initially emphasized that

posterior fossa migraine was prevalent in adolescent girls and commonly occurred in association with their menstrual periods. Others have described a more widespread distribution.[6, 27, 51] It is estimated to affect 10 to 24 percent of patients suffering from migraine. One must be alert for the possibility of posterior fossa migraine in any patient presenting with transient vertigo and other posterior fossa symptoms. In some individuals the headache is not severe and is adequately managed by aspirin, sleep, or mild analgesics and sedatives. Some of these patients are unaware that migraine is the cause of their headaches and are much more concerned about the aura. If vertigo is prominent, the patient may not mention the headache—thinking it is unimportant. Similarly, other transient manifestations may be given less importance to concentrate on the vertigo. Such patients may be misdiagnosed as having peripheral labyrinthine disease if the physician is not alert to the possibility of posterior fossa migraine.

Migraine Equivalents

BENIGN PAROXYSMAL VERTIGO OF CHILDHOOD

Basser[7] described an episodic disorder in children under the age of 4 that he called benign paroxysmal vertigo. The physician is consulted because the child exhibits spells of peculiar behavior. A completely normal child suddenly becomes frightened, cries out, clings to the parent, or staggers as though drunk and exhibits pallor, diaphoresis, and often vomiting. Symptoms are accentuated by head movements, and sometimes nystagmus and torticollis are observed. Some children report a true spinning sensation, but most have difficulty describing what they are experiencing. The spells typically last for several minutes. Afterward, the child is immediately normal and can resume playing as though nothing had happened.

The spells typically begin before the age of 4 and occur up to several times a month. After a period 2 to 3 years they decrease in number and gradually disappear. Most children have no further spells after the age of 7 or 8. The cause of benign paroxysmal vertigo of childhood is unknown, although most authors suspect a vascular disturbance affecting the posterior circulation. Follow-up studies of patients with typical benign paroxysmal vertigo during childhood indicate that more than 50 percent subsequently develop classic migraine.[37, 54] When the clinical picture is clear neither treatment nor extensive evaluation is necessary.

BENIGN RECURRENT VERTIGO

Slater[49] and Moretti and colleagues[40] described patients who, between the ages of 7 and 55 years, began to experience repeated episodes of vertigo, nausea, vomiting, and diaphoresis. The attacks often occurred on awakening in the morning, being particularly common around menstrual periods in women. Duration varied from a few minutes to as long as 3 to 4 days, with the vertigo becoming primarily positional toward the end of the spell. Nearly all patients were asymptomatic between spells. During the episodes there were no auditory symptoms, specifically no hearing loss, tinnitus, or ear pressure or fullness. Most patients either had migraine themselves or a strong family history of migraine. Furthermore, the episodes of vertigo had several features in common with migraine, including precipitation by alcohol, lack of sleep, emotional stress, and a female preponderance.

OTHERS

In young children the manifestations of migraine are protean, and headache is not always present.[18] So-called migraine equivalents may appear as cyclic vomiting, attacks of abdominal pain, or even ophthalmoplegia. As the child matures these nonspecific and other puzzling symptoms may cease and are supplanted by more typical paroxysmal head pain.

Symptoms of migraine equivalents can also begin in adulthood. Isolated episodes of scintillating scotomas are not uncommon after the age of 40. Fisher[20] reported 60 patients with what he called "transient migrainous accompaniments" which were attacks of paresthesias, aphasia, dysarthria, paresis, diplopia with or without the visual manifestations of migraine. None of these patients had headache. Normal angiography, long-term follow-up, and, in a few cases, necropsy, suggested a migrainous syndrome despite the absence of associated headaches.

Pathophysiology

The mechanism of migraine is incompletely understood, but the headache most likely results from dilatation of extracranial and dural arteries, causing stretching of sensitive pain fibers in the walls of the arteries.[16] The aura phenomena are—at least in part—due to constriction of intracranial arteries, resulting in transient ischemia in the area supplied by the constricted vessels.

Abnormalities in the release and uptake of vasoactive amines have been implicated in the pathogenesis of migraine. Plasma serotonin levels fall during an attack of classic or common migraine, and because serotonin is platelet bound, the fall in serotonin must be preceded by a release from platelets and a subsequent degradation by monoamine oxidase. One simple hypothesis is that the initial release of serotonin causes transient vasoconstriction, which is followed by vasodilitation coincident with destruction of plasma serotonin. Many of the complex aura phenomena seen in classic migraine, however, are not explained by ischemia confined to the distribution of a single cerebral blood vessel (e.g., the scintillating scotoma).

The mechanism for the vertigo associated with migraine is equally poorly understood. Constriction of the internal auditory artery could explain some symptoms, although one might expect a higher incidence of hearing loss accompanying the vertigo. Although hearing loss does occur with migraine, it is infrequent compared with the incidence of vertigo. Phonophobia and tinnitus are much more common than hearing loss, with the former being particularly prominent during the period of severe headache.[32] The possible association between migraine and Meniere's syndrome initially suggested by Meniere himself complicates the situation even further.[32] Numerous case reports show migraine and

Meniere's attacks occurring in the same patient. Typically the patient had classic migraine episodes for many years before developing symptoms and signs of Meniere's syndrome. There is a correspondence in the laterality of the hearing loss and migrainous headache and in the occurrence of headache and attacks of vertigo. Atkinson[3] postulated a common vascular etiology for both disorders. This hypothesis deserves further attention, but no well-controlled studies have been conducted to demonstrate an increased incidence of the combined occurrence of migraine and Meniere's syndrome.

Diagnosis

The diagnosis of migraine is relatively easy when headaches are the major feature and there is a strong family history. In patients in which headache is less prominent or in patients with migraine equivalents, the diagnosis can be missed if one is unaware of the diversity of this syndrome. We have seen numerous patients who presented with a primary complaint of vertigo and mentioned associated headaches only after being questioned.

Prensky and Sommer[44] suggested the following diagnostic criteria for migraine headaches: (1) recurrent headaches separated by symptom-free intervals; and (2) any three of the following six symptoms: abdominal pain, nausea, or vomiting during the headache; hemicrania; a throbbing pulsate quality of pain; complete relief after a brief period of rest; an aura—visual, sensory, or motor; and a history of migraine headaches in one or more members of the immediate family. Motion sickness has been reported in up to 55 percent of adults[26] and 45 percent of children[5] with migraine and has been recommended for inclusion as another minor criterion for diagnosis.

Management

Treatment of migraine can be divided into two general categories: symptomatic and prophylactic.[57] Certain drugs are useful in ameliorating the symptoms of the acute attack, whereas others are effective in reducing the frequency and severity of attacks or eliminating their occurrence entirely. Symptomatic treatment includes analgesics, antiemetics, antivertiginous drugs, sedatives, and vasoconstrictors. The decrease in gastric motility that occurs during migraine attacks can decrease the absorption of oral drugs as well as contribute to the nausea and vomiting. Metoclopramide (Reglan) promotes normal gastric motility and may improve absorption of oral drugs. For many patients, aspirin and rest are adequate to relieve the headache. The many combination preparations for symptomatic treatment of migraine contain sedatives that are effective partially because they enhance sleep. Fiorinal (a combination containing aspirin, caffeine, and butalbital) and Midrin (which contains the sympathomimetic amine isometheptene—a mild sedative—dichloralphenazone, and acetaminophen) are examples.

Ergotamine, an alpha-adrenergic blocking agent with direct action on smooth muscle fibers of peripheral and cranial vessels, is probably the most effective drug for relief of migraine headache. It acts as a vasoconstrictor if the vascular resistance is low but induces vasodilitation if there is increased resistance.[28] It also affects serotonin turnover in the brain.[50] The major side effect is severe nausea and vomiting, which may preclude the use of the drug if it cannot be improved by metoclopramide. Pregnancy is an absolute contraindication to the use of ergotamine because of its uterine effects. Hypertension, hepatitis, and renal disease are also relative contraindications for the use of ergotamine preparations. Ergotamines should be given as soon as possible after the onset of symptoms, either at the beginning of the aura in classic or posterior fossa migraine or with the first prodromal symptoms of headache in common migraine. Ergotamine may be prescribed for oral use (Gynergen and others), sublingually (Ergostat and others), or rectally with caffeine (Cafergot suppositories). The total daily dosage of oral or rectal ergotamines should not exceed 4 to 5 mg per day or 10 mg per week. Vascular occlusion and gangrene have been recorded with higher doses, and the risk of severe rebound headache is significant. Ergotamine preparations are gener-

ally restricted to persons over 10 years of age but are occasionally used in younger children who have very well recognized migraine aura.

Antivertiginous and antiemetic medications are useful in patients in whom vertigo and nausea are prominent features (see Table 11–1). Promethazine, 25 or 50 mg orally or via suppository, is particularly effective for relief of both vertigo and nausea. These drugs also have a sedative effect, which is usually acceptable in a patient who is eager to sleep.

Prophylactic treatment is necessary when migraine attacks are frequent or the severity cannot be ameliorated by symptomatic medicines. It is the only treatment effective for treating migraine equivalents, particularly episodic vertigo. At the present time propranolol (Inderol) is the drug of choice for the prevention of migraine episodes. It is contraindicated in patients with asthma, congestive heart failure, peripheral vascular disease, diabetes, and hypothyroidism. Propranolol is the only beta-adrenergic blocking agent approved by the US Food and Drug Administration for use in migraine. Up to 70 percent of treated patients respond to the drug.[14, 58] The mechanism of action in migraine is not known, but it may be related to interference with serotonin metabolism at several levels rather than with beta-adrenergic blockade. The principal side effects are fatigue and lethargy; but weakness, nonspecific dizziness, insomnia, depression, gastrointestinal symptoms, and weight gain have occasionally been seen. Side effects can be minimized by slowly increasing the dosage from a low starting level. Adults usually require between 120 and 360 mg per day for maximum effect (average 180 mg per day); the most common first sign of effectiveness is a decrease in the severity of individual attacks or an improved response to symptomatic medication during an acute attack rather than an actual decrease in the frequency of episodes. A trial of propranolol should be continued for at least 2 to 3 months at the highest level of tolerance before it is considered a failure. Discontinuation should be gradual over several days.

Amitriptyline also has been demonstrated to decrease the frequency and severity of migraine attacks.[58] It is especially useful when the episodes are triggered by tension or are closely associated with tension headache. It also is effective for treating the nonspecific lightheaded dizziness that accompanies the headache. A single nocturnal dose of 50 to 100 mg is often effective and avoids the major side effects of sedation and anticholinergic activity. Methysergide (Sansert), an ergot alkaloid, can effectively prevent migraine headaches, but it can cause retroperitoneal pleuropericardial and subendocardial fibrosis. Because of these dangerous side effects it is now rarely used—and never for longer than 6 months at a time.

Calcium channel blockers (nifedipine, verapamil) also can reduce the frequency of migraine attacks, probably by stabilizing blood vessels. Whether they are as effective or more effective than propranolol is yet to be established because long-term evaluation is lacking. Preliminary assessment has been encouraging, and side effects have been minimal. In those women whose migraines are periodic and premenstrual, naproxen (a nonsteroidal anti-inflammatory agent) or acetazolamide (Diamox) can be taken for a few days each month, when the migraine is expected, to prevent its appearance.

It has been our experience that a trial of migraine prophylaxis is warranted in any patient with episodic vertigo of unknown cause who has a past history of migraine or strong family history of migraine.

REFERENCES

1. Adams, R: Occlusion of the anterior inferior cerebellar artery. Arch Neurol Psychiatr 49:765, 1943.
2. Andrews, J, Hoover, LA, Lee, RS, and Honrubia, V: Vertigo in the hyperviscosity syndrome. Otolaryngol Head Neck Surg 98:144, 1988.
3. Atkinson, M: Meniere's syndrome and migraine: Observations on a causal relationship. Ann Intern Med 18:797, 1943.
4. Baloh, RW, Yee, RD, and Honrubia, V: Eye movements in patients with Wallenberg's syndrome. Ann NY Acad Sci 374:600, 1981.
5. Barabas, G, Matthews, WS, and Ferrari, M: Childhood migraine and motion sickness. Pediatrics 72:188, 1983.
6. Bartleson, JD: Transient and persistent neurological manifestations of migraine. Stroke 15:383, 1984.
7. Basser, LS: Benign paroxysmal vertigo of childhood. Brain 87:141, 1964.
8. Bickerstaff, ER: Basilar artery migraine. Lancet 1:15, 1961.
9. Bjerner, K and Silfverskiöld, BP: Lateropulsion and imbalance in Wallenberg's syndrome. Acta Neurol Scand 44:91, 1968.
10. Bogousslavsky, J, Fox, AJ, Barnett, HJM, Hachinski, VC, Vinitski, S, and Carey, LS: Clinico-topographic correlation of small vertebrobasilar infarct using magnetic resonance imaging. Stroke 17:929, 1986.
11. Brennen, RW and Bergland, RM: Acute cerebellar hemorrhage. Analysis of clinical findings and outcome in 12 cases. Neurology 27:527, 1977.
12. Caplan, LR: Treatment of patients with vertebrobasilar occlusive disease. Comprehensive Therapy 12:23, 1986.
13. Caplan, LR: Vertebrobasilar disease. In Barnett, HJM, Mohr, JP, Stein, BM, Yatsu, FM (eds): Stroke: Pathophysiology, Diagnosis and Management. Churchill Livingstone, New York, 1986.
14. Diamond, S, et al: Long-term study of propranolol in the treatment of migraine. Headache 22:268, 1982.
15. Dinsdale, HB: Spontaneous hemorrhage in the posterior fossa: A study of primary cerebellar and pontine hemorrhage with observations on the pathogenesis. Arch Neurol 10:200, 1964.
16. Drummond, PD and Lance, JW: Extracranial vascular changes and the source of pain in migraine headache. Ann Neurol 13:32, 1983.
17. Duncan, GW, Parker, SW, and Fisher, CM: Acute cerebellar infarction in the PICA territory. Arch Neurol 32:364, 1975.
18. Fenichel, GM: Migraine in children. Neurologic Clinics 3:77, 1985.
19. Fields, WS: Arteriography in the differential diagnosis of vertigo. Arch Otolaryngol 85:111, 1967.
20. Fisher, CM: Late-life migraine accompaniments as a cause of unexplained transient ischemic attacks. J Can Sci Neurol 7(1):9, 1980.
21. Fisher, CM: Vertigo in cerebrovascular disease. Arch Otolaryngol 85:855, 1967.
22. Fisher, CM, Karnes, WE, and Kubik, CS: Lateral medullary infarction—the pattern of vascular occlusion. J Neuropath Exp Neurol 20:323, 1961.
23. Freeman, RE, et al: Spontaneous intracerebellar hemorrhage. Diagnosis and surgical treatment. Neurology 23:84, 1973.
24. Friedman, AP: The infinite variety of migraine. In Smith, R (ed): Background to Migraine. William Heinemann, London, 1970.
25. Grad, A and Baloh, RW: Vertigo of vascular origin: Clinical and ENG features in 84 cases. Arch Neurol 46:281, 1989.
26. Graham, JR: The natural history of migraine: Some observations and a hypothesis. Trans Am Clin Climatol Assoc 64:61, 1952.
27. Harker, LA and Rassek, HC: Episodic vertigo in basilar migraine. Otolaryngol Head Neck Surg 96:239, 1987.
28. Hellig, WH and Berde, B: Studies of the effect of natural and synthetic polypeptide-type ergot

compounds on a peripheral vascular bed. Br J Pharmacol 36:561, 1969.

29. Huang, CY and Yu, YL: Small cerebellar strokes may mimic labyrinthine lesions. J Neurol Neurosurg Psych 48:263, 1985.

30. Igarashi, M and Ishikawa, K: Post-labyrinthectomy balance compensation with preplacement of cerebellar vermis lesion. Acta Otolaryngol 99:452, 1985.

31. Jaffe, B: Sudden deafness—a local manifestation of systemic disorders: Fat emboli, hypercoagulation and infections. Laryngoscope 80:788, 1970.

32. Kayan, A and Hood, JD: Neuro-otological manifestations of migraine. Brain 107:1123, 1984.

33. Kirikae, I, et al: Sudden deafness due to Buerger's disease. Arch Otolaryngol 75:502, 1962.

34. Kistler, JP, Ropper, AH, and Heros, RC: Therapy of ischemic cerebral vascular disease due to atherothrombosis. N Engl J Med 311:27, 100, 1984.

35. Kommerell, G and Hoyt, WF: Lateropulsion of saccadic eye movements. Electro-oculographic studies in a patient with Wallenberg's syndrome. Arch Neurol 28:313, 1973.

36. Kushner, MJ and Bressman, SB: The clinical manifestations of pontine hemorrhage. Neurology 35:637, 1985.

37. Lanzi, G, et al: Benign paroxysmal vertigo in childhood: A longitudinal study. Headache 26:494, 1986.

38. Lindsay, JR and Hemenway, WG: Postural vertigo due to unilateral sudden partial loss of vestibular function. Ann Otol Rhinol Laryngol 65:692, 1956.

39. Manzoni, GC, Farina, S, Lanfranchi, M, and Solari, A: Classic migraine—clinical findings in 164 patients. Eur Neurol 24:163, 1985.

40. Moretti, G, et al: Benign recurrent vertigo and its connection with migraine. Headache 20:344, 1980.

41. Naritomi, H, Sakai, F, and Meyer, JS: Pathogenesis of transient ischemic attacks within the vertebrobasilar arterial system. Arch Neurol 36:121, 1979.

42. Ott, KH, et al: Cerebellar hemorrhage: Diagnosis and treatment. Arch Neurol 31:160, 1974.

43. Polus, K: The problem of vascular deafness. Laryngoscope 82:24, 1972.

44. Prensky, AL and Sommer, D: Diagnosis and treatment of migraine in children. Neurology 29:506, 1979.

45. Ruben, R, et al: Sudden sequential deafness as the presenting symptom of macro-globulinemia. JAMA 209:1364, 1969.

46. Schuknecht, H: Cupulolithiasis. Arch Otolaryngol 90:765, 1969.

47. Schuknecht, HF: Pathology of the Ear. Harvard University Press, Cambridge, MA, 1974.

48. Selby, G and Lance, JW: Observations on 500 cases of migraine and allied vascular headaches. J Neurol Neurosurg Psychiatry 23:23, 1960.

49. Slater, R: Benign recurrent vertigo. J Neurol Neurosurg Psychiatry 42:363, 1979.

50. Sofia, RD and Vassan, HB: The effect of ergotamine and methysergide on serotonin metabolism in the rat brain. Arch Int Pharmacodyn Ther 216:40, 1975.

51. Sturzenegger, MH and Meienberg, O: Basilar artery migraine: A follow-up study of 82 cases. Headache 25:408, 1985.

52. Sypert, GW and Alvord, EG: Cerebellar infarction. Arch Neurol 32:357, 1975.

53. Waters, EE and O'Connor, PJ: Prevalence of migraine. J Neurol Neurosurg Psychiatry 38:613, 1975.

54. Watson, P and Steele, JC: Paroxysmal disequilibrium in the migraine syndrome of childhood. Arch Otolaryngol 99:177, 1974.

55. Williams, D and Wilson, TG: The diagnosis of the major and minor syndromes of basilar insufficiency. Brain 85:741, 1962.

56. Zee, DS: Perspectives on the pharmacotherapy of vertigo. Arch Otolaryngol 111:609, 1986.

57. Ziegler, D: Headache syndromes. In Rosenberg, RN (ed): The Clinical Neurosciences, Vol 1. Harper & Row, Philadelphia, 1983.

58. Ziegler, DK, et al: Migraine prophylaxis: A comparison of propranolol and amitriptyline. Arch Neurol 44:486, 1987.

Chapter 13

TUMORS

TUMORS OF THE MIDDLE EAR AND TEMPORAL BONE

A wide variety of benign and malignant tumors involve the middle ear and temporal bone. Tumors involving the middle ear produce symptoms of fullness or conductive hearing loss early, whereas tumors in the temporal bone outside the middle ear can become quite large without producing symptoms. The tumor may not become apparent until it erodes into the external auditory canal (producing a conductive hearing loss) or through the mastoid cortex into the skin. Anterior extension into the cavernous sinus produces ophthalmoplegia from involvement of the third, fourth, and sixth nerves. Malignant tumors in this region tend to spread locally to the regional lymph nodes; distant metastasis is unusual. Ultimately the tumor can be seen in the nasopharynx, middle ear, or neck.

Malignant Tumors

Squamous cell carcinoma is the most frequent histologic type of malignant tumor involving the middle ear and mastoid.[2] It typically arises from epidermal cells of the auricle, external auditory canal, or the middle ear and mastoid. The prognosis is good for tumors confined to the auricle and external canal but not for those invading the middle ear and mastoid.[28] The latter are frequently associated with prominent ear symptoms which include vertigo, hearing loss, pain, otorrhea, mastoid swelling, and facial paralysis. Squamous cell carcinomas often begin in an ear with previous otologic disease, particularly chronic suppurative otitis media with a mastoid cavity. Other, less common, tumors originating in the external auditory canal and middle ear include adenoid cystic carcinoma, basal cell carcinoma, mucoepidermoid carcinoma, and ceruminoma. In general, these tumors are less malignant but occasionally will be locally invasive. Adenoid cystic carcinoma arises from glandular tissue of the external canal and middle ear; it typically has severe pain as an early symptom and may be associated with distant metastasis.

Generally, carcinomas occur in an elderly age group, whereas sarcomas occur in the young. Both osteogenic sarcoma and chondrosarcoma occur as primary tumors of the temporal bone, running fulminant courses in older children and young adults. Rhabdomyosarcoma is the most common middle ear malignant tumor in the young, typically occurring in children under the age of 5.[13] The initial symptom is often facial paralysis, which may be misdiagnosed as idiopathic Bell's palsy. In later stages, the tumor extends beyond the middle ear to involve the petrous apex and may invade the posterior or middle cranial fossi. Rhabdomyosarcoma should be considered in any infant presenting with idiopathic facial paralysis.

Metastatic involvement of the temporal bone is common with several different tumor types but, because of the enchondral layers' resistance, neoplasms rarely invade the bony labyrinth. The most common sites of origin for metastatic tumors in order of frequency are breast, kidney, lung, stomach, larynx, prostate, and thyroid gland.[25] Metastatic tumors from the breast and prostate commonly incite new bone formation.

Glomus Body Tumors

Glomus tumors are the most common tumor of the middle ear, and next to schwannomas they are the most common tumor of the temporal bone.[5] Glomus tumors arise in the glomera of the chemoreceptor system, which may be found along the vagus nerve, glossopharyngeal nerve, Jacobson's nerve (tympanic branch of the ninth nerve) and the nerve of Arnold (postauricular branch of the tenth nerve). The most common tumor sites are the glomus jugulare (jugular bulb), glomus tympanicum (middle ear), and glomus vagale (along the course of the vagus nerve). Glomus vagale and jugulare tumors often involve the labyrinth and cranial nerves, whereas glomus tympanicum tumors usually produce only local symptoms such as conductive hearing loss, pulsatile tinnitus, and rhinorrhea because of the tumor bulk in the middle ear. Invasion of the labyrinth is an uncommon but serious prognostic sign and is often associated with extension to the petrous apex and into the middle and posterior cranial fossae. The jugular foramen syndrome consisting of ninth, tenth, and eleventh nerve involvement occurs with glomus jugulare and vagale tumors.[17, 27] Involvement of the twelfth nerve is an ominous sign, indicating destruction of the jugular foramen with tumor extension into the hypoglossal canal and usually into the posterior fossa.

Diagnosis

Tumors of the middle ear space and temporal bone can often be identified on careful physical examination. A malignant tumor may be visible after it has eroded into the external auditory canal or through the mastoid cortex into the skin. Nearby lymph nodes are often enlarged. A biopsy of these lesions should lead to the correct histologic diagnosis. Glomus body tumors are often visible through the tympanic membrane (see Fig. 5–1C). If not all the borders are visible, the tumor may be either a large glomus tympanicum tumor or a much larger glomus jugulare tumor that has extended from the jugular bulb into the middle ear. If cranial nerve deficits are present, the tumor is most likely a glomus jugulare type.

Although physical examination can often identify the presence of a tumor involving the middle ear or temporal bone, computerized tomography (CT) and magnetic resonance (MR) scanning are necessary to assess the extent of the tumor. CT is the diagnostic procedure of choice for determining bony involvement, and MR is most useful for determining the soft tissue extent. Angiography and jugular venography can be helpful for diagnosing glomus body tumors. Arteriography may identify a characteristic vascular blush, and venography provides information about whether the tumor involves the jugular bulb and whether it has extended into the jugular vein.

Management

As suggested above, malignant tumors confined to the ear and external auditory canal can often be surgically resected with minimal cosmetic and functional disability. Much more extensive surgical procedures with greater cosmetic and functional disabilities are required for tumors invading the middle ear and mastoid, and often only subtotal resection is possible. Most patients are treated with postsurgical radiation, but the long-term prognosis in these patients is poor.

Although some small glomus tympanicum tumors, when the borders are clearly demarcated, can be removed via the external auditory canal, more extensive procedures are usually required for these tumors. Glomus jugulare and vagale tumors are much more difficult to remove because they are highly vascular and closely interrelated with key neural and vascular structures.[17, 27] Radiation therapy has been proposed for management of tumor recurrences and for unresectable lesions.

TUMORS OF THE INTERNAL AUDITORY CANAL AND CEREBELLOPONTINE (CP) ANGLE

Tumors arising in the narrow confines of the internal auditory canal typically produce a gradual compression of the seventh and eighth cranial nerves. Sensorineural hearing loss, tinnitus, and facial paresis insidiously evolve usually over months to years. Vertigo is uncommon with such lesions because the nervous system is able to adapt to the gradual loss of vestibular function. Lesions within the CP angle produce a similar, slowly progressive compression of the seventh and eighth cranial nerves, although if the tumor arises in the angle, it can grow to a much larger size before critical compression occurs. Most often, tumors begin in the internal auditory canal and grow outward into the CP angle, inasmuch as it is the path of least resistance. Next to the seventh and eighth nerves, the fifth nerve is most commonly involved with CP angle tumors, causing ipsilateral facial numbness. In later stages of progression, involvement of the sixth, ninth, and tenth nerves may give rise to diplopia, dysphonia, and dysphagia. Compression of the brain and cerebellum results in ipsilateral gaze dysfunction and dysmetria of the extremities.

In a series of over 2000 tumors of the CP angle reported by Brackman and Bartels,[3] 92 percent were vestibular schwannomas (acoustic neuromas); 3 percent, meningiomas; 2.5 percent, epidermoid cysts; and 1 percent, facial nerve schwannomas.

Schwannomas

Tumors arising from the sheaths of the cranial and peripheral nerves have been called neuromas, neurilemmomas, and neurofibromas, but convincing evidence that they represent a proliferation of the sheath-producing schwann cells make schwannoma a more appropriate term.[25] These tumors comprise about 5 percent of intracranial neoplasms and are by far the most common tumor found in the temporal bone.[3] They arise from the vestibular nerve in more than 90 percent of cases, and much less frequently from the facial, acoustic, or trigeminal nerves. The general term *acoustic neuroma*, therefore, is inappropriate on two accounts.

Mostly, schwannomas are circumscribed and encapsulated, encroaching on and displacing neural structures as they grow, without direct invasion of tissue. Vascu-

larity is variable, but they are usually less vascular than meningiomas. Vestibular schwannomas typically arise at the myelinglial junction near the porous acousticus, producing symptoms by exerting pressure on surrounding neurovascular structures. Infrequently, the tumor arises from the vestibular nerve terminals near the end-organ, in which case end-organ destruction occurs, or it may arise from the nerve after it leaves the canal in the CP angle, in which case it can be relatively large before producing symptoms and signs. Schwannomas usually grow very slowly but occasionally hemorrhage into the tumor, cyst formation or associated edema produces clinical evidence of more rapid growth. Malignant schwannomas are rare; approximately half of them occur with neurofibromatosis.

VESTIBULAR SCHWANNOMAS (ACOUSTIC NEUROMA)

By far the most common symptom associated with a vestibular schwannoma is a slowly progressive unilateral hearing loss.[7, 19] Occasionally, patients will experience fluctuating or sudden hearing loss, apparently from compression of the labyrinthine vasculature. Often patients will complain of an inability to understand speech when using the telephone even before they are aware of a loss of hearing. Unilateral tinnitus is the next most common symptom. Vertigo occurs in less than 20 percent of patients, although about half will complain of some mild impairment of balance. Next to the auditory nerve, the most commonly involved cranial nerves (by compression) are the seventh and fifth, producing facial weakness and numbness, respectively. Involvement of the sixth, ninth, tenth, eleventh, and twelfth nerves occurs only in the late stages of disease with massive tumors. Large vestibular schwannomas may also produce increased intracranial pressure from obstruction of cerebrospinal fluid outflow, resulting in severe headaches and vomiting.

FACIAL NERVE SCHWANNOMAS

Facial nerve schwannomas typically present with a slowly progressive facial paralysis developing over months to years—although rare cases with sudden onset of paralysis, fluctuating paresis, and facial tic have been reported. Hearing loss from compression of the cochlear nerve in the internal auditory canal is the second most common presenting symptom. Conductive hearing loss can occur when the tumor arises in the middle ear where it can disrupt the ossicular chain. In these cases the tumor mass may be visible behind the posterior superior tympanic membrane.

Neurofibromas

Neurofibromas involving the eighth cranial nerve are invariably a manifestation of neurofibromatosis—either the generalized variety or a central variety, which has virtually none of the peripheral stigmata but has multiple central nervous system (CNS) tumors.[14] With the latter the most common intracranial manifestation is bilateral neurofibromas of the eighth nerve.[34] Although both neurofibromas and schwannomas are derived from schwann cells, schwannomas begin in one area and grow as an expanding mass, pushing the rest of the nerve away, whereas neurofibromas grow from many fascicles of the nerve and are intimately involved with the nerve. Despite these histologic differences the clinical presentation of schwannomas and neurofibromas of the eighth nerve are identical; they both produce a slowly progressive hearing loss and tinnitus. As with schwannomas, malignant degeneration of neurofibromas is also rare.

Meningiomas

Meningiomas comprise about 14 percent of intracranial tumors and after schwannomas are the most common primary tumor of the CP angle.[11] Meningiomas arise from arachnoid fibroblasts, usually in the posterior aspect of the petrous pyramid near the sigmoid and petrosal sinuses.[21] They displace cranial nerves and compress the brainstem and cerebellum but do not invade brain tissue. In the posterior fossa, the lobulated variety is more common than the flat (en-plaque) type. Meningiomas in the CP angle are frequently calcified and induce osteoblastic

reaction in adjacent bone. Because these tumors arise outside of the internal auditory canal, they often become very large before producing symptoms and signs. As with schwannomas the most common symptoms are auditory—hearing loss and tinnitus. Large tumors compress the brainstem and cerebellum and stretch the fifth and seventh cranial nerves, producing facial numbness and weakness.

Epidermoid Cysts (Primary Cholesteatomas)

Epidermoid cysts arise from congenital epithelial inclusion rests in the area of the petrous apex.[15] They slowly enlarge to fill the CP angle, stretching nearby cranial nerves and eventually compressing the brainstem and cerebellum. Because these cysts are slow growing, the symptoms do not become manifest until the second to fourth decade of life. As with other CP angle tumors, involvement of the eighth nerve is a common early feature, but unlike other tumors in this area hemifacial spasm is a frequent early distinguishing feature.

Cholesterol Granulomas

Cholesterol granulomas arise in the pneumatized spaces of the temporal bone when a small hemorrhage into the air cells causes a foreign body reaction and progressive granuloma formation.[9] The lesion within the temporal bone expands and can produce compression of the structures in the CP angle. As with other CP angle lesions, eighth nerve involvement is most common, with hearing loss being the most frequent presenting symptom. This is an important lesion to recognize because the surgical management is quite different from that of other CP angle tumors (see below).

Metastatic Tumors

The internal auditory canal is a frequent site of metastatic tumor growth. From this site tumor cells destroy the seventh and eighth nerves and extend into the inner ear or into the CP angle. The rapid onset of hearing loss and vertigo followed by other signs of cranial nerve compression and brainstem dysfunction suggests the likelihood of a malignant tumor rather than the more common benign CP angle tumors. The lung and breast are the most common sites for the primary neoplasm.[24]

Differential Diagnosis

By far the most common presentation of a cerebellar pontine angle tumor is a slowly progressive unilateral sensorineural hearing loss (Fig. 13–1). Unilateral tinnitus is the next most common symptom, with vertigo being an infrequent symptom. The sudden onset of vertigo and unilateral

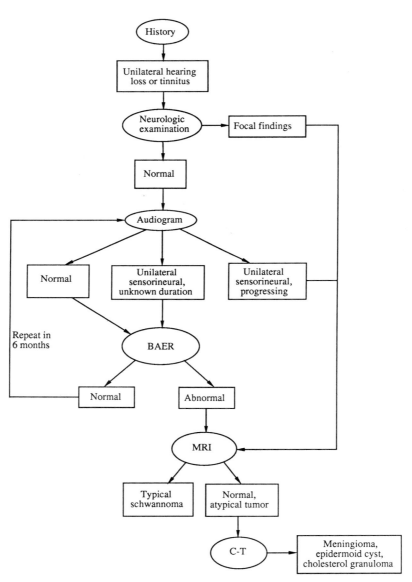

Figure 13–1. Algorithm for diagnosis of tumors of the cerebellopontine angle. *BAER*, brain stem auditory evoked response; *MRI*, magnetic resonance imaging; *C-T*, computerized tomography.

hearing loss can occasionally be seen with benign tumors but should suggest the possibility of a malignant tumor. The neurologic examination should focus on the nearby cranial nerves—particularly the fifth and seventh nerves. If there are findings localizing to the internal auditory canal or CP angle, one would proceed directly to neuroimaging, beginning with an MR scan. In those cases in which the neurologic examination is nonlocalizing, the first diagnostic test should be an audiogram. If a progressing unilateral sensorineural hearing loss is documented, then one would proceed directly to an MR scan because there is a high likelihood of an expanding lesion. If the audiogram is normal or if there is a unilateral sensorineural hearing loss of unknown duration, then one would proceed with a brainstem auditory-evoked response (BAER) inasmuch as this is the most sensitive special audiometric test for documenting eighth nerve involvement. The BAER is abnormal in 95 to 98 percent of patients with vestibular schwannomas.[20, 26] If the BAER is normal, then the patient should be followed with at least one repeat audiogram in 6 months. Whether further repeat studies are necessary should the second audiogram be normal depends on whether the patient notes a subjective progression of either the hearing loss or tinnitus. If the BAER is abnormal, then one would proceed directly to an MR scan with emphasis on the internal auditory canal and CP angles.

The relative merit of MR and CT scanning for identifying tumors in this region is still being defined, although there is no question that MR scanning is superior to CT scanning for identifying vestibular schwannomas.[1, 31] MR scanning can identify small tumors confined to the internal auditory canal (Fig. 13–2)—tumors that are missed with CT scanning. Even with contrast infusion CT will identify only 90 to 95 percent of vestibular schwannomas.[30] CT scanning is most useful for identifying bony erosion and/or calcification within tumors. Meningiomas are usually more dense than vestibular schwannomas on CT. With contrast infusion they appear very dense and homogeneous, a feature that differentiates them from schwannomas.[11] There may be calcifica-

tion within the tumor, and the nearby temporal bone may be thickened. Epidermoid cysts also have a characteristic profile on CT; they are less dense than brain and do not enhance after intravenous contrast material. They have an irregular scalloped surface contour and are usually eccentric to the opening of the internal auditory canal. Cholesterol granulomas appear as a punched-out lesion in the temporal bone with a central density the same as brain and with a rim of enhancement after contrast infusion.[9] The lesions are smooth walled and the contralateral petrous bone is always well pneumatized. On MR imaging they give a high-intensity signal in both T_1 and T_2 weighted images.[31]

Management

With few exceptions management of tumors in the internal auditory canal and CP angle is surgical. Occasionally, one might follow a patient with a small vestibular schwannoma, particularly if the patient is elderly or has underlying medical problems.[32] These tumors can remain confined to the internal auditory canal for years, and symptoms may be restricted to those of the eighth nerve.

There are three general surgical approaches to the CP angle: (1) translabyrinthine, (2) suboccipital, and (3) middle fossa.[19] The translabyrinthine approach destroys the labyrinth but often allows complete removal of the tumor without endangering other nearby neural structures, particularly the facial nerve. This would be the procedure of choice for a patient with severe hearing loss and a tumor under 3 cm in size. With the suboccipital and middle fossa approaches, residual hearing can be saved inasmuch as the labyrinth is not destroyed during the surgical procedure. With the introduction of the modern operating microscope, preservation of hearing is now a distinct possibility with either of these procedures.[29] Traditionally, the suboccipital approach is performed by neurosurgeons, whereas the middle fossa approach was developed by otologic surgeons. The middle fossa approach is more likely to save hearing and avoid damage to the facial nerve when the tumor is under 3

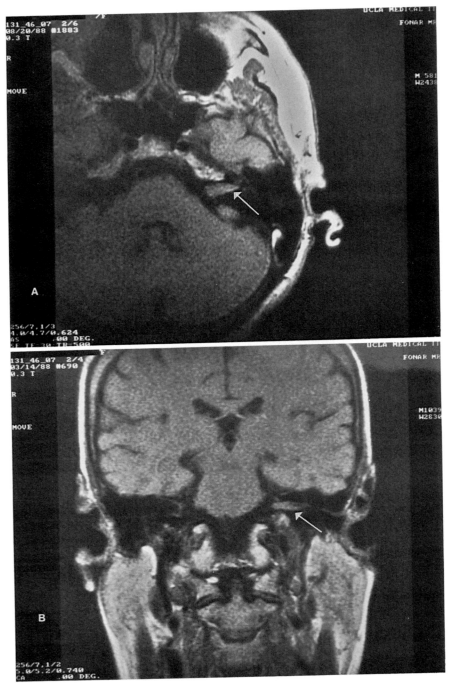

Figure 13—2. MR scans (T_1 weighted) demonstrating a small acoustic neuroma confined to the internal auditory canal. *(A)* Transverse section. *(B)* Coronal section. *Arrows* point to tumor.

cm in size. For tumors larger than 3 cm in diameter a combined translabyrinthine-suboccipital approach is commonly used. This procedure allows the surgeon to reduce the size of the tumor from behind by working between the tumor capsule and the brainstem. Furthermore, large tumors are often adjacent to or attached to the basilar artery; with the combined approach the surgeon can dissect the artery from the tumor capsule under direct vision.

BRAIN TUMORS

Brainstem

Gliomas of the brainstem usually grow slowly and infiltrate the brainstem nuclei and fiber tracts, producing multiple symptoms and signs. Although these tumors are five to ten times more common in children than in adults, they still make up approximately 1 percent of adult intracranial tumors.[33] The neurologic symptoms and signs of childhood brainstem gliomas do not differ in essence from those of adults. The typical history is that of relentless progressive involvement of one brainstem center after another, often ending with destruction of the vital cardiorespiratory centers of the medulla. Vestibular and cochlear symptoms and signs are common (occurring in approximately 50 percent of cases), the brainstem origin of which is usually obvious because of the multiple associated findings. Tumors originating in the pons or midbrain usually cause long tract signs, cranial nerve deficits, and ataxia. Spontaneous, gaze-evoked, and central paroxysmal positional nystagmus all occur, and impairment of saccade and pursuit eye movements further suggests an intrinsic brainstem disorder. Although less common, gliomas originating in the medulla may present with recurrent vertigo and vomiting.

Many tumors arising in the fourth ventricular region compress the vestibular nuclei and produce vestibular symptoms. *Medulloblastomas*, occurring primarily in children and adolescents, are rapidly growing, highly cellular tumors that arise in the posterior midline or vermis of the cerebellum and invade the fourth ventricle and adjacent cerebellar hemispheres.[23] Vertigo and disequilibrium are common initial complaints. Headaches and vomiting also occur early from an obstructive hydrocephalus and associated increased intracranial pressure. An attack of headache, vertigo, vomiting, and visual loss may result from a change in head position, producing transient cerebrospinal fluid (CSF) obstruction (Bruns' symptom). In Nylen's study[22] of patients with subtentorial tumors, 17 of 27 patients with medulloblastoma demonstrated positional nystagmus, and in two cases it was the only focal neurologic sign. Grand[10] reported two cases of medulloblastoma in which paroxysmal positional nystagmus was the initial abnormal neurologic sign. Other fourth ventricular tumors that produce similar clinical pictures include ependymomas, papillomas, teratomas, epidermoid cysts, and, in endemic areas, cysticercosis.

Cerebellum

Gliomas of cerebellum may be relatively silent until they become large enough to obstruct CSF circulation or compress the brainstem.[6] The most common symptoms are headache, vomiting, and gait imbalance. Approximately 90 percent of patients have papilledema from increased intracranial pressure.[8] As with medulloblastoma, positional vertigo is occasionally the initial symptom of a cerebellar glioma.[12] The associated paroxysmal positional nystagmus is central in type because it is induced in several positions and is nonfatigable. Other tumors that produce identical symptoms and signs include teratomas, hemangiomas, and hemangioblastomas.

Diagnosis and Management

MR imaging is the diagnostic procedure of choice for identifying brainstem and cerebellar tumors (Fig. 13–3).[4] Despite the recent technical improvements in CT scanning, the posterior fossa is difficult to visualize and even in cases where the tumor is seen, its true extent and precise relationship with adjacent structures cannot

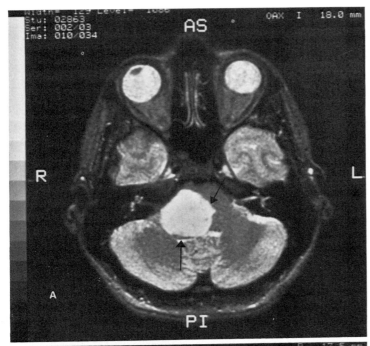

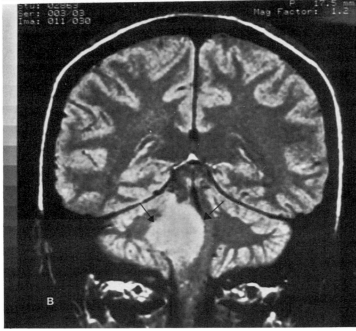

Figure 13–3. MR scans (T_2 weighted) showing a brainstem glioma *(arrows)* involving the root entry zone of the right eighth nerve. *(A)* Transverse section. *(B)* Coronal section.

be fully appreciated. Gliomas of the posterior fossa are particularly difficult to identify with CT because they are often isodense; the only evidence for a lesion is enlargement of the brainstem or compres-

sion of the fourth ventricle (the tumor shown in Fig. 13–3 was not seen on CT scanning). MR imaging, on the other hand, can reliably identify both brainstem and cerebellar gliomas as well as the other tumor types mentioned above. In some cases, CT scanning can complement MR imaging by helping differentiate between tumor and associated edema.

When possible, biopsy and surgical resection of the tumor is the treatment of choice. For nonresectable tumors radiation therapy is often beneficial. Prolonged survival (more than 5 years) is not uncommon with more benign astrocytomas.[16] Medulloblastomas are also very sensitive to radiation therapy.[18]

REFERENCES

1. Baker, HL: The application of magnetic resonance imaging in otolaryngology. Laryngoscope 96:18, 1986.
2. Batsakis, JG: Tumors of the Head and Neck, ed 2. Williams & Wilkins, Baltimore, 1979.
3. Brackman, DE and Bartels, LJ: Rare tumors of the cerebellopontine angle. Otolaryngol Head Neck Surg 88:555, 1980.
4. Bradac, GB, Schorner, W, Bevder, A, and Felix, R: MRI (NMR) in the diagnosis of brain stem tumors. Neuroradiology 27:208, 1985.
5. Brown, JS: Glomus jugulare tumors revisited: A ten-year statistical follow-up of 231 cases. Laryngoscope 95:284, 1985.
6. Bucy, PC and Thieman, PW: Astrocytomas of the cerebellum. Arch Neurol 24:125, 1971.
7. Erickson, L, Sorenson, G, and McGavran, M: A review of 140 acoustic neurinomas (neurilemmomas). Laryngoscope 75:601, 1965.
8. Geissinger, JD and Bucy, PC: Astrocytomas of the cerebellum in children. Long-term study. Arch Neurol 24:125, 1971.
9. Gherini, SG, et al: Cholesterol granuloma of the petrous apex. Laryngoscope 95:6, 1985.
10. Grand, W: Positional nystagmus: An early sign of medulloblastoma. Neurology 21:1157, 1971.
11. Granick, MS, et al: Cerebellopontine angle meningiomas: Clinical manifestations and diagnosis. Ann Otol Rhinol Laryngol 94:34, 1985.
12. Gregorius, FK, Crandall, PH, and Baloh, RW: Positional vertigo in cerebellar astrocytoma: Report of two cases. Surgical Neurol 6:283, 1976.
13. Jaffe, B, Fox, J, and Batsakis, J: Rhabdomyosarcoma of the middle ear and mastoid. Cancer 27:29, 1971.
14. Kanter, W, et al. Central neurofibromatosis: Genetic, chemical, and biochemical distinctions from peripheral neurofibromatosis. Neurology 30:851, 1980.
15. Keville, FJ and Wise, BL: Intracranial epidermoid and dermoid tumors. J Neurosurg 16:564, 1959.
16. Kim, TH, et al: Radiotherapy of primary brain-stem tumors. Int J Radiat Oncol Biol Phys 6:51, 1980.
17. Kinney, SE: Glomus jugulare tumors with intracranial extension. Am J Otolaryngol 1:67, 1979.
18. Landberg, TG, et al: Improvements in the radiotherapy of medulloblastoma: 1946–1975. Cancer 45:670, 1980.
19. Mattox, DE: Vestibular schwannomas. Otolaryngol Clin North Am 20:149, 1987.
20. Musiek, FE, Josey, AF, and Glasscock, ME: Auditory brain stem response in patients with acoustic neuromas. Arch Otolaryngol 112:186, 1986.
21. Nager, G: Meningiomas involving the temporal bone: Clinical and pathological aspects. Charles C Thomas, Springfield, IL, 1964.
22. Nylen, CO: The oto-neurological diagnoses of tumors of the brain. Acta Otolaryngol (Suppl 33):81, 1939.
23. Pobereskin, L and Treip, C: Adult medulloblastoma. J Neurol Neurosurg Psych 49:39, 1986.
24. Schuknecht, H, Allam, A, and Murakami, Y: Pathology of secondary malignant tumors of the temporal bone. Ann Otol Rhinol Laryngol 77:5, 1968.
25. Schuknecht, HF: Pathology of the Ear. Harvard University Press, Cambridge, MA, 1974.
26. Selters, WA and Brackman, DE: Brain stem electric response audiometry in acoustic tumor detection. In House, WF and Luetje, CM (eds): Acoustic Tumors in Diagnosis. University Park Press, Baltimore, 1979, p 225.
27. Spector, GJ, et al: Neurologic implications of glomus tumors in the head and neck. Laryngoscope 85:1387, 1975.
28. Stell, PM and McCormick, MS: Carcinoma of the external auditory meatus and middle ear. Prognostic factors and a suggested staging system. J Laryngol Otol 99:847, 1985.
29. Tator, CH and Nedzelski, JM: Preservation of hearing in patients undergoing excision of acoustic neuromas and other cerebellopontine angle tumors. J Neurosurg 63:168, 1985.
30. Thomsen, J, Gyldensted, C, and Lester, J: Computer tomography of cerebellopontine angle lesions. Arch Otolaryngol 103:65, 1977.
31. Valvassori, GE: Diagnosis of retrocochlear and central vestibular disease by magnetic resonance imaging. Ann Otol Rhinol Laryngol 97:19, 1988.
32. Wazen, J, Silverstein, H, Norrell, H, and Besse, B: Preoperative and postoperative growth rates in acoustic neuromas documented with CT scanning. Otolaryngol Head Neck Surg 93:151, 1985.
33. White, HH: Brain stem tumors occurring in adults. Neurology 13:292, 1963.
34. Young, D, Eldridge, R, and Gardner, W: Bilateral acoustic neuroma in a large kindred. JAMA 214:347, 1970.

Chapter 14

TRAUMA

TRAUMA TO THE TEMPORAL BONE

Fractures

Fractures of the temporal bone most commonly result from direct lateral blunt trauma to the skull in the parietal region of the head.[6] Because the otic capsule surrounding the inner ear is very dense bone, the fracture usually courses around it to involve the major foramina in the skull base, the most common being that of the carotid artery and the jugular bulb. Fractures commonly occur near the roof of the external auditory canal and run parallel along the petrous apex, extending anteriorly to the foramen lacerum and the carotid artery. They may also extend into the temporal mandibular joint region.

Longitudinal fractures account for between 70 and 90 percent of temporal bone fractures. They pass parallel to the anterior margin of the petrous pyramid and usually extend medially from the region of the gasserian ganglion to the middle ear and laterally to the mastoid air cells. Typically the fracture line transverses the tympanic annulus, lacerating the tympanic membrane and producing a steplike deformity in the external auditory canal (see Fig. 5–1D). Cerebrospinal and hemorrhagic otorrhea are common, and the combination of laceration of the tympanic membrane, ossicular damage, and hemotympanum produces a conductive hearing loss. Sensorineural hearing loss and vertigo, characteristic of inner ear concussion, frequently accompany a longitudinal temporal bone fracture, but the bony labyrinth is rarely fractured.[23] Damage to the seventh and eighth cranial nerves is infrequent.

Transverse fractures of the temporal bone account for less than 20 percent of fractures in this region. They run orthogonal to the long axis of the petrous pyramid. In contrast to longitudinal fractures they usually pass through the vestibule of the inner ear, tearing the membranous labyrinth and lacerating the vestibular and cochlear nerve and producing complete loss of vestibular and cochlear function. Vertigo, nausea, and vomiting are prominent for several days after the fracture typical of acute unilateral vestibular loss. The facial nerve is lacerated in about 50 percent of cases, and the loss of function may be permanent unless surgical repair is instituted.[11] Examination of the ear reveals hemotympanum, but bleeding from the ear occurs infrequently because the tympanic membrane usually remains intact. Cerebrospinal fluid (CSF) often fills the middle ear and drains through the eustachian tube into the nasopharynx. Meningitis is a late complication of both types of temporal bone fractures.[1]

Labyrinthine Concussion

Auditory and vestibular symptoms (either isolated or in combination) frequently follow blows to the head that do not result in temporal bone fracture. Voss suggested the name labyrinthine concussion for these symptoms.[14] The absence of associated brainstem symptoms and signs and the usual rapid improvement in symptoms following injury support a peripheral localization for the lesion. Although protected by a bony capsule, the delicate labyrinthine membranes are susceptible to blunt trauma.[24] Of 57 cases of labyrinthine concussion reported by Davy,[8] 51 percent resulted from blows to the occipital region; 26 percent, to the frontal region; and 23 percent, to other areas. In the majority of cases the blow resulted in loss of consciousness.

Sudden deafness following a blow to the head without associated vestibular symptoms is often partially or completely reversible. It is probably caused by intense acoustic stimulation from pressure waves created by the blow which are are transmitted through the bone to the cochlea just as pressure waves are transmitted from air through the conduction mechanism.[13] Supporting this suggestion, the pathologic changes in the cochlea produced by experimental headblows in animals are similar to those produced by intense airborne sound stimuli.[24] These changes consist of degeneration of hair cells and cochlear neurons in the middle turns of the cochlea. Pure-tone hearing loss is usually most pronounced at 4000 and 8000 Hz.

Posttraumatic Positional Vertigo

The most common neurotologic sequela to head injury is so-called benign positional vertigo. The patient develops sudden brief attacks of vertigo and nystagmus precipitated by changing head position (see Chapter 10). Barber[3] reported positional vertigo with 47 percent of head injuries associated with longitudinal temporal bone fractures and with 21 percent of head injuries of a comparable severity without skull fracture. In over 90 percent of patients typical paroxysmal positional nystagmus was induced with a rapid positional change (see Fig. 5–5). Presumably, the trauma results in dislodgement of calcium carbonate crystals from the macula of the utriculus which become attached to the cupula of the posterior semicircular canal (see Fig. 10–1).[22] The prognosis for patients with posttraumatic benign positional vertigo is good; spontaneous remission occurs in most within 3 months and almost all have a remission within 2 years of the head injury.[3, 23] Multiple recurrences are not infrequent, however.[2]

Diagnosis and Management

High-resolution computerized tomography (CT) scanning with bone windows is the radiologic procedure of choice for evaluating trauma to the temporal bone and skull base. With CT scanning, one often is able to identify multiple fracture lines spreading throughout the base of the skull (Fig. 14–1). Magnetic resonance (MR) scanning can be of some use for identifying soft tissue lesions but is of little use for identifying fractures. Once the patient stabilizes, a systematic evaluation of the auditory, vestibular, and facial nerves should be undertaken. There is no treatment for sensorineural hearing loss secondary to temporary bone trauma unless there is evidence for a perilymphatic fistula (discussed below). If, based on the audiometric testing and tympanometric studies, a conductive hearing loss is identified, surgical intervention may lead to restoration of normal hearing. Separation of the incudostapedial joint with or without dislocation of the body of the incus from the articulation with the malleus head is the most common type of ossicular dislocation seen with temporal bone injury.[12] The surgeon can usually deal with these problems through a transcanal route under local anesthesia using a tympanomeatal flap.

Damage to the vestibular apparatus results in acute symptoms, with gradual improvement as central compensation occurs. Symptomatic treatment of vertigo is helpful initially, and the patient is encouraged to begin vestibular exercises as soon as possible to accelerate the compensation process (see Table 11–2). Posttraumatic positional vertigo responds to positional exercises similar to other varieties of benign positional vertigo (see Fig. 10–2). Persistent fluctuating vestibular symptoms may indicate the presence of a perilymphatic fistula and necessitate exploration of the middle ear (see below). The decision regarding surgical intervention in patients with facial nerve injury secondary to temporal bone trauma is often difficult.[9] As suggested above, longitudinal fractures usually do not interrupt the continuity of the facial nerve. In these cases it is appropriate to observe the facial weakness closely with regular follow-up from the time of the accident. If function does not return within 4 to 6 months, surgical intervention is probably indicated. As a general rule regeneration of a damaged but

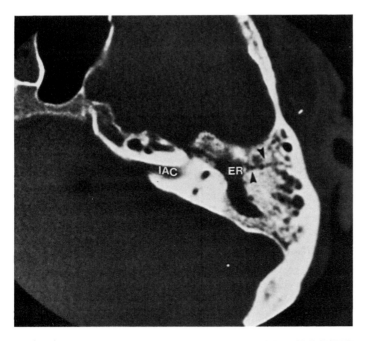

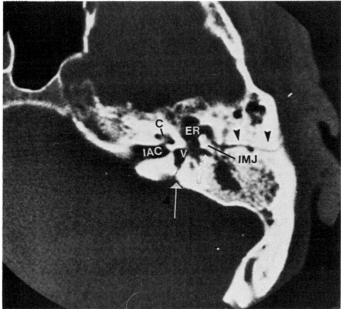

Figure 14–1. CT scans of the temporal bone showing longitudinal and transverse fractures in the same patient *(arrows)*. The longitudinal fracture crosses the middle ear, disrupting the ossicular chain, and the transverse fracture enters the vestibule, damaging the membranous labyrinth. *C,* cochlea; *ER,* epitympanic recess; *IMJ,* incudomalleal joint; *V,* vestibule; *IAC,* internal auditory canal.

uninterrupted nerve occurs at a rate of about 1 millimeter a day. There is marked variability in this rate, however; some patients show evidence of continued improvement for a year or longer after injury. In cases of transverse fracture of the temporal bone with associated severe auditory and vestibular loss, the likelihood of me-

chanical disruption of the facial nerve is great, so the decision regarding surgical intervention is easier. In these cases, translabyrinthine decompression and repair of the facial nerve may be achieved because there is already a total loss of auditory and vestibular function. Some cases of severe blunt head injury may result in a tear of the facial nerve at the root entry zone into the brainstem. These patients invariably have a prolonged period of unconsciousness at the time of the accident, and there are nearly always associated symptoms and signs of brainstem injury. Obviously, there is little prospect for recovery of facial nerve function with this type of lesion.

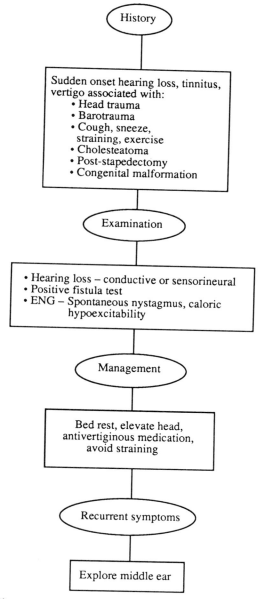

Figure 14-2. Algorithm for diagnosis and management of a perilymph fistula.

PERILYMPH FISTULA

With this disorder there is a disruption of the limiting membranes of the labyrinth—usually at the oval or round windows. The symptoms and signs are remarkably variable; a perilymph fistula must be considered in the differential diagnosis of sudden hearing loss, recurrent vestibulopathy, Meniere's syndrome, congenital sensorineural hearing loss, post-traumatic hearing loss and vertigo, and stapedectomy failure (Fig. 14-2).[15]

Causes of Perilymph Fistulae

The cause of a fistula is obvious when there is a disruption of the otic capsule or a tear in the membranous labyrinth associated with trauma, surgery, or infection; spontaneous fistulae are more difficult to explain. A sudden negative or positive pressure change in the middle ear from violent nose blowing, sneezing, or barotrauma, or a sudden increase in cerebrospinal fluid (CSF) pressure associated with lifting, straining, coughing, or vigorous activity could lead to rupture of the round window.[10] In the latter case, the change in CSF pressure is transmitted to the inner ear via the cochlear aqueduct and/or internal auditory canal (see Chapter 2). Perilymph fistulae may also be associated with developmental abnormalities of the middle ear and otic capsule (e.g., defects in the stapes footplate or other malformations of the stapedial arch).

Pathophysiology

How leakage of perilymph leads to fluctuating vestibular and auditory symptoms is unclear. Removal of the round window in animals has little effect on cochlear electrical potentials,[29] and the perilymphatic space is routinely entered during stapedectomy surgery, usually without sequelae. The cochleosacculotomy operation for Meniere's syndrome produces a round window membrane puncture, yet the incidence of postoperative sensorineural hearing loss is low (less than 25 percent).[25] Although the sensorineural hearing loss associated with perilymph fistulae is usually not reversible, patients occasionally have been reported with dramatic recovery of hearing as long as 10 years after the onset of hearing loss.[26] Obviously, such patients could not have had irreversible damage of their sensory epithelium. Presumably, the perilymph fistula leads to aberrant or inefficient transmission of mechanical energy within the cochlea.

Vestibular symptoms are even more difficult to explain on the basis of perilymph fistulae. How would such a leakage lead to stimulation of the vestibular receptors? Pressure changes in the middle ear would be transmitted through the labyrinthine windows to the cochlea but not the semicircular canals. Transient displacement of the otolithic membrane in the sacculus might be produced, but this could not explain a prolonged episode of vertigo and nystagmus.

Diagnosis

The classical presentation of an acute perilymph fistula is a sudden audible pop in the ear immediately followed by hearing loss, vertigo, and tinnitus. The key to the diagnosis is to identify the characteristic precipitating factors listed in Figure 14–2.

Nonspecific imbalance and disequilibrium aggravated by quick head movements or sudden turning may result from chronic perilymph fistulae. Patients report aggravation of these symptoms in certain head positions, preferring to sleep on one side rather than on the other to avoid an ill-defined uncomfortable "dizzy" sensation. The latter feature might suggest benign positional vertigo, although the positional dizziness with perilymph fistulae is not as intense and is more persistent than that associated with benign positional vertigo. Occasionally, perilymph fistulae are discovered during middle ear exploration for other reasons in a patient with auditory or vestibular symptoms.

Unfortunately, there is no pathognomonic test for a perilymphatic fistula.[27] A positive fistula test (see Chapter 5) is suggestive but not specific. False-negatives are common, and false-positives occur with Meniere's syndrome and after stapedectomy. Furthermore, dizziness and imbalance are occasionally reported by normal subjects when the air pressure is changed in the external auditory canal during routine pneumatoscopy. Auditory examination may identify either a conductive or sensorineural hearing loss and electronystagmography, a unilateral caloric hypoexcitability; but these findings are not unique to a perilymph fistula. Because of the nonspecificity of diagnostic tests the decision as to whether to perform an exploratory tympanotomy is guided by the clinical history.

Management

The great majority of perilymph fistulae spontaneously heal without intervention. For this reason, most authors advocate conservative management with an initial period of bedrest, sedation, head elevation, and measures to decrease straining.[15] The one exception to this conservative approach might be acute barotrauma in which immediate exploration has been advocated.[20] Persistent auditory and vestibular symptoms are indications for exploration of the middle ear after an initial trial of conservative management. Even in these cases, however, only about half to two thirds of ears are found to have fistulae.

The goal of surgery is to stabilize the hearing loss and relieve vestibular symptoms. The middle ear is typically explored through a posterior tympanotomy.[10] Most often the fistula is in the area of the oval window. The perilymphatic leak can be very subtle; the surgeon may have difficulty distinguishing between a fluid leak and the accumulation of normal secretions. The perilymph leak may become apparent only when the patient is placed in the Trendelenburg position, after performing a Valsalva maneuver, after jugular vein compression, or with manipulation of the ossicular chain. Recurrence of symptoms after repair occurs in at least 10 percent of cases; rarely, intractable symptoms will necessitate destructive surgery with labyrinthectomy or nerve section.

BRAIN TRAUMA

The most common mechanism of brain injury with blunt head trauma is movement and deformation of the brain within the skull. When the rapidly moving head is suddenly stopped, the viscoelastic brain continues to move and may rotate in the skull around the axis of the brainstem. The internal shearing and stress forces traumatize neurons and disrupt axons and blood vessels. The latter may cause multifocal petechial hemorrhages or even massive intracerebral hemorrhage. The term *concussion* refers to a brief loss of consciousness after head trauma unassociated with focal neurologic signs or radiologic evidence of structural brain damage. Usually the loss of consciousness lasts for only a few minutes, although residual symptoms may last for months to years (see below). The mechanism for such a brief loss of consciousness and rapid recovery is unknown, but a diffuse release of neurotransmitters has been postulated.[7]

Most patients who suffer concussion probably have some irreversible injury to brain cells, but nearly all rapidly regain function within minutes of the injury. They can usually remember the events up to a few moments before the injury and have little or no retrograde amnesia. The blow itself is rarely recalled, and there is invariably a brief period of memory loss following the injury (posttraumatic amnesia). The duration of postconcussion symptoms and signs varies with the intensity of the blow and the degree of brain deformity.[4]

Dizziness due to Brainstem Trauma

Brainstem injury from blunt head trauma is not a common cause of isolated auditory and vestibular symptoms.[8] Severe head blows may produce hemorrhage or infarction in the brainstem, but these pathologic changes are invariably associated with alteration in the level of consciousness and multiple neurologic signs. Mitchell and Adams[18] studied serial sections of the brainstem in 100 cases of fatal blunt head injury. Only 18 patients showed no evidence of increased intracranial pressure, and of these only 7 had abnormalities in the brainstem attributable to the primary impact. In these seven, other areas of the brain were damaged, suggesting to the authors that so-called primary

brainstem injury does not exist but, rather, is one aspect of diffuse brain damage. As a general rule, isolated episodes of vertigo occurring after brain trauma should not be attributed to brainstem injury.

Caloric examination can be particularly helpful in evaluating the brainstem status in patients who are comatose from blunt head injuries. These patients do not produce saccades, so a "normal" response is a conjugate tonic deviation of the eyes toward the side of a cold stimulus or away from the side of a warm stimulus. Absence of this tonic deviation affirms that the brainstem vestibulo-ocular reflex pathways have been damaged, assuming that the eighth nerve and end-organs are intact. Unilateral loss of tonic deviation or nonconjugate deviation indicates focal involvement of the reflex pathways. The absence of caloric responses after an acute head injury is a poor prognostic sign.[17, 19]

Postconcussion Syndrome

The postconcussion syndrome has long been the center of medical-legal controversy.[5, 28] Symptoms include dizziness, headache (usually diffuse), increased irritability, insomnia, forgetfulness, mental obtuseness, and loss of initiative—all of which occur after a concussion. Because of the ill-defined nature of these symptoms it is difficult to localize the site of lesion and the patient is frequently diagnosed as being psychoneurotic (compensation neurosis).[16] The dizziness associated with the postconcussion syndrome is nearly always nonspecific; patients use terms such as swimming, light-headed, floating, rocking, and disoriented to describe the sensations they feel. If vertigo is present, an additional labyrinthine lesion should be suspected.

Rutherford and coworkers[21] followed 145 patients with concussion from minor head injuries to assess the type and frequency of symptoms and to evaluate whether the symptoms correlated with the severity of injury, associated neurologic signs, or other circumstances related to the injury. Concussion was defined as a period of amnesia—no matter how brief— caused by a blow to the head. All of the patients were released from the hospital after a brief observation. Table 14–1 lists the symptoms and their frequency of occurrence reported by the 145 patients 6 weeks after the concussion. Approximately one half were symptom free, but the other half complained of one or more symptoms. In those patients with multiple symptoms no consistent pattern was found to support the concept of a postconcussion syndrome. A significant correlation existed between the presence of multiple symptoms at 6 weeks and the occurrence of positive neurologic signs and symptoms within 24 hours of the concussion. Postconcussion symptoms were more frequent in women and in patients who blamed their employers or large impersonal organizations for their accidents. The authors concluded that both organic and psychosomatic fac-

tors were involved in the pathogenesis of postconcussion symptoms.

Diagnosis and Management

Persistent dizziness after a blunt head injury often poses a difficult diagnostic dilemma (Table 14–2). A careful neurotologic examination should identify most specific syndromes that require individualized treatment. Examination of the ear may reveal evidence of a temporal bone fracture or perilymph fistula, positional testing may reveal benign positional nystagmus, and neurologic examination may identify signs of brainstem damage. Standard audiometric, brainstem auditory-evoked response (BAER), and electronystagmographic (ENG) testing are useful to assess the functional status of the auditory and vestibular systems. Neuroimaging is usually helpful only when there are focal findings on the neurologic examination.

CT scanning is most useful for evaluating the base of the skull, and MR scanning provides the best assessment of brainstem and cerebellar structures.

Treatment of the postconcussion syndrome begins by providing the patient with reassurance that there is no evidence of structural damage, that the symptoms are not unusual after head injury, and that they nearly always disappear spontaneously. The patient should be encouraged to return to a normal exercise level gradually, even though initially the dizziness and other symptoms may be aggravated. Tranquilizers such as diazepam and alprazolam can be useful for a transient period, but prolonged use should be avoided inas-

Table 14–1. SYMPTOMS REPORTED 6 WEEKS AFTER A CONCUSSION IN 145 PATIENTS[21]

Symptom	Number	Percentage
Headache	36	24.8
Anxiety	28	19.3
Insomnia	22	15.2
Dizziness	21	14.5
Irritability	13	9.0
Fatigue	13	9.0
Loss of concentration	12	8.3
Loss of memory	12	8.3
Hearing defect	10	6.9
Sensitivity to alcohol	9	6.2
Depression	8	5.5
Visual defect	7	4.8
Anosmia	4	2.8
Epilepsy	3	2.1
Diplopia	2	1.4
Other	16	11.0
No symptoms	71	49.0

Table 14–2. DIFFERENTIAL DIAGNOSIS OF PERSISTENT DIZZINESS AFTER HEAD TRAUMA

	Dizziness	Exam	Laboratory
Benign positional vertigo	Brief episodes, position induced	Fatigable positional nystagmus	Normal
Labyrinthine concussion	Severe initially, gradual improvement	Peripheral spontaneous nystagmus	Caloric vestibular paresis, unilateral hearing loss
Perilymph fistula	Fluctuating, induced by coughing, sneezing, straining	Positive fistula test	Caloric vestibular paresis, unilateral hearing loss
Brainstem contusion	Severe, associated brainstem symptoms	Focal neurologic signs	MR scan shows focal lesions
Postconcussion syndrome	Continuous, associated headaches, irritability, etc.	Normal	Normal

much as dependency is common. Endogenous depression is a common sequela after brain injury, and antidepressant medications (e.g., imipramine and desipramine) may be helpful in severe cases. Although recovery is the rule, some patients will have persistent symptoms for years after a concussion. Although there is a positive correlation between the severity of head injury and the length of postconcussion symptoms, one cannot reliably judge the prognosis for recovery based on the nature of the head injury.

REFERENCES

1. Applebaum, E: Meningitis following trauma to the head and face. JAMA 173:1818, 1960.
2. Baloh, RW, Honrubia, V, and Jacobson, K: Benign positional vertigo: Clinical and oculographic features in 240 cases. Neurology 37:371, 1987.
3. Barber, H: Positional nystagmus especially after head injury. Laryngoscope 74:891, 1964.
4. Becker, DP, Miller, JD, and Gade, G: Diagnosis and treatment of head injury in adults. In Youmans, JR (ed): Neurological Surgery, ed 3. WB Saunders, Philadelphia, 1988.
5. Binder, LM: Persisting symptoms after mild head injury: A review of the post concussive syndrome. J Clin Exp Neuropsych 8:323, 1986.
6. Cannon, CR and Jahrsdoerfer, RA: Temporal bone fractures. Review of 90 cases. Arch Otolaryngol 109:285, 1983.
7. Cooper, P (ed): Head Injury, ed 2. Williams & Wilkins, Baltimore, 1987.
8. Davey, LM: Labyrinthine trauma in head injury. Conn Med 29:250, 1965.
9. Fisch, U: Facial paralysis in fractures of the petrous bone. Laryngoscope 84:2141, 1974.
10. Goodhill, V: Leaking labyrinth lesions, deafness, tinnitus, and dizziness. Ann Otol Rhinol Laryngol 90:99, 1981.
11. Grove, WE: Skull fractures involving the ear: A clinical study of 211 cases. Laryngoscope 49:678, 1939.
12. Hongli, J and Stuart, W: Middle ear injuries in skull trauma. Laryngoscope 78:899, 1968.
13. Igarashi, M, Schuknecht, H, and Myers, E: Cochlear pathology in humans with stimulation deafness. J Laryngol 78:115, 1964.
14. JAMA: Is there a labyrinthine concussion? In Foreign Letters, JAMA 103:1721, 1934.
15. Mattox, DE: Perilymph fistulas. In Cummings, CW, Fredrickson, JM, Harker, LA, Krause, CJ, and Schuller, DE (eds): Otolaryngology—Head and Neck Surgery. CV Mosby, St Louis, 1986, p 3113.
16. Miller, H: Mental sequelae of head injury. Proc Roy Soc Med 59:257, 1966.
17. Minderhoud, JM, Van Woerkom, TC, and Van Weerden, TW: On the nature of brain stem disorders in severe head injured patients. II. A study on caloric vestibular reactions and neurotransmitter treatment. Act Neurochirugica 34:23, 1976.
18. Mitchell, DE and Adams, JH: Primary focal impact damage to the brain stem in blunt head injuries. Does it exist? Lancet 2:215, 1973.
19. Poulsen, J and Zilstrorff, K: Prognostic value of the caloric vestibular test in the unconscious patient with cranial trauma. Acta Neurol Scand 48:282, 1972.
20. Pullen, FW, Rosenberg, GH, and Cabeza, CH: Sudden hearing loss in divers and fliers. Laryngoscope 84:1373, 1979.
21. Rutherford, WH, Merrett, JD, and McDonald, JR: Sequelae of concussion caused by minor head injuries. Lancet 1:1, 1977.
22. Schuknecht, H: Cupulolithiasis. Arch Otolaryngol 90:765, 1969.
23. Schuknecht, H and Davison, R: Deafness and vertigo from head injury. Arch Otolaryngol 63:513, 1956.
24. Schuknecht, H, Neff, W, and Perlman, H: An experimental study of auditory damage following blows to the head. Ann Otol Rhinol Laryngol 60:273, 1951.
25. Schuknecht, HF: Cochleosacculotomy for Meniere's disease: Theory, technique and results. Laryngoscope 92:853, 1982.
26. Shannon, DA and Blum, SL: Surgical treatment of long term sensorineural hearing loss due to labyrinthine fistula. J Am Aud Soc 5:1, 1979.
27. Simmons, FB: Perilymph fistula: Some diagnostic problems. Adv Otorhinolaryngol 28:68, 1982.
28. Symonds, C: Concussion and its sequelae. Lancet 1:1, 1962.
29. Weisskopf, A, Murphy, JT, and Merzenich, MM: Genesis of the round window rupture syndrome; some experimental observations. Laryngoscope 88:389, 1978.

Chapter 15

METABOLIC DISORDERS

DIZZINESS AND SYSTEMIC METABOLIC DISORDERS

Diabetes Mellitus

Vestibular symptoms and signs are common in patients with diabetes mellitus, but convincing evidence does not exist for a specific vestibular lesion.[39] In those diabetic patients with vestibular dysfunction whose temporal bones and nervous systems have been studied at necropsy, pathologic changes can be explained on the basis of associated vascular disease.[48, 68] Three types of vascular changes occur with diabetes mellitus: (1) endothelial proliferation narrowing the lumens of arterioles, capillaries, and venules; (2) arteriosclerotic narrowing of small arteries and arterioles; and (3) atherosclerotic narrowing of the large arteries. These vascular changes may damage the vestibular system from the peripheral end-organ and vestibular nerve to its diffuse central nervous system (CNS) connections. The most common finding in the labyrinth at necropsy in patients with diabetes mellitus is a PAS positive thickening of the capillary walls—most prominent in the vascular stria of the cochlea, where it probably accounts for the progressive bilateral high-frequency hearing loss characteristic of the disease.[40] Similar changes are found in the vestibular end-organs, which, along with degeneration of vestibular nerve and ganglion, could explain the frequent complaints of chronic dysequilibrium and dizziness in diabetic patients.[56]

Sudden onset of hearing loss and/or vertigo in patients with diabetes mellitus can result from occlusion of the vessels to the labyrinth or the eighth nerve.[39] Cranial nerve mononeuropathies are a well-known clinical phenomenon associated with diabetes mellitus; they are most likely due to arteriosclerotic occlusion of arterioles supplying the cranial nerve. Atherosclerosis of larger vessels predisposes the patient to transient vertebrobasilar insufficiency and to specific occlusive syndromes, such as the anterior vestibular artery syndrome and the lateral medullary syndrome (see Chapter 12).

Uremia

Multiple causes of auditory and vestibular symptoms can be identified in patients with chronic renal disease.[5] The same pathologic process can affect both the kidneys and the labyrinths, as seen in Alport's syndrome (hereditary nephritis and deafness), diabetes mellitus, and Fabry's disease. Immunosuppressive treatment either of the primary renal disorder or to avoid transplant rejection predisposes the patient to otologic infections, often with exotic or saprophytic organisms. Patients with renal disease are particularly vulnerable to the ototoxic effects of aminoglycoside antibiotics and loop diuretics because of their inability to clear these substances from the blood; ototoxicity is probably the most common cause of auditory and vestibular symptoms in uremic patients.

Hyponatremia causes reversible hearing loss and tinnitus in patients undergoing chronic hemodialysis. Yassin and coworkers[86] found a high degree of correlation between hearing loss and serum sodium levels irrespective of the blood urea level. The hearing loss could be corrected by returning the serum sodium level to normal in 80 percent of patients with acute renal failure and in 52 percent of those with chronic renal failure. Patients undergoing chronic hemodialysis and those receiving kidney transplants often experience ill-defined fluctuating auditory and vestibular symptoms. Oda and coworkers[57] performed necropsy studies on temporal bones of eight patients with chronic uremia who had undergone long-term hemodialysis therapy (24 to 546 treatments). At least one kidney transplant was performed in seven of the eight patients. Vestibular symptoms occurred in five patients and auditory symptoms in three; all symptoms began after the start of hemodialysis. Abnormal concretions were found in the vascular stria of the cochlea and in the subepithelial connective tissue of the maculae and cristae in seven of the eight patients. The source of these abnormal deposits is unknown.

Hypothyroidism

A symmetrical, mild to moderate sensorineural hearing loss is commonly associated with sporadic, nonendemic hypothyroidism.[53, 62] Vertigo also may occur in hypothyroid patients, although there is no vertiginous syndrome that is characteristic of this disorder. Some investigators have found a high incidence of hypothyroidism in patients with idiopathic Meniere's syndrome, but others have not. Auditory and vestibular abnormalities have also been documented in animals who have been made hypothyroid.[85] Because the temporal bones in these animals were normal, the auditory and vestibular losses were presumably on a biochemical basis. In only 1 of 11 animals the hearing loss, identified by cochlear microphonic potentials, returned to normal after hormone replacement.

Alcohol and Thiamine Deficiency

ACUTE EFFECTS OF ALCOHOL

Acute alcohol intoxication is regularly associated with unsteadiness of gait, slurring of speech, and occasionally vertigo. The gait ataxia and slurring of speech suggest cerebellar dysfunction, but an additional vestibular component may be involved. In animal studies alcohol selectively interferes with synaptic transmission within the vestibular nuclei.[41] Vestibular function testing with rotational stimulation in patients with alcohol intoxication has revealed normal vestibulo-ocular reflex gain in the dark, but impaired fixation-suppression of vestibular nystagmus consistent with cerebellar dysfunction.[27, 31] Slowing of saccades and smooth pursuit is consistently found in subjects after only moderate alcohol ingestion.[43, 44, 84] Gaze-evoked nystagmus is a reliable sign of intoxication, the magnitude of which is highly correlated with the blood alcohol concentration.[28]

Positional vertigo is another well-documented effect of alcohol on the vestibular system.[1] Within 30 minutes after ingesting a moderate amount of alcohol (e.g., 100 ml of whiskey), the subject develops a direction-changing static positional nystagmus often associated with vertigo. The positional nystagmus beats to the right in the right lateral position, to the left in the left lateral position, and is inhibited by fixation. The primary phase of the positional nystagmus reaches its peak in about 2 hours, at approximately the time of peak blood alcohol level (0.1 percent for the above example). Four to five hours after alcohol ingestion, when the blood alcohol level is below 0.01 percent, positional nystagmus is still present, but now it is right-beating in the left lateral position and left-beating in the right lateral position (secondary phase). The positional nystagmus can last up to 12 hours, at which time alcohol cannot be detected in the blood.

The studies of Money and Myles[54] provide a reasonable explanation for alcohol positional nystagmus. These investigators produced a direction-changing positional nystagmus in the reverse direction of primary alcohol positional nystagmus by giving the subject heavy water—H_3O. When subjects with alcohol direction-changing positional nystagmus (primary phase) were given H_3O, the nystagmus disappeared. The authors interpreted these findings to indicate that alcohol and heavy water direction-changing positional nystagmus were due to a different rate of diffusion of alcohol and heavy water into the cupula and the surrounding endolymph. In the primary phase of alcohol positional nystagmus, alcohol rapidly diffuses into the base of the cupula because of the latter's proximity to blood capillaries while it slowly diffuses into the endolymph. The cupula then has a lower specific gravity than the endolymph and acts as a gravity-sensing organ, maintaining a slight deflection as long as the position is held. After approximately 3 hours, the endolymph and cupula have approximately the same alcohol concentration, and the positional nystagmus disappears. As the blood alcohol level falls, the reverse situation occurs with the cupula being heavier than the surrounding endolymph, and the secondary phase of positional nystagmus occurs.

WERNICKE'S ENCEPHALOPATHY

This is a common clinical syndrome caused by thiamine deficiency (usually secondary to malnutrition from chronic alcoholism).[81] It is characterized by the subacute onset of confusion, ophthalmoplegia, and ataxia of stance and gait. Vertigo and hearing loss are not common complaints.The truncal ataxia is often dramatic, with the patient being unable to take even a few steps without support, and yet standard cerebellar function testing with finger-to-nose and heel-knee-shin is often normal or minimally impaired.The ataxia is increased with eye closure or darkness. These findings suggest a combination of midline cerebellar and either proprioceptive or vestibular impairment. Two reports have documented impaired bithermal caloric responses in patients with acute Wernicke's encephalopathy.[26, 29] Some patients did not respond even to ice water.

Experimental studies in thiamine-deficient rats[75] and monkeys[15] revealed that the earliest pathologic changes originate in the vestibular nuclei, particularly in the lateral nucleus. The nerve terminals and axons degenerate without evidence of damage to the neuronal parikaria. Neurologic signs appear even before these early pathologic changes. Loss of transketolase activity (a thiamine-dependent enzyme) in the lateral pontine tegmentum, including the lateral vestibular nuclei, correlates better with the onset of clinical signs. Injection of thiamine promptly restores transketolase activity and improves clinical signs. Pathologic changes are common in the vestibular nuclei of patients with thiamine deficiency studied at necropsy. In the report by Victor and coworkers,[81] the medial vestibular nucleus was involved in 71 percent of cases with the lateral, superior, and descending nuclei being involved in 50, 36, and 30 percent of cases respectively. The changes in the vestibular nuclei were relatively mild, however, compared with the frank necrosis and demyelination occurring in other areas. Apparently, the majority of clinical findings (including impaired vestibular function) are secondary to thiamine-dependent enzyme loss in the brainstem, and only after prolonged and/or repeated episodes of deficiency do irreversible structural changes occur.

CEREBELLAR DEGENERATION

In 1959, Victor and associates[82] reported a dramatic clinical syndrome in 50 alcoholics manifested by severe truncal ataxia with relative sparing of the upper extremities. On clinical examination all patients exhibited severe ataxia of stance and gait, with instability of the trunk while standing and severe incoordination on the heel-knee-shin test. On neuropathologic examination, atrophy was remarkably localized to the superior cerebellar vermis, paramedian superior cerebellar hemispheres, and the flocculi. More recently, computerized tomographic (CT) scans have documented shrinkage of the cerebellum, particularly the vermis in chronic alcoholics.[33] The cerebellar atrophy is most likely due to malnutrition rather than direct alcohol toxicity, inasmuch as similar cellular changes have been seen in malnourished nonalcoholics[49] and some of the symptoms and signs seen with acute cerebellar degeneration can be reversed with massive doses of thiamine.[30]

Management

There is no specific treatment for the neurotologic manifestations of diabetes mellitus. Presumably the likelihood of vascular occlusion (small and large vessel) decreases with good control of blood glucose levels.[77] Although it has been suggested that auditory and vestibular dysfunctions occur in the prediabetic state, similar to the retinal and renal changes, there have been no controlled studies to support this supposition. The single most important aspect in preventing auditory and vestibular dysfunctions in patients with uremia is to avoid the use of potential ototoxic drugs. Careful management of electrolytes in patients undergoing chronic renal dialysis will prevent fluctuating auditory and vestibular symptoms. The bilateral sensorineural hearing loss associated with acquired hypothyroidism improves in a small percentage of patients after thyroid hormone replacement.[53]

With Wernicke's encephalopathy the ophthalmoplegia, confusion, and ataxia usually respond rapidly to thiamine replacement.[15] Some patients are left with a chronic memory disorder (Korsakoff's syndrome) as well as mild ataxia due to midline cerebellar degeneration. In patients receiving thiamine replacement vestibular function as measured by serial caloric testing slowly returns toward normal over several weeks, although in some cases recovery is asymmetric and incomplete. As suggested above, alcoholic cerebellar degeneration also may respond to thiamine replacement. Diener and colleagues[17] demonstrated that patients with alcoholic cerebellar degeneration who stopped drinking exhibited a significant and sometimes dramatic decrease of body sway measured with posturography, compared with patients who continued drinking. This improvement after abstinence from alcohol may have resulted from central plastic changes or to recovery of function where structural damage was not complete. Ron and associates[60] reported that the cortical shrinkage and ventricular dilation seen on CT scanning of the cerebellum was partially reversible with abstinence from alcohol.

METABOLIC DISORDERS OF THE TEMPORAL BONE

Otosclerosis

Otosclerosis is a metabolic disease of the bony labyrinth that usually manifests itself by immobilizing the stapes and thereby producing a conductive hearing loss.[36, 42] Seventy percent of patients with clinical otosclerosis note hearing loss between the ages of 11 and 30. The disorder is most common in whites (clinically evident in 0.5 to 2 percent), infrequent in blacks, and almost nonexistent in Asians and American Indians. A positive family history for otosclerosis is reported in between 50 and 70 percent of cases. The sporadic cases may represent autosomal recessive inheritance, spontaneous mutation, or they may be nongenetic in origin.

Although otosclerosis is primarily a disorder of the auditory system, vestibular symptoms and signs are more common than generally appreciated. Cody and Baker[13] found that 46 percent of 500 patients with nonsurgically treated otosclerosis complained of vestibular symptoms. The most common symptoms were recurrent attacks of vertigo (26 percent) and postural imbalance (22 percent). Those patients with more severe sensorineural hearing loss were more likely to have vestibular complaints. Abnormalities on electronystagmography (ENG) testing have been found in about 50 percent of patients tested, with the most common abnormality being unilateral hypoexcitability to caloric stimulation.[83] ENG abnormalities are more common in patients with greater sensorineural hearing loss, but they are not necessarily seen in the poorer hearing ear.

The basic pathologic process of otosclerosis is a resorption of normal bone particularly around blood vessels, and its replacement by cellular fibrous connective tissue.[46] With time immature basophilic bone is produced in the resorption space; after several cycles of resorption and new bone formation a mature acidophilic bone with a laminated matrix is produced. Bilateral involvement is usual, but about a fourth of cases are unilateral. Areas of predilection for otosclerotic foci include the oval window region, the round window niche, the anterior wall of the internal auditory canal, and within the stapedial footplate. Although conductive hearing loss is the hallmark of otosclerosis, a combined conductive-sensorineural hearing loss pattern is frequent. The sensorineural component is perhaps caused by foci of otosclerosis next to the spiral ligament of the cochlea, producing atrophy of the spiral ligament.

The mechanism for the production of dizziness in patients with otosclerosis is poorly understood. Direct mechanical deformation of the labyrinth or biochemical abnormalities of inner ear fluids are likely possibilities. Endolymphatic hydrops has been identified in a few temporal bones with multiple foci of otosclerosis.[47] Sando and co-workers[65] studied four temporal bones of two patients with otosclerosis who complained of prominent vestibular symptoms and found otosclerotic foci in opposition to the superior vestibular nerve in each. Vestibular nerve degeneration distal to these foci was also present, and three of the four temporal bones exhibited a marked degeneration of the sensory epithelium of the cristae of the lateral semicircular canals.

Paget's Disease

Paget's disease is a metabolic disorder of bone marked by pronounced osteoclastic resorption of old fully calcified bone and deposition of new osteoid layers that calcify normally.[58] The clinical picture varies from the classic one of an enlarged skull, progressive kyphosis, and short stature to the more common restricted forms confined to the skull, spine, pelvis, and femur. Hearing loss is a common symptom, initially described by Paget in his early reports and subsequently studied in detail by numerous investigators.[12, 16] A progressive combined sensorineural and conducting hearing loss is usually found. The vestibular labyrinth may also be progressively destroyed, resulting in unsteadiness of gait and, in rare cases, episodic vertigo. In the late stages, complete destruction of the bony labyrinth may occur with invasion of the inner ears, fractures, and degeneration of the membranous labyrinth. Paget's disease is inherited as an autosomal dominant disorder, usually becoming clinically manifest in the sixth decade. It affects men four times more commonly than women.

Other Disorders

Other, less common, metabolic disorders of the temporal bone that are associated with hearing loss and dizziness include osteogenesis imperfecta,[78] fibrous dysplasia,[69] and osteopetrosis.[32] The clinical presentation of these disorders is often indistinguishable from that of otosclerosis and of Paget's disease.

Diagnosis

The diagnosis of otosclerosis is based on finding a conductive hearing loss in a patient with the clinical picture outlined above. A flat tympanogram with maximum compliance near zero pressure is characteristic (see Fig. 8–4C). As the disease progresses, a mixed conductive, sensorineural hearing loss is common. About 10 percent of patients exhibit hyperemia of the promontory mucosa of the middle ear visible through the tympanic membrane (Schwartze's sign).[36] Conventional and computed x-ray tomography may show changes in the otic capsule (ranging from a small dehiscence in the normal, crisp outline of the capsule to entire loss of anatomic details), but these changes are not specific for otosclerosis inasmuch as they are also found in osteogenesis imperfecta, fibrous dysplasia, and even some normal subjects.[79]

The diagnosis of Paget's disease rests on finding the characteristic roentgenographic findings of increased density of bone with loss of the normal architecture, mingled with areas of decreased bone density.[58] The skull is enlarged, with indistinct margins giving a "cotton wool" appearance. High-resolution CT scans of the temporal bone typically reveal poor definition of the cortical margins of the inner ear and internal auditory canals.

Management

There is now convincing evidence that sodium fluoride retards the progression of otosclerosis.[73] A recent controlled study from Denmark and France documented both biochemical and audiometric changes in a treated group of patients with otosclerosis compared with a control group.[8] The usual dosage is 40 to 50 mg sodium fluoride per day given most conveniently as Florical (8.5 mg sodium fluoride and 364 mg calcium carbonate per capsule) plus 500 mg of vitamin D daily. The calcium and vitamin D prevent secondary hyperparathyroidism from developing. Side effects occur in as many as 20 percent of patients, with the most common being gastrointestinal upset and musculoskeletal pain. Whether sodium fluoride can reverse the vestibular abnormalities associated with otosclerosis is unproven, but at the present time it is the only therapy with promise.

Surgical treatment of otosclerosis is directed at improving the conductive hearing loss. Many different operations have been developed, and most have a high success rate. Although data on the results of surgical therapy in patients with vestibular symptoms are not available, there is little reason to expect improvement in such patients. In fact, surgical therapy may aggravate the vestibular symptoms. Smyth[72] detected decreased caloric responses 3 months postoperatively in 30 percent of 26 ears with normal values preoperatively.

Calcitonin, a peptide that inhibits calcium release from bone, has been effective in the treatment of Paget's disease, although reversibility of auditory and vestibular symptoms and signs is yet to be demonstrated.[11]

FAMILIAL ATAXIA SYNDROMES

Auditory and vestibular symptoms and signs occur with several of the hereditary ataxia syndromes, for example, Friedreich's ataxia,[10, 19, 25] olivopontocerebellar degeneration,[4] Refsum's disease,[59] cerebellar atrophy,[89] and familial periodic vertigo and ataxia.[20] In addition, isolated families with atypical ataxia syndromes associated with hearing loss and abnormal vestibular function have been reported.[7, 67, 80] Clinically, however, cerebellar findings usually overshadow the loss of vestibular function; patients present with ataxia and incoordination. In most, the symptoms are slowly progressive, although in some they are episodic. Head-movement-induced oscillopsia and dizziness occur because of the patient's inability to suppress the vestibulo-ocular reflex with fixation (see Oscillopsia, Chapter 4). Often, only after performing caloric or rotational testing can the physician recognize impaired vestibular function. Vertigo is usually not present because the vestibular loss occurs gradually in a bilateral symmetrical fashion. Many types of pathologic nystagmus are encountered, including gaze-evoked, central spontaneous (particularly upbeat and downbeat), rebound, and central paroxysmal positional.

Differential Diagnosis

The diagnosis of the familial ataxia syndromes is primarily clinical, based on the characteristic profile for each syndrome (Table 15–1).

FRIEDREICH'S ATAXIA

This is the most common variety of spinocerebellar degeneration, typically presenting in childhood or early adolescence

Table 15–1. DIFFERENTIAL FEATURES OF THE COMMON ATAXIA SYNDROMES

	Clinical	ENG	Neuroimaging
Friedreich's	Early onset, muscle atrophy, areflexia	Saccade dysmetria, ocular flutter, decreased calorics	Mild cerebellar atrophy
Olivopontocerebellar atrophy (OPCA)	Early to midlife onset, spasticity, hyperreflexia	Slow saccades, impaired pursuit, and fixation suppression of VOR	Prominent atrophy of pons and cerebellum (diffuse)
Cerebellar cortical atrophy (Holmes; Marie, Foix Alajouanine)	Late onset, predominantly truncal, dysarthria	Downbeat and rebound nystagmus, central positional nystagmus, impaired pursuit, and fixation suppression of VOR	Prominent cerebellar vermion atrophy
Familial periodic vertigo and ataxia	Early onset, episodes induced by exercise, stress	Usually normal, may have downbeat or rebound nystagmus	Usually normal, may have vermion atrophy

as an insidiously progressive truncal and extremity ataxia. It can be inherited as an autosomal recessive or dominant trait; sporadic cases are not infrequent. Skeletal (kyphoscoliosis and pes cavus) and cardiac (cardiomyopathy, murmurs, conduction defects) abnormalities are common. The combination of slowly progressive ataxia, dysarthria, loss of position and vibratory sense in the lower extremities, muscle weakness, atrophy and areflexia and symmetrical loss of auditory and vestibular function complete the clinical profile.

Spoendlin[74] studied the temporal bones in two sisters with Friedreich's ataxia and found extensive degeneration of the neurons of the eighth nerve (both auditory and vestibular), with preservation of the peripheral receptor organs. These changes correlated with the clinical findings of progressive bilateral deafness and caloric hypoexcitability for several years prior to death.

REFSUM'S DISEASE

This autosomal recessively inherited disorder is characterized by a combination of retinitis pigmentosa, bilateral sensorineural hearing loss, cerebellar ataxia, and peripheral neuropathy. Patients with Refsum's disease have an elevated serum phytanic acid, the result of a defect in lipid alpha-oxidase.[35] The disorder typically begins in the first decade, is slowly progressive, and, like Friedreich's ataxia, can be associated with cardiac conduction defects and cardiomyopathy. A specific laboratory test is available for identifying the defect in lipid alpha-oxidase activity.[61]

OLIVOPONTOCEREBELLAR DEGENERATION

This syndrome represents a group of adult-onset degenerative disorders clinically manifested by cerebellar, brainstem, and spinal cord findings. Sporadic cases outnumber those with a positive family history, but the pathologic changes of atrophy primarily involving the cerebellum, cerebellar peduncles, and basis pontis are common to all varieties.[4] The diagnosis rests on finding the onset in early to mid adult life of progressive ataxia, dysarthria, dys-

metria, and nystagmus. Later in the course, patients may develop spasticity, optic nerve atrophy, distal sensory involvement, and even loss of cognitive function. CT and magnetic resonance (MR) studies document atrophy of the cerebellum and pons early in the disease process; later there are enlarged ventricles and cerebral atrophy.

LATE-ONSET CORTICAL CEREBELLAR ATROPHY

This disorder is characterized by the gradual onset of ataxia beginning in mid to late life. It can be sporadic[3] or inherited[89] (as an autosomal dominant trait). Both varieties show a highly localized atrophy of the cerebellum, particularly the archicerebellum and paleocerebellum. There is extensive loss of Purkinje cells in the vermis (especially the anterior vermis) and the flocculonodular lobe, with relatively little neuronal loss in other areas of the brain. Cerebellar eye signs are common, including several types of pathologic nystagmus (especially spontaneous downbeat or upbeat). MR scans of the brain identify atrophy remarkably localized to the midline cerebellum (Fig. 15–1).[3]

FAMILIAL PERIODIC VERTIGO AND ATAXIA

These patients manifest recurrent episodes of vertigo and/or ataxia, sometimes associated with other brainstem symptoms such as diplopia, weakness, and dysarthria.[22, 88] The attacks typically begin in early childhood or early adulthood, last for hours to days at a time, and often recur several times a year. The inheritance pattern is usually autosomal dominant, although some sporadic cases have been identified. Most of the patients are normal between the episodes, although some have persistent spontaneous or gaze-evoked nystagmus and a few have been described with a slowly progressive ataxia.[20] Neuroimaging is usually normal, although one family had midline cerebellar atrophy on MR scanning similar to that seen in patients with late-onset cortical cerebellar atrophy.[24] The differential diagnosis includes other causes of episodic ataxia,

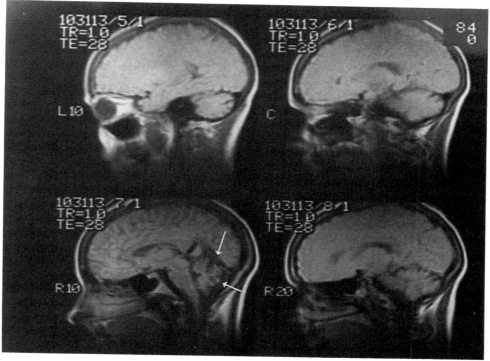

Figure 15—1. MR scans (T₁ weighted, sagittal sections) demonstrating midline cerebellar atrophy in a 37 year-old woman with slowly progressive truncal ataxia. The section through the vermis shows atrophic folia *(arrows)*, and the sections through the lateral hemispheres are normal.

including the aminoacidemias and disorders of the pyruvate dehydrogenase complex.[88] This disorder represents one of the few treatable causes of episodic vertigo and ataxia (see below).

Management

Because the specific enzymatic defect is unknown in most of these degenerative disorders, treatment is symptomatic. Patients with ataxia are encouraged to use a cane or walker to improve sensory input and to avoid falls. Regular physical therapy to maintain range of motion about all joints is critical to avoid painful contractions. A special diet low in long-chain fatty acids can be effective in controlling the progression of symptoms and signs with Refsum's disease.[18] Acetazolamide (Diamox) is remarkably effective for relieving the episodic symptoms in patients with familial periodic vertigo and ataxia.[88] The

usual dosage is 250 mg twice a day. The most common side effect is paresthesias of the extremities, a symptom that may spontaneously disappear with continued use. How acetazolamide benefits this disorder is unknown. It inhibits carbonic anhydrase, which catalyzes the interconversion of CO_2 to H_2CO_3. It also reduces the amount of brain lactate and pyruvate and produces brain acidosis. A therapeutic trial of acetazolamide should be undertaken in any patient with early-onset episodic vertigo and/or ataxia who has a family history of similar episodes.

OTOTOXINS

Patients who receive ototoxic drugs are often bedridden and suffer from multiple symptoms of systemic illness, so additional symptoms of auditory and vestibular dysfunction may be easily overlooked. Vestibular symptoms are particularly difficult to identify in this setting. Only after the patient begins to recover do the devastating effects of vestibular loss become apparent. By this time, the damage is irreversible. The examining physician must be keenly aware of the potential auditory and vestibular toxicity of any drug that is used, if ototoxicity is to be prevented.

Aminoglycosides

The commonly used aminoglycosides are listed in Table 15–2. Although each of these drugs can produce both auditory and vestibular damage, streptomycin and gentamycin are relatively specific for the vestibular system whereas kanamycin, tobramycin, and amikacin produce more damage to the auditory system.[23, 71] The newer aminoglycosides dibekacin and netilmicin are overall less ototoxic than the older aminoglycosides.[63]

The pharmacologic and biochemical characteristics are similar for all of the aminoglycoside antibiotics.[45] They are excreted almost exclusively by glomerular filtration; they are not metabolized. Patients with renal impairment cannot excrete the drugs, so the aminoglycosides accumulate in the blood and inner ear tissues. The ototoxicity of the aminoglycosides has been shown convincingly to be due to hair cell damage in the inner ear. Unlike penicillin and other common antibiotics, aminoglycosides are concentrated in the perilymph and endolymph. The earliest effect of the vestibulotoxic compounds such as streptomycin and gentamycin is a selective destruction of type I hair cells in the crista. Later type II hair cells are destroyed, but

Table 15–2. RELATIVE VESTIBULAR AND AUDITORY OTOTOXICITIES OF COMMONLY USED AMINOGLYCOCIDES

	Vestibular	Auditory
Streptomycin	+ + +	+
Gentamicin	+ + +	+
Tobramycin	+ +	+ +
Kanamycin	+	+ + +
Amikacin	+	+ + +
Dibekacin	+	+
Netilmicin	+	+

Key:
+ = mild, + + = intermediate, + + + = severe

the supporting cells remain unaffected. With the cochleotoxic agents such as kanamycin and amikacin there is first a selective destruction of the outer hair cells in the basal turn of the cochlea, followed by total hair cell loss throughout the cochlea as the dose and duration of treatment are increased. Consistent with these pathologic changes, the sensorineural hearing loss caused by the aminoglycosides usually begins in the high frequencies and progresses to a flat 60 to 70 dB loss across all frequencies. Degeneration of neurons may occur years after the loss of inner and outer hair cells caused by the aminoglycosides. This secondary degeneration of cochlear neurons is so extensive that the use of cochlear implant devices for tonotopic stimulation of the distal ends of the cochlear neurons may be impossible.[63] Even after treatment is terminated some of the aminoglycosides (dihydrostreptomycin, gentamycin, and tobramycin, in particular) have been shown to produce continued damage to the sensory structures of the organ of corti.

Because streptomycin was the first antibiotic found to be effective against tuberculosis, there is a large body of clinical literature regarding its ototoxic effects. Many of the early clinical reports documented that parenteral streptomycin in a dose of 2 to 3 grams per day usually resulted in complete loss of vestibular function in 2 to 4 weeks.[9, 21] More prolonged treatment resulted in progressive auditory impairment. Although some patients did complain of vertigo (presumably due to asymmetric involvement of the vestibular system), most complained of an unsteady gait, particularly at night or in a darkened room. Head-movement-induced oscillopsia was also common. Serial caloric and rotational examinations documented a progressive bilateral loss of vestibular responsiveness. Because of this highly selective effect on the vestibular end-organ, streptomycin has been used to produce a chemical vestibulectomy in patients with episodic vertigo from Meniere's syndrome.[70]

"Loop" Diuretics

The two main ototoxic diuretics, furosemide and ethacrynic acid, act by inhibiting active resorption of chloride in the loop of Henle, thereby preventing the renal resorption of sodium that passively follows chloride.[63] The mechanism of their ototoxic effect is not completely known, although these drugs clearly influence ion pumps in the kidney and in the cochlear duct. The ototoxic effects of the loop diuretics appear to be confined to the cochlea, although detailed studies of vestibular function in such patients are lacking. About 6 percent of patients receiving furosemide develop a temporary hearing loss that is nearly always reversible. The newer loop-inhibiting diuretics, bumetanide and piretanide, appear to have a much lower rate of cochleotoxic effects in both animal and human studies.[64, 76]

Salicylates

Patients receiving high-dose salicylate therapy frequently complain of hearing loss, tinnitus, dizziness, loss of balance, and occasionally vertigo. Sensorineural hearing loss involves all frequencies and is associated with recruitment, suggesting a cochlear rather than a nervous system etiology.[51, 55] The tinnitus is high pitched and frequently precedes the onset of hearing loss. Both hearing loss and tinnitus invariably occur when the plasma salicylate level approaches 0.35 mg per ml. Caloric testing often reveals bilateral depressed responses consistent with bilateral vestibular endorgan damage.[6] All symptoms and signs are rapidly reversible after the cessation of salicylate ingestion (usually within 24 hours). As with the aminoglycosides, salicylates are highly concentrated in the perilymph, and preliminary evidence suggests that they interfere with enzymatic activity of the hair cells and/or the cochlear neurons.

Cis-platinum

Cis-platinum is commonly associated with both auditory and vestibular toxicity. By way of comparison, the incidence of aminoglycoside ototoxicity is about 10 percent, whereas the incidence of cis-platinum ototoxicity is in the range of 50 percent.[63] Tinnitus and hearing loss are

extremely common. Typically, the tinnitus is transient, lasting from a few hours to up to a week after cis-platinum therapy. The hearing loss is usually bilateral, beginning in the high frequencies and progressing to involve all frequencies; it may not appear until several days after the cis-platinum treatment. The hearing loss usually has some degree of reversibility, although when it is severe and involves all frequencies it is often permanent. Vestibular loss identified with caloric or rotational testing parallels the hearing loss. The critical cumulative ototoxic dose of cis-platinum has been reported to be in the range of 3 to 4 mg per kg of body weight.[34] The ototoxic effects can be decreased by using slow infusions and dividing the doses over several months.[66] As with the aminoglycosides, vestibular toxicity may be overlooked because the patient has multiple systemic symptoms due to the underlying malignancy. Morphologic studies in animals who have been given cis-platinum show hair cell damage similar to that seen with the aminoglycosides. Cis-platinum ototoxicity may result from inhibition of the activity of adenylate cyclase in the inner ear tissues.[2]

Diagnosis

The clinician must be constantly on the alert for the early symptoms of ototoxic drugs. This is particularly important in a patient who is seriously ill and confined to bed or in any patient who has renal impairment, particularly renal failure. Bedside audiometric assessment is available in most hospitals; bedridden patients can be tested with reproducible auditory stimuli. Although less satisfactory than conventional testing in a sound-proof room, earphones help exclude ambient noise. Because the hearing loss due to ototoxic drugs usually begins in the high-frequency range, a screen of the high frequencies will predict future low-frequency loss. Bedside vestibular testing is less satisfactory for the reasons outlined in Chapter 5, but spontaneous and positional nystagmus can sometimes be identified when fixation is inhibited with Frenzel glasses. In patients who can cooperate, the dynamic visual acuity test (see Tests of the Vestibulo-ocular Reflexes, Chapter 5) will identify early functional impairment of the vestibulo-ocular reflex. In our experience, bedside caloric tests are of little use for identifying early ototoxic effects. Ambulatory patients can be assessed with quantitative caloric and rotational testing as part of the ENG examination. Rotational testing is ideally suited for identifying early vestibular ototoxic effects, because the normal response variability is much less than that seen with caloric testing (see Chapter 7).

Management

The key to the management of the ototoxicity is prevention. Kidney function should be measured prior to beginning any potentially ototoxic drug. Patients in high-risk groups (Table 15–3) should be monitored with periodic auditory and vestibular testing. All patients should be questioned on a regular basis to identify early symptoms of auditory or vestibular loss. When the earliest effects of ototoxicity are identified, adjustments in the dosage schedule often can reduce the likelihood of symptom progression. Sometimes different drugs can be used that have less ototoxic potential.

As with other vestibular disorders, management of patients with permanent bilateral vestibular loss due to ototoxins should be directed at retraining the nervous system to use other sensory signals to replace the lost vestibular signals. Practical suggestions on how to avoid head-movement-induced oscillopsia (stopping and holding the head still when attempting to read a sign) and gait unsteadiness (always have a light on throughout the night) are useful along with an active exercise program to force central compensation (see Table 11–2). Younger patients often will return to nearly normal activity over a period of

years, but elderly patients are rarely able to compensate fully for the vestibular loss.

AUTOIMMUNE DISORDERS OF THE INNER EAR

Clinical Patterns

Autoimmune inner ear disease is an uncommon but important cause of progressive bilateral loss of auditory and vestibular functions.[37, 38] It can occur in children (although it is much more common in adults) and can be confined to the inner ears (although it is more often part of a systemic immune complex disorder involving the inner ear and other target organs). The inner ear dysfunction may begin on one side, but invariably it progresses to involve both sides, leading to profound deafness and vestibular loss if treatment is not instituted. Three characteristic clinical syndromes have been recognized: (1) inner ear involvement as part of a systemic autoimmune disorder—e.g., polyarteritis, rheumatoid arthritis, ulceritive cholitis, (2) inner ear involvement plus interstitial keratitis (Cogan's syndrome),[14] and (3) isolated inner ear involvement. Often patients will move from one category to another, with the most typical progression being from 3 to 2 to 1. Clinical symptoms often begin with fluctuating hearing loss, ear pressure, and tinnitus, along with vertigo, suggesting the diagnosis of endolymphatic hydrops. Unlike idiopathic Meniere's syndrome, however, these symptoms rapidly progress to involve the opposite ear over weeks to months. Occasionally, there is a slowly progressive bilateral sensorineural hearing loss accompanied by a progressive bilateral loss of vestibular function (i.e., loss of response to caloric and rotational stimulation).

Pathophysiology

The blood-labyrinth barrier is analogous to the blood-brain barrier with respect to immunoglobulin equilibrium, and the inner ear is capable of responding to an antigen challenge just as the brain is.[37] Probably both cellular and humoral mediated

Table 15–3. MAJOR RISK FACTORS FOR DRUG OTOTOXICITY

Impaired renal function	Course >14 days
High serum levels	Pre-existing sensorineural hearing loss
Prior use of ototoxic drugs	Age >65

immune pathways are involved in the production of autoimmune inner ear disease. Yoo and associates[87] were able to produce an animal model of autoimmune inner ear disease by immunizing rats with type 2 collagen. Hearing was assessed with brainstem auditory-evoked responses (BAER), and the temporal bones were studied with immunofluorescent techniques to detect antibody deposition. Immunized animals develop auditory and vestibular dysfunction not seen in controls. Immune complexes were found in the cochlear artery wall, perivascular fibrous tissue, and surrounding bone in the immunized rats. Although one must be careful in extrapolating these animal experiments to human inner ear pathology, there is abundant clinical evidence demonstrating that the human inner ear is capable of mounting an immune response.[37]

A few pathologic studies have been performed on the temporal bones from patients with Cogan's syndrome.[68] Surprisingly, they have not shown localized vasculitis even in patients with prominent vasculitis in other organs. The most consistent finding has been diffuse degeneration of all neural elements in the inner ear. Endolymphatic hydrops was found in one case.

Diagnosis

The diagnosis of autoimmune inner ear disease is based on finding the characteristic clinical course (described above), along with laboratory tests of altered immune function. It should be considered in any patient with progressive bilateral inner ear disease, particularly those with features of endolymphatic hydrops but rapidly progressing and not responding to conventional therapy. The history and examination should search for symptoms and signs of associated systemic autoimmune disorders and for evidence of interstitial keratitis (using a slitlamp). Blood tests for an elevated sedimentation rate, cryoglobulins, or serum complement are helpful but not diagnostic. Hughes and colleagues[37] suggested that lymphocyte transformation with pooled inner ear antigens is the most specific test for autoim-

mune inner ear disease. They reported, however, that the test could be false-negative (normal) even in patients with acute symptoms. Because whole fresh blood is required for this type of cellular autoimmune testing and because test centers are not yet widely available, the diagnosis is usually made on clinical grounds alone. A trial of therapy (see below) should be considered in any patient with a progressive audiovestibular dysfunction not responding to conventional therapy.

Management

Therapeutic guidelines for the treatment of autoimmune inner ear disease are controversial. Many different therapeutic regimens have been tried, and reported results vary. There is general agreement, however, that initial treatment should be with high-dose steroids (60 to 100 mg of prednisone or 12 to 16 mg of dexamethazone per day in divided doses for a minimum of 10 days) followed by gradual tapering to a maintenance dose (10 mg prednisone or 2 to 4 mg dexamethazone every other day for 3 to 6 months). Response to treatment seems to be more effective if the steroids are begun early in the course, although there have been reports of recovery of hearing in patients with near total deafness.[38, 52] Not infrequently, the disease process will become reactivated after a period of stability off steroids. A subsequent course of steroids may or may not be effective in such patients. Hughes and others[38] recommend a course of cytotoxic drugs if the patient fails to respond to steroids. McCabe[50] combines high-dose steroids and cyclophosphamide from the start. Reported responses to therapy are variable; there are many well-documented cases with dramatic improvement of hearing that remain stable for long periods, either on low-dose maintenance steroids or after therapy has been discontinued.

Recently, plasmapheresis has been used for the treatment of autoimmune inner ear disease when patients have not responded to steroids and cytotoxic drugs.[37] Dramatic responses in individual patients have been reported, but there are no large-scale studies of the effectiveness of this type of therapy. Presumably, plasmapheresis removes acute phase immune complexes but does not treat the underlying disease process. Therefore, it would not replace steroids or cytotoxic drugs but, rather, would be used in conjunction with these drugs.

REFERENCES

1. Aschan, G and Bergstedt, M: Positional alcoholic nystagmus (PAN) in man following repeated alcohol doses. Acta Otolaryngol (Suppl 330):15, 1975.
2. Bagger-Sjöbäck, D, Filipek, CS, and Schacht, J: Characteristics and drug responses of cochlear and vestibular adenylate cyclase. Arch Otolaryngol 228:217, 1980.
3. Baloh, RW, Yee, RD, and Honrubia, V: Late cortical cerebellar atrophy. Clinical and oculographic features. Brain 109:159, 1986.
4. Berciano, J: Olivopontocerebellar atrophy—a review of 117 cases. J Neurol Sci 53:253, 1982.
5. Bergstrom, L, et al: Hearing loss in renal disease: Clinical and pathological studies. Ann Otol Rhinol Laryngol 82:555, 1973.
6. Bernstein, JM and Weiss, AD: Further observations on salicylate ototoxicity. J Laryngol Otol 81:915, 1967.
7. Bogaert, L Van and Martin, L: Optic and cochleovestibular degenerations in the hereditary ataxias. I. Clinico-pathological and genetic aspects. Brain 97:15, 1974.
8. Bretlaw, P, et al: Otospongiosis and sodium fluoride. Ann Otol Rhinol Laryngol 94:103, 1985.
9. Brown, H and Hinshaw, H: Toxic reaction of streptomycin on the eighth nerve apparatus. Proc Staff Meeting, Mayo Clinic 21:347, 1946.
10. Cassandro, E, et al: Otoneurological findings in Friedreich's ataxia and other inherited neuropathies. Audiology 25:84, 1986.
11. Chen, J-R, Rhee, RSC, Wallach, S, Avramides, A, and Flores, A: Neurologic disturbances in Paget disease of bone: Response to calcitonin. Neurology 29:448, 1979.
12. Clemis, J, et al: The clinical diagnosis of Paget's disease of the temporal bone. Ann Otol Rhinol Laryngol 76:611, 1967.
13. Cody, DTR and Baker, HL: Otosclerosis: Vestibular symptoms and sensorineural hearing loss. Ann Otol Rhinol Laryngol 87:778, 1978.
14. Cogan, DG: Syndrome of nonsyphilitic interstitial keratitis and vestibuloauditory symptoms. Arch Ophthalmol 33:144, 1945.
15. Cogan, DG, Witt, ED, and Goldman-Rakic, PS: Ocular signs in thiamine-deficient monkeys and in Wernicke's disease in humans. Arch Ophthalmol 103:1212, 1985.
16. Davies, D: Paget's disease of the temporal bone: A clinical and histopathological survey. Acta Otolaryngol (Suppl 242):7, 1968.
17. Diener, HC, et al: Improvement of ataxia in alcoholic cerebellar atrophy through alcohol abstinence. J Neurol 231:258, 1984.
18. Djupesland, G, Flottorp, G, and Refsum, S: Phytanic acid storage disease: Hearing maintained after 15 years of dietary treatment. Neurology (NY) 33:237, 1983.
19. Ell, J, Prasher, D, and Rudge, P: Neuro-otological abnormalities in Friedreich's ataxia. J Neurol Neurosurg Psychiatr 47:26, 1984.
20. Farmer, TW and Mustian, VM: Vestibulocerebellar ataxia. Arch Neurol 8:21, 1963.
21. Farrington, R, et al: Streptomycin toxicity: Reactions to highly purified drug on long-continued administration to human subjects. JAMA 134:679, 1947.
22. Farris, BK, Smith, JL, and Ayyar, DR: Neuroophthalmologic findings in vestibulocerebellar ataxia. Arch Neurol 43:1050, 1986.
23. Fee, WE: Aminoglycoside ototoxicity in the human. Laryngoscope 24(Suppl):1, 1980.
24. Froment, JC, Trillet, M, and Aimard, G: Magnetic resonance imaging in familial paroxysmal ataxia. Arch Neurol 45:547, 1988.
25. Furman, JM, Perlman, S, and Baloh, RW: Eye movements in Friedreich's ataxia. Arch Neurol 40:343, 1983.
26. Ghez, C: Vestibular paresis: A clinical feature of Wernicke's disease. J Neurol Neurosurg Psychiatr 33:134, 1969.
27. Gilson, RD, et al: Effects of different alcohol dosages and display illumination on tracking performance during vestibular stimulation. Aerospace Med 43:656, 1972.
28. Goding, GS and Dobie, RA: Gaze nystagmus and blood alcohol. Laryngoscope 96:713, 1986.
29. Goor, C, Endtz, LJ, and Muller Kobold, MJP: Electronystagmography for the diagnosis of vestibular dysfunction in Wernicke-Korsakoff syndrome. Clin Neurol Neurosurg 78:112, 1975.
30. Graham, JR and Woodhouse, D: Massive thiamine dosage in an alcoholic with cerebellar cortical degeneration. Lancet 2:107, 1971.
31. Guedry, FE, et al: Some effects of alcohol on various aspects of oculomotor control. Aviat Space Environ Med 46:1008, 1975.
32. Hamersma, H: Osteopetrosis (marble bone disease) of the temporal bone. Laryngoscope 80:1518, 1970.
33. Haubek, A and Lee, K: Computed tomography in alcoholic cerebellar atrophy. Neuroradiology 18:77, 1979.
34. Hayes, DM, et al: High dose cis-dichlorodiamineplatinum: Amelioration by mannitol diuresis. Cancer 39:1372, 1977.
35. Herndon, JH, Steinberg, D, and Vhlendorf, BW: Refsum's disease: Defective oxidation of phytanic acid in tissue cultures derived from homozygotes and heterozygotes. N Engl J Med 281:1034, 1969.
36. Houck, JR and Harker, LA: Otosclerosis. Diagnosis and nonsurgical management. In Cummings, CW, Fredrickson, JM, Harker, LA, Krause, CJ, and Schuller, DE (eds): Otolaryngology—Head and Neck Surgery. CV Mosby, St Louis, 1986, p 3095.
37. Hughes, GB, Barna, BP, and Calabrese, LH: Immune mechanisms in auditory and vestibular disease. In Cummings, CW, Fredrickson,

JM, Harker, LA, Krause, CJ, and Schuller, DE (eds): Otolaryngology—Head and Neck Surgery. CV Mosby, St Louis, 1986, p 3149.

38. Hughes, GB, Kinney, SE, Barna, BP, and Calabrese, LH: Practical versus theoretical management of autoimmune inner ear disease. Laryngoscope 94:758, 1984.

39. Jorgensen, M and Buch, N: Studies on inner-ear function and cranial nerves in diabetics. Acta Otolaryngol 53:350, 1961.

40. Jorgensen, M: The inner ear in diabetes mellitus. Arch Otolaryngol 74:373, 1961.

41. Kashii, S, et al: Effects of ethanol applied by electrosmosis on neurons in the lateral and medial vestibular nuclei. Jpn J Pharmacol 36:153, 1984.

42. Larsson, A: Otosclerosis: A genetic and clinical study. Acta Otolaryngol (Suppl 154):6, 1960.

43. Lehtinen, I, et al: Acute effects of alcohol on saccadic eye movements. Psychopharmacology 63:17, 1979.

44. Lehtinen, I, et al: Quantitative effects of ethanol infusion on smooth pursuit eye movements in man. Psychopharmacology 77:74, 1982.

45. Lerner, SA and Matz, GJ: Aminoglycoside ototoxicity. Am J Otolaryngol 1:169, 1980.

46. Lim, DJ: Pathogenesis and pathology of otosclerosis: A review. In Nomura, Y (ed): Hearing Loss and Dizziness. Igaku-Shoin, Tokyo, 1985, p 43.

47. Liston, SL, Paparella, MM, Mancini, F, and Anderson, JH: Otosclerosis and endolymphatic hydrops. Laryngoscope 94:1003, 1984.

48. Makishima, K and Tanaka, K: Pathological changes of the inner ear and central auditory pathways in diabetics. Ann Otol Rhinol Laryngol 80:218, 1971.

49. Mancall, EL and zMcentee, WJ: Alterations of the cerebellar cortex in nutritional encephalopathy. Neurology 15:303, 1965.

50. McCabe, BF: Autoimmune sensorineural hearing loss. Ann Otol Rhinol Laryngol 88:585, 1979.

51. McCabe, BF and Dey, F: The effect of aspirin upon auditory sensitivity. Ann Otol Rhinol Laryngol 74:312, 1965.

52. McDonald, TJ, Vollersten, RS, and Younger, BR: Cogan's syndrome: Audiovestibular involvement and prognosis in 18 patients. Laryngoscope 95:650, 1985.

53. Meyerhoff, WL: The thyroid and audition. Laryngoscope 86:483, 1976.

54. Money, KE and Myles, WS: Heavy water nystagmus and effects of alcohol. Nature 247:404, 1974.

55. Myers, E, Bernstein, J, and Fostiropolous, G: Salicylate ototoxicity: A clinical study. N Engl J Med 273:587, 1965.

56. Myers, SF, et al: Morphological evidence of vestibular pathology in long-term experimental diabetes mellitus. I. Microvascular changes. Acta Otolaryngol (Stockh) 100:351, 1985.

57. Oda, M, et al: Labyrinthine pathology of chronic renal failure patients treated with hemodialysis and kidney transplantation. Laryngoscope 84:1489, 1974.

58. Proops, D, Bayley, D, and Hawke, M: Paget's disease and the temporal bone—a clinical and histopathological review of six temporal bones. J Otolaryngol 14:20, 1985.

59. Refsum, S: Heredopathia atactica polyneuritiformis. Acta Genet 7:344, 1957.

60. Ron, MA, et al: Computerized tomography of the brain in chronic alcoholism: A survey and follow-up study. Brain 105:497, 1982.

61. Rosenberg, RN and Pettegrew, JW: Genetic neurologic disease. In Rosenberg, RN (ed): The Clinical Neurosciences, Vol 1. Harper & Row, Philadelphia, 1983.

62. Rubenstein, N, Rubenstein, C, and Theodor, R: Hearing dysfunction associated with congenital sporadic hypothyroidism. Ann Otol Rhinol Laryngol 83:814, 1974.

63. Rybak, LP and Matz, GJ: Auditory and vestibular effects of toxins. In Cummings, CW, Fredrickson, JM, Harker, LA, Krause, CJ, and Schuller, DE (eds): Otolaryngology—Head and Neck Surgery. CV Mosby, St Louis, 1986, p 3161.

64. Rybak, LP and Whitworth, C: Comparative ototoxicity of furosemide and piretanide. Acta Otolaryngol 101:59, 1986.

65. Sando, I, et al: Vestibular pathology in otosclerosis temporal bone histopathological report. Laryngoscope 84:593, 1974.

66. Schaefer, SD, Post, JD, Close, LG, and Wright, CG: Ototoxicity of low- and moderate-dose cisplatinum. Cancer 56:1934, 1985.

67. Schmidley, JW, Levinsohn, MW, and Manetto, V: Infantile X-linked ataxia and deafness: A new clinicopathologic entity? Neurology 37:1344, 1987.

68. Schuknecht, HF: Pathology of the Ear. Harvard University Press, Cambridge, MA, 1974.

69. Sharp, M: Monostotic fibrous dysplasia of the temporal bone. J Laryngol 84:697, 1970.

70. Singleton, E and Schuknecht, H: Streptomycin sulfate in the management of Meniere's disease. Otolaryngol Clin North Am October: 531, 1968.

71. Smith, CR, et al: Double blind comparison of the nephrotoxicity and auditory toxicity of gentamicin and tobramycin. N Engl J Med 302:1106, 1980.

72. Smyth, GDL: Recent and future trends in the management of otosclerotic conductive hearing loss. Clin Otolaryngol 7:153, 1982.

73. Snow, JB, Jr: Current status of fluoride therapy for otosclerosis. Am J Otol 6:56, 1985.

74. Spoendlin, H: Optic and cochleovestibular degenerations in the hereditary ataxias. II. Temporal bone pathology in two cases of Friedreich's ataxia with vestibulo-cochlear disorders. Brain 97:41, 1974.

75. Tellez, I and Terry, RD: Fine structure of the early changes in the vestibular nuclei of the thiamine-deficient rat. Am J Pathol 52:777, 1968.

76. Tnzel, IJ: Comparison of adverse reactions of bumetanide and furosemide. J Clin Pharmacol 21:615, 1981.

77. Troni, W, et al: Peripheral nerve function and metabolic control in diabetes mellitus. Ann Neurol 16:178, 1984.

78. Tsipouras, P, Barabas, G, and Matthews, WS:

Neurologic correlates of osteogenesis imperfecta. Arch Neurol 43:150, 1986.

79. Valvassori, GE: New imaging tests for otology. Am J Otol 5:434, 1984.

80. Verhagen, WIM, Huygen, PLM, and Joosten, EMG: Familial progressive vestibulocochlear dysfunction. Arch Neurol 45:766, 1988.

81. Victor, M, Adams, RD, and Collins, CH: The Wernicke-Korsakoff Syndrome. FA Davis, Philadelphia, 1971.

82. Victor, M, Adams, RD, and Mancall, EL: A restricted form of cerebellar cortical degeneration occurring in alcoholic patients. Arch Neurol 1:579, 1959.

83. Virolainen, E: Vestibular disturbances in clinical otosclerosis. Acta Otolaryngol (Suppl 306):7, 1972.

84. Wilkinson, IMS, Kime, R, and Purnell, M: Alcohol and human eye movement. Brain 97:785, 1974.

85. Withers, BT, Reuter, S, and Janeke, J: The effects of hypothyroidism on the ears of cats and squirrel monkeys: A pilot study. Laryngoscope 82:779, 1972.

86. Yassin, A, Badry, A, and Fatt-Hi, A: The relationship between electrolyte balance and cochlear disturbances in cases of renal failure. J Laryngol 84:429, 1970.

87. Yoo, TJ, et al: Type II collagen-induced autoimmune sensorineural hearing loss and vestibular dysfunction in rats. Ann Otol 92:267, 1983.

88. Zasorin, NL, Baloh, RW, and Myers, LB: Acetazolamide-responsive episodic ataxia syndrome. Neurology 33:1212, 1983.

89. Zee, DS, et al: Ocular motor abnormalities in hereditary cerebellar ataxia. Brain 99:207, 1976.

Chapter 16

DEVELOPMENTAL DISORDERS

MALFORMATIONS OF THE INNER EAR

Although congenital deafness is usually recognized during infancy, congenital vestibular impairment is not, because the manifestations are more subtle. Children learn to use other sensory information to compensate for vestibular loss and appear normal on standard developmental tests. Congenital deafness has therefore received extensive study, whereas congenital vestibular loss has been relatively neglected.

Congenital deformities of the inner ear are divided into two major categories: hereditary and acquired. Hereditary disorders result from abnormal genes, and acquired disorders from abnormal development of a normal fertilized egg.

Hereditary Disorders

It has been estimated that more than one half of all congenital deafness is inherited, with more than three quarters being inherited in an autosomal recessive fashion.[24] Despite the large number of recognizable syndromes that have been described (more than 60 with congenital hearing loss as a feature), the majority of cases of genetically determined hearing loss are not associated with malformations of other organs or body systems. Families with congenital vestibular loss have been described less frequently probably because the vestibular loss is relatively silent.[30]

Although it is beyond the scope of this monograph to review all of the hereditary syndromes that may produce sensorineu-ral deafness and vestibular loss, a few common disorders deserve mention. Alport's syndrome is manifested by a sex-linked dominantly inherited sensorineural deafness and interstitial nephritis. Miller and coworkers[16] found decreased vestibular responses in several patients with Alport's syndrome and suggested an associated vestibular system disorder. The inner ear histology is normal; abnormalities of lipid and amino acid metabolism have been reported, but the exact enzyme defect or defects are yet to be identified.[23] Waardenburg's syndrome is a dominantly inherited sensorineural deafness associated with (1) lateral displacement of the medial canthae and lacrimal punctii, (2) hyperplastic high nasal root, (3) hyperplasia of the medial portions of the eyebrows, (4) partial or total heterochromia iridis, and (5) circumscribed albinism of the frontal head hair (white forelock).[31] Vestibular function is usually impaired bilaterally, and computerized tomography (CT) studies of the temporal bone reveal bony abnormalities of the inner ear. Ophthalmologic evaluation can be helpful in defining the characteristic eye signs. Of note, Marcus[12] studied a large family with Waardenburg's syndrome and found several children who had vestibular malfunction despite normal hearing, with minimal or no other signs of the syndrome. A combination of recessively inherited retinitis pigmentosa and sensorineural deafness is known as Usher's syndrome.[29] Hearing loss is present at birth, but the retinitis pigmentosa is not recognized until about the age of 10, when the patient develops night blindness and/or contraction of the visual fields.[9] Caloric responses are usually diminished bilaterally.

Extra or transposed chromosomes result in multiple congenital defects. Trisomy 13 and trisomy 18 are associated with malformations of the inner ear and decreased auditory and vestibular function. The more common trisomy 21 (Down's syndrome) does not produce ear deformities.

Acquired Disorders

The most common cause of acquired congenital malformations of the inner ear is maternal rubella infection during the critical developmental period (the first 9 weeks of gestation for vestibular development and the first 25 weeks for auditory development). Infants born to mothers who acquire rubella in the first trimester of pregnancy may have multiple congenital defects, including cataracts, patent ductus arteriosus, microcephaly, dental defects, and generally impaired growth and development.[4] Hearing loss is more common than vestibular loss (apparently because of the longer critical developmental period). Although less common, the infant's fully developed inner ear can be damaged by a maternal rubella infection in the last two trimesters.[17] Other important causes of acquired congenital inner ear defects include maternal drug or toxin ingestion, hyperbilirubinemia, anoxia associated with difficult birth, and cretinism.[23]

Pathophysiology

The first pathologic study of an inner ear congenital malformation was reported by Mundini in 1791. The Mundini malformation consists of subtotal development of the osseous and membranous labyrinth with only the basal turn of the cochlea being completely formed.[5] The endolymphatic duct system is dilated and the vestibular labyrinth is underdeveloped. This deformity occurs with many different syndromes—both hereditary and acquired—and is invariably associated with some (and often complete) loss of auditory and vestibular function. Cochleosaccular dysgenesis initially described by Scheibe consists of dysplasia of the pars inferior (coch-

lea and sacculus) with a fully developed bony labyrinth and normal pars superior (semicircular canals and utriculus).[23] The Scheibe deformity is frequently produced by congenital rubella, accounting for the relative sparing of vestibular function in many of these children. A rare deformity characterized by complete failure of development of the inner ear (Michel deformity) is associated with total loss of auditory and vestibular function. This deformity has been found in several patients with Thalidomide anomalies of the ear.[27]

Diagnosis and Management

As noted above, although inherited loss of auditory and/or vestibular function may be part of a well-described multiorgan syndrome, the majority of cases occur in isolation with an autosomal recessive inheritance. Even with the well-defined syndromes, variability in gene penetrance can complicate the clinical picture. For example, with Waardenburg's syndrome penetrance for deafness is only 20 percent. Thus, although this dominant disorder is passed to 50 percent of progeny, only 20 percent of this 50 percent will be deaf.[24]

Identification of hearing loss or vestibular loss in an infant requires objective measurements, inasmuch as behavioral testing is usually impractical. Brainstem auditory evoked responses (BAER) reflect the electrical activity of the auditory pathways in the brainstem and therefore provide an objective measure of whether the end-organ and peripheral nerve generate signals to transmit through the brainstem pathways.[21] One must keep in mind, however, that the presence of BAER does not mean that the infant is able to discriminate sounds. Rotational testing can be performed on infants by rotating the child on the mother's lap while eye movements are recorded with electronystagmography (ENG). Caloric testing is more difficult to quantify but can be used to identify the presence of unilateral vestibular dysfunction.

Most malformations of the inner ear do not affect the otic capsule, and therefore the inner ear appears normal even with high-resolution CT scans of the temporal bone. The main exception is the Mundini malformation; it is readily identified with high-resolution CT scans. Also, the abnormally developed membranous labyrinth can usually be seen on T_2-enhanced magnetic resonance (MR) scans.

Congenital hearing loss is obviously important to identify as early as possible because of the ramifications regarding early language development and learning abilities. Infants with siblings or parents with known hereditary deafness should be screened for hearing loss immediately after birth. Genetic counseling is an important part of the management of these families. Detailed probability charts have been developed to estimate the occurrence of hearing impairment in future offspring.[24]

DISORDERS OF THE CRANIAL VERTEBRAL JUNCTION

Patients with disorders of the cranial vertebral junction present with a range of brainstem and lower cranial nerve symptoms, including tinnitus, vertigo, hearing loss, pharyngeal dysfunction, hoarseness, or even airway obstruction.[6] The basic pathophysiologic mechanism for these symptoms is compression of the nervous system at the upper spinal cord and medulla. The rostrocaudal extent of the compression is variable, and the impingement can be ventral, dorsal, or (rarely) both. A second, less common, cause of symptoms is vascular insufficiency due to angulation, stretching, or extrinsic compression of the anterior spinal or vertebral arteries.

Basilar Impression

Basilar impression is an upward indentation or invagination of the ridged cervical spine into the normally convex skull base.[8] The odontoid projects intracranially to compress the ventral aspect of the medulla; the cerebellum is compressed posteriorly by the first and second cervical vertebrae. Disorders known to cause basilar impression include Paget's disease, rheumatoid arthritis, osteomalacia, osteogenesis imperfecta, cretinism, and rickets.[15] The term platybasia has been used syn-

onymously with basilar impression by some authors. Technically, it is not a measure of basilar impression and although the two often coexist, platybasia by itself causes no symptoms.

Bony Fusions

Assimilation of the atlas (also called occipitalization of the atlas) is a bony union between the first cervical vertebra and the skull. The amount of union varies, but motion between the two structures does not occur. As a result, the odontoid impinges on the effective anterior posterior diameter of the foramen. Frequently, there is associated fusion of the axis to the third cervical vertebra. Many different varieties of cervicovertebral fusion have been reported. Klippel and Feil initially described a patient with only four cervical vertebrae that were fused into a single column of bone. These anatomic features were associated with a clinical triad of short neck, low hairline, and limitation of neck movements. Although partial coalescence of two or more cervical vertebrae occurs in many patients, few develop the syndrome originally described by Klippel and Feil. Spillane and coworkers[25] suggested that fusion of cervical vertebrae should be called congenital cervical synostosis and that the term Klippel-Feil should be used to describe only typical clinical syndromes associated with either complete fusion of the cervical spine or reduction in the number of cervical vertebrae. Patients with classic Klippel-Feil syndrome have a high incidence of deafness. McLay and Maran[13] studied the temporal bone of one such patient and found a vestigial inner ear having a rudimentary cystic cavity for a cochlea and only one semicircular canal incompletely formed. The inner ear abnormalities with Klippel-Feil syndrome may be unilateral or bilateral and may be appreciated on high-resolution CT scans of the temporal bone.

Atlantoaxial Dislocation

During flexion and extension of the neck, congenital fusion of the occiput to the atlas increases the strain on the structures that normally restrict the motion of the atlas on the axis, especially if there is fusion of other cervical vertebrae as well. The transverse ligament that normally secures the odontoid against the anterior aspect of the arch of the atlas may weaken because of this repeated strain, and the resultant laxity allows the odontoid to move posterior into the lumen of the foramen magnum. Flexion or extension of the neck may then produce symptoms, depending on whether the predominant neural compression is anterior from the odontoid or posterior from the posterior arch of C1. When the atlas or congenital cervical fusion has been assimilated, the transverse odontoid ligament is sometimes hypoplastic, which makes laxity and atlantoaxial dislocation even more likely. Atlantoaxial instability is also known to be associated with a number of congenital and acquired disease processes. It occurs in 18 to 30 percent of individuals with Down's syndrome[19] and is frequently seen with spondyloepiphyseal dysplasia, Hurler's syndrome, Morquio's syndrome, and in achondroplastic dwarfs. Of patients with rheumatoid arthritis, 25 percent have atlantoaxial instability secondary to destruction of normal stabilizing mechanisms by inflammatory rheumatoid tissue in the synovial membrane.[7, 18] Similarly, ligamentous laxity can result from inflammatory conditions affecting retropharyngeal soft tissue or cervical bony structures such as tuberculosis (or other bacterial) osteitis, retropharyngeal abscess, or lymphadenitis.

Chiari Malformation

In 1895, Chiari described a congenital malformation of the hindbrain in which the brainstem and cerebellum were elongated downward into the cervical canal. Most frequently, the deformity manifests itself in the first few months of life and is associated with hydrocephalus and other nervous system malformations (Chiari type II malformation). Less frequent but more important to the neurotologist are those cases in which the onset of symptoms and signs is delayed until adult life (Chiari type I malformation). These cases

often present with subtle neurologic symptoms and signs and are usually unassociated with other developmental defects.[3] The most common neurologic symptom is slowly progressive unsteadiness of gait, which the patient frequently describes as dizziness. Vertigo and hearing loss occur in about 10 percent of patients.[22] On neurologic examination the patient is ataxic, suggesting midline cerebellar involvement. Pathologic nystagmus is nearly always present. Spontaneous downbeat nystagmus is particularly common,[2] but other forms of central spontaneous nystagmus and rebound nystagmus also occur. Oscillopsia is nearly always associated with the spontaneous nystagmus. Dysphagia, hoarseness, and dysarthria result from stretching of the lower cranial nerves, and obstructive hydrocephalus results from occlusion of the basilar cisterns.[20]

Syringobulbia

Syrinx formation in the medulla (syringobulbia) damages any of the lower cranial nerve nuclei but most often involves the twelfth nuclei and the descending tract and nucleus of the fifth nerve, producing atrophy and fasciculations of the tongue and loss of pain and temperature sensation on one or both sides of the face. Dysphonia and dysphagia are also prevalent because of the damage to the ninth and tenth nuclei. As with Chiari malformation, pathologic nystagmus is a common finding in nearly all reported series, and occasionally it is the only abnormal neurologic sign.[28] A pure torsional nystagmus either in the primary position or on lateral gaze is particularly characteristic of syringobulbia. Any adult presenting with oscillopsia and central spontaneous nystagmus should be suspected of having either syringobulbia or a Chiari type I malformation.

Diagnosis

Patients with congenital abnormalities of the craniovertebral junction often exhibit associated morphologic abnormalities of the neck, such as low hairline, short neck, abnormal head position, limitation

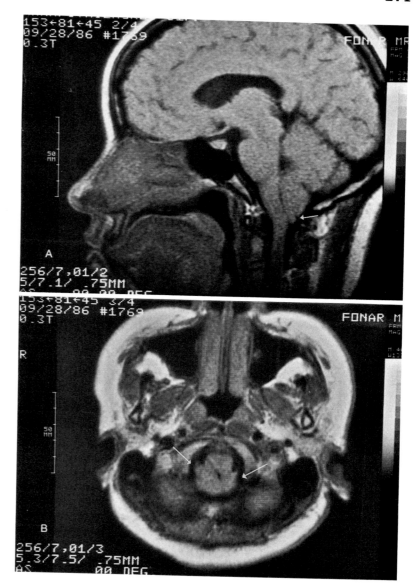

Figure 16-1. MR scans (T$_1$ weighted) showing a Chiari type I malformation. (A) midline sagittal section. (B) Transverse section at C$_1$ level. *Arrows* point to cerebellar tonsils.

of motion, and painful torticollis. Accentuation of symptoms by coughing, straining, or change in neck position is common. Clinical manifestations of cervicomedullary compression are usually relentless and severe, progressing over months to years. Occipital pain with radiation toward the vertex is a common presenting symptom. Other symptoms can be related to brainstem and cranial nerve dysfunction from compression.

The diagnosis of basilar impression is confirmed when lateral radiographs of the skull demonstrate that the tip of the odontoid either extends above Chamberlain's line (a line drawn from the posterior edge of the hard palate to the posterior lip of the foramen magnum) or projects posterior to Wackenheim's clivus-canal line. With assimilation of the atlas or atlantoaxial dislocation, the critical assessment is whether the abnormality is reducible and the direction of encroachment on the cervical medullary junction. High-resolution CT scanning is performed in the frontal and lateral projections, the lateral with the patient's head in both neutral and extended positions (with the attending neurosurgeon supervising the procedure).[10] MR scanning is now the procedure of choice for assessing the degree of soft tissue compression and for identifying Chiari malformations and syrinx formation.[1] Midline saggital sections are ideal for identifying the level of the cerebellar tonsils (Fig. 16–1) and syrinx formation in the medulla and high cervical cord.

Management

A series of operations have been developed to correct bony deformities at the craniovertebral junction, to eliminate the cervical medullary compression, and to prevent its recurrence. They are designed to reduce the odontoid from its cranial position; to remove any bony ligamentous or inflammatory soft tissue compression of the cervicomedullary junction; and to fix the skull to the cervicovertebral column in the reduced position when necessary. In patients with Chiari type I malformations, suboccipital decompression of the foramen magnum region can stop the progression and occasionally lead to improvement in neurologic symptoms and signs.[11, 26] Special emphasis should be given to patients with rheumatoid arthritis because up to 25 percent of them have significant cranial vertebral abnormalities. In a series of 45 patients surgically treated for cervical medulllary compression secondary to rheumatoid arthritis and cranial settling, there were no operative deaths and no infections.[14] All the patients improved to a functional class two grades above the preoperative level, and some improvement in cranial nerve function occurred in patients who had preoperative deficits.

REFERENCES

1. Aubin, ML, Vignand, J, Iba-Zizen, MT, and Stoffels, C: NMR imaging of the cranio-cervical junction and cervical spine. Normal and pathologic features. J Neuroradiol 11:229, 1984.
2. Baloh, RW and Spooner, JW: Down beat nystagmus: A type of central vestibular nystagmus. Neurology 31:304, 1981.
3. Banerji, NK and Millar, JHD: Chiari malformation presenting in adult life. Brain 97:157, 1974.
4. Barr, B and Lundström, R: Deafness following maternal rubella. Acta Otolaryngol 53:413, 1961.
5. Beal, D, Davey, P, and Lindsay, J: Inner ear pathology of congenital deafness. Arch Otolaryngol 85:134, 1967.
6. Bertrand, G: Anomalies of the craniovertebral junction. In Youmans, JR (ed): Neurological Surgery, Vol 3, ed 2. WB Saunders, Philadelphia, 1982.
7. Bland, JH: Rheumatoid arthritis of the cervical spine. J Rheumatol 1:319, 1974.
8. Elies, W and Plester, D: Basilar impression. Arch Otolaryngol 106:232, 1980.
9. Kumar, A, Fishman, G, and Torok, N: Vestibular and auditory function in Usher's syndrome. Ann Otol Rhinol Laryngol 93:600, 1984.
10. Kumar, A, Jafar, J, Mafu, M, and Glick, R: Diagnosis and management of anomalies of the craniovertebral junction. Ann Otol Rhinol Laryngol 95:487, 1986.
11. Levy, WJ, Mason, L, and Hahn, JF: Chiari malformation presenting in adults: A surgical experience in 127 cases. Neurosurgery 12:377, 1983.
12. Marcus, R: Vestibular function and additional findings in Waardenburg's syndrome. Acta Otolaryngol (Suppl 229):7, 1968.
13. McLay, K and Maran, A: Deafness and Klippel-Feil syndrome. J Laryngol 83:175, 1969.
14. Menezes, AH, et al: Odontoid upward migration in rheumatoid arthritis or "cranial settling": An analysis of 45 patients. J Neurosurg 63:500, 1985.
15. Menezes, AH, et al: Craniocervical abnormalities: A comprehensive surgical approach. J Neurosurg 53:444, 1980.
16. Miller, GW, et al: Alport's syndrome. Arch Otolaryngol 92:419, 1970.
17. Monif, G, Hardy, J, and Sever, J: Studies in congenital rubella, Baltimore 1964–1965. I. Epidemiologic and virologic. Bull Johns Hopkins Hosp 118:85, 1966.
18. Nakano, KK, Schoene, WC, Baker, RA, and Dawson, DM: The cervical myelopathy associated with rheumatoid arthritis: Analysis of 32 patients, with 2 post mortem cases. Ann Neurol 3:144, 1978.
19. Nordt, JC and Stauffer, ES: Sequelae of atlantoaxial stabilization in two patients with Down's syndrome. Spine 6(5):437, 1981.
20. Paul, KS, Lye, RH, Strang, FA, and Dutton, J: Arnold-Chiari malformation: Review of 71 cases. J Neurosurg 58:183, 1983.
21. Riko, K, Hyde, ML, and Alberti, PW: Hearing loss in early infancy: Incidence, detection, and assessment. Laryngoscope 95:137, 1985.
22. Saez, RJ, Onofrio, BM, and Yanagihara, T: Experience with Arnold-Chiari malformation: 1960 to 1970. J Neurosurg 45:416, 1976.
23. Schuknecht, HF: Pathology of the Ear. Harvard University Press, Cambridge, MA, 1974.
24. Smith, RJ: Medical diagnosis and treatment of hearing loss in children. In Cummings, CW,

Fredrickson, JM, Harker, LA, Krause, CJ, and Schuller, DE (eds): Otolaryngology—Head and Neck Surgery. CV Mosby, St Louis, 1986, p 3225.

25. Spillane, JD, Pallis, C, and Jones, AM: Developmental abnormalities in the region of the foramen magnum. Brain 80:11, 1957.

26. Spooner, JW and Baloh, RW: Arnold-Chiari malformation: Improvement in eye movements after surgical treatment. Brain 104:51, 1981.

27. Takemori, S, Tanaka, Y, and Suzuki, J: Thalidomide anomalies of the ear. Arch Otolaryngol 10:425, 1976.

28. Thrush, DC and Foster, JB: An analysis of nystagmus in 100 consecutive patients with communicating syringomyelia. J Neurol Sci 20:381, 1973.

29. Usher, C: On the inheritance of retinitis pigmentosa, with notes of case. Roy London Ophth Hosp Rep 19:130, 1914.

30. Verhagen, WIM, Huygen, PLM, and Horstink, N: Familial congenital vestibular areflexia. J Neurol Neurosurg Psychiatr 50:933, 1987.

31. Waardenburg, P: A new syndrome combining developmental anomalies of the eyelids, eyebrows, and nose root with pigmentary defects of the iris and head hair and with congenital deafness. Am J Hum Genet 3:195, 1951.

Chapter 17

OTHER NEUROLOGIC DISORDERS

MULTIPLE SCLEROSIS

Multiple sclerosis is a demyelinating disease of the central nervous system (CNS) of unknown cause with onset usually in the third and fourth decades of life.[22] The key to the diagnosis is the finding of disseminated signs of CNS dysfunction manifested in an alternating remitting and exacerbating course. Although many symptoms occur with multiple sclerosis, certain ones deserve emphasis because of their consistent appearance. Blurring or loss of vision caused by demyelination of the optic nerve (retrobulbar neuritis) is an initial symptom of multiple sclerosis in approximately 20 percent of patients. Diplopia, weakness, numbness, and ataxia also occur early in the disease process. Vertigo is the initial symptom in about 5 percent of patients and is reported sometime during the disease in as many as 50 percent.[15] Hearing loss occurs in about 10 percent of patients.[24] No apparent relationship exists between the severity or duration of multiple sclerosis and the hearing loss; auditory impairment may be part of the initial episode or may occur more than 10 years after the onset.[12] The hearing loss can be acute (hours to a few days), subacute (over months), or insidious in onset. Partial or complete remission after the onset of hearing loss is common. A typical bout of vertigo associated with multiple sclerosis lasts from hours to days, although positional vertigo lasting seconds is also a common feature.

Pathophysiology

The demyelination in multiple sclerosis is confined to CNS myelin; the myelin produced by oligodendrogliocytes.[22] Peripheral nerve myelin produced by Schwann cells is minimally affected. Because both peripheral and cranial nerves contain CNS myelin at their root entry zones, a demyelinated plaque involving the root entry zone may produce signs of peripheral nerve dysfunction. Plaques involving the vestibular and auditory nerve root entry zones can explain the frequent findings of unilateral caloric hypoexcitability and hearing loss in patients with multiple sclerosis. In a typical demyelinated plaque the majority of myelin sheaths are destroyed, and those that remain become swollen and fragmented. The axis cylinders and neurons are relatively spared so that conduction of nerve impulses still occurs but at a decreased frequency and rate. Whether the remissions and exacerbations of symptoms and signs are related to repair of demyelinated regions or changes in the physiology of nerve conduction unrelated to demyelination is currently debated. It has been repeatedly shown, however, that there is a poor correlation between the clinical symptoms experienced during life and the pathologic findings at necropsy.

Diagnosis

The findings on examination in a patient with multiple sclerosis are as diverse as the symptoms. In most long-standing cases there are signs of involvement of the pyramidal tracts (hyperreflexia, extensor plantar responses), cerebellum (intention tremor, ataxia, slurred speech), sensory tracts (impaired vibratory and position sense), and visual pathways (decreased visual acuity and pallor of the optic disk). The finding of dissociated nystagmus on

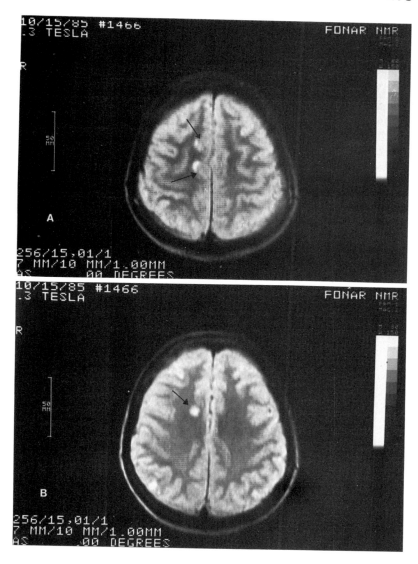

Figure 17–1. MR scans (T_2 weighted) demonstrating deep white matter lesions (*arrows*) in a patient with multiple sclerosis.

lateral gaze or acquired spontaneous pendular nystagmus is particularly helpful in the diagnosis of multiple sclerosis because these are common with multiple sclerosis and relatively unusual with other disease processes.[3, 7] All varieties of positional nystagmus can be seen with multiple sclerosis, and caloric examination is abnormal in about 25 percent of patients.[11] Puretone hearing levels, when abnormal, have no characteristic pattern with multiple sclerosis. Special audiometric studies (speech discrimination, tone decay, acoustic reflex) indicate a neural site for the lesion. Brainstem auditory-evoked re-

sponses (BAER) can detect subclinical lesions of multiple sclerosis even when hearing is normal (see Auditory-Evoked Responses, Chapter 8).[12, 30] Electronystagmography (ENG) with computerized eye tracking tests also can be helpful for identifying subclinical signs in patients with multiple sclerosis.[19, 29]

No specific laboratory test for multiple sclerosis exists, but abnormalities in the cerebrospinal fluid (CSF) can be identified in about 80 to 90 percent of patients at some time in the disease course. Findings include elevated gamma globulin, increased gamma globulin synthesis, ologoclonal banding of gamma globulin, and elevated myelin basic protein.[32] Unfortunately, none of these findings are specific for multiple sclerosis. Magnetic resonance (MR) scanning of the brain will identify white matter lesions (on T_2 weighted images) in about 95 percent of patients with multiple sclerosis (Fig. 17-1), although similar lesions are sometimes seen in patients without the clinical criteria for the diagnosis of multiple sclerosis.[18]

Management

No definitive treatment of multiple sclerosis exists. Steroids and adrenocorticotropic hormone may hasten the remission of symptoms and signs after an acute exacerbation, but no evidence indicates that these drugs alter the natural history of multiple sclerosis.[9] The potential benefit of other immunosuppressent drugs, such as cyclophosphamide and azathioprine, are still being investigated, particularly regarding the risk-benefit ratio.

VERTIGO AND FOCAL SEIZURE DISORDERS

Because there are well-documented projections from the vestibular nuclei to the cerebral cortex, it could be predicted that focal epileptic discharge from some areas of the cortex would result in a sensation of altered orientation and vertigo (see Anatomy and Physiology of Vestibular Sensation, Chapter 3). In Penfield and Kristiansen's[25] series of 222 patients with focal seizures in which the irritable focus was identified at the time of surgery, nine reported an ictal sensory experience of vertigo. In eight of these patients the causal lesion was found in the posterior half of the superior temporal gyrus or at the parietotemporal junction. Electrical stimulation of these areas produced vertiginous experiences similar to those experienced during a spontaneous seizure. Other investigators reported vertiginous auras with lesions in other parts of the temporal and parietal lobes, suggesting that cortical vestibular projections were more diffuse

than suggested by Penfield and Kristiansen's studies.

Smith[28] studied 120 patients with focal seizures who experienced vestibular symptoms as part of their aura. He attempted to define the cortical focus of origin on the basis of associated symptoms. The most common vestibular symptom was a sense of spinning (occurring in 55 percent of cases), followed by a sense of linear movement occurring in 30 percent of cases. Common associated symptoms and their frequency of occurrence were visceral and autonomic in 62 percent, visual in 45 percent, auditory in 28 percent, and somatosensory in 22 percent. Of the visceral and autonomic complaints, an abnormal epigastric sensation was most frequent, followed by nausea, mastication, and salivation. Visual illusions and hallucinations occurred frequently, suggesting a close functional relationship between cortical visual and vestibular projections. Auditory symptoms included tinnitus, auditory hallucinations, and auditory illusions. Maping the suspected cortical foci on the basis of these associated symptoms indicated that lesions of the frontal, parietal, and temporal cortex can result in vestibular symptoms as part of the aura phenomena.

Diagnosis and Management

As in the evaluation of most patients with dizziness, the history is critical for determining whether the dizziness could be due to a focal seizure disorder. One must obtain an accurate description of the typical ictal event; an eyewitness is often the key. Was the patient unresponsive? Were there associated stereotyped motor phenomena? Episodic vertigo as an isolated manifestation of a focal seizure disorder is a rarity if it occurs at all.

An electroencephalogram (EEG) is the most useful diagnostic test for evaluating patients with suspected seizures. Patients with temporal lobe seizures often show unilateral or bilateral independent anterior temporal lobe spikes. They may also have memory deficits and psychiatric symptomatology. Unfortunately, complex partial seizures are often difficult to control with anticonvulsive medications, even when patients are maintained on high therapeutic blood levels.

CERVICAL DIZZINESS AND VERTIGO

Although the term cervical vertigo has been used as a specific diagnosis, it is an ill-defined entity that may have several different pathophysiologic mechanisms.

Vascular Occlusion

Because of their long course through the bony canal of the cervical vertebrae, the vertebral arteries are vulnerable to compression (e.g., by cervical osteoarthritic spurs[16] or occipitoatlantal instability[10]). Compression results from head movements such as lateral rotation or hyperextension. The latter can occlude the vertebral arteries even in normal subjects, but collateral circulation via the carotid arteries usually prevents symptoms.[14] In patients with atherosclerotic vascular disease the already compromised cerebral circulation may be further impaired by vertebral compression, producing vertebrobasilar insufficiency (see Chapter 12). Precipitating maneuvers include, for example, (1) reaching for an item from a high overhead shelf, (2) backing a vehicle from a loading dock, and (3) therapeutic neck manipulations.

The so-called posterior cervical sympathetic syndrome of Barré is a disputed cause of vertigo arising from cervical lesions. Barré[4] proposed that cervical lesions might irritate the sympathetic vertebral plexus and result in a decreased blood flow to the labyrinth due to constriction of the internal auditory artery. Although numerous clinical reports of Barré syndrome have been published, few objective data exist to support an association between episodic vertigo and cervical sympathetic dysfunction. Because intracranial circulation is autoregulated independently of cervical sympathetic control, it is unlikely that lesions in the vertebrosympathetic plexus could produce focal constriction of the vasculature to the inner ear.

Altered Proprioceptive Signals

The role of lesions involving the deep neck proprioceptive afferents in the production of vertigo and disequilibrium is controversial (see Neck Vestibular Interaction, Chapter 3). Some investigators feel that cervical lesions are a common cause of vertigo, whereas others feel they are a rare cause. Interruption of unilateral neck afferent input in normal human subjects by injection of a local anesthetic near the upper cervical joints results in vertigo and ataxia.[13] Subjects report a sensation of falling or tilting toward the side of the injection, and when walking they deviate toward the injected side. Although animals consistently develop spontaneous nystagmus after unilateral cervical anesthesia, human subjects have not done so despite prominent vertigo and ataxia. This may be due either to a species specificity or to some difficulty with injecting local anesthetics near the upper cervical vertebrae in humans.

Biemond[5] described five patients with unilateral cervicobrachial radiculoneuritis who developed vertigo and positional nystagmus when assuming a particular position. The positional nystagmus beat toward the side of the diseased brachial plexus. In four of these patients the vertigo and nystagmus cleared as the radiculoneuritis cleared. The same author reported a patient who developed positional vertigo and nystagmus after unilateral section of the third and fourth cervical sensory routes in the course of removal of multiple neuromas.[6] For several days after the operation the patient developed nystagmus when rotating the head with respect to the trunk and on turning the entire body about its longitudinal axis. In these and other reports of vestibular symptoms and signs associated with neck lesions a concomitant vestibular lesion cannot be ruled out. For example, the same etiologic factor might produce a radiculoneuritis and a labyrinthitis, and surgical procedures involving cervical dorsal roots often result in loss of large quantities of cerebrospinal fluid (CSF) that might in turn affect labyrinthine function. Despite these reservations, however, convincing reports suggest that certain acute lesions of the high cervical dorsal roots may lead to symptoms indistinguishable from those produced by labyrinthine disease.

Whiplash Injuries

A perplexing problem because of the frequency of occurrence and the medicolegal ramifications is the role of soft tissue injuries of the neck in producing dizziness and disequilibrium. Patients often describe the dizziness in nonspecific terms such as lightheaded, swimming, off-balance, floating, and rocking; as with psychophysiologic dizziness they may describe a sensation of spinning inside the head unassociated with an illusion of movement or with spontaneous nystagmus (see Chapter 4). The dizziness may last for months or years after the injury, although it usually disappears as the swelling and pain subside. Some reports indicate a high incidence of positional and spontaneous nystagmus on ENG examination in such patients.[8, 31] These findings must be interpreted with caution, however, inasmuch as normal subjects frequently have both spontaneous and positional nystagmus when tested with eyes closed (see Recording Pathologic Nystagmus, Chapter 6). The occasional finding of unilateral caloric hypoexcitability is likely due to associated labyrinthine trauma.

From the known anatomic substrate for neck-vestibular interaction (see Chapter 3), it is unlikely that lesions involving only soft tissues of the neck could produce vertigo and disequilibrium. The major neck afferent input to the vestibular nuclei arises from the paravertebral joints and capsules, with a relatively minor input from the paravertebral muscles. The skin and superficial muscles do not appear to provide any input to the vestibular system. In addition, the relative contribution of neck afferent input to the vestibular nuclei is small compared with the direct labyrinthine and indirect visual signals transmitted via other brainstem nuclei and the cerebellum. Lesions involving the neck afferents in primates are rapidly compensated, and therefore prolonged dizziness after neck injuries of any type would be difficult to explain on the basis of damage to the neck afferent input to the vestibular nuclei.

Diagnosis and Management

Angiography can occasionally identify occlusion of the vertebral arteries with neck rotation or extension in patients who report episodes of vertebrobasilar insufficiency with extreme neck movements. Common sense dictates that elderly patients with known diffuse atherosclerotic vascular disease should avoid extreme rotations or hyperextension of the neck; manipulations should be performed only with the greatest care. Rarely, nystagmus can be induced by turning the neck while the patient is sitting or lying. We routinely record for positional nystagmus in the lateral positions first by turning just the patient's head and then the entire head and body. Although positional nystagmus (present with both head and body turning) is commonly seen with eyes open in darkness, neck-rotation-induced nystagmus (present with head turned only) is extremely rare, having been identified in less that 0.01 percent of patients tested. Similarly, rotational tests in which the body is turned sinusoidally while the head is fixed have not proved clinically useful because of the large variability in normal responses.[17]

Soft tissue injuries of the neck are usually associated with focal muscle tenderness and spasm. Initial management consists of rest and immobilization with a soft collar to allow the muscle contusions to heal. Once serious problems have been ruled out, the patient should be reassured that there is no evidence of neurologic damage and that the symptoms nearly always spontaneously disappear. As in patients with postconcussion syndrome, it is important to begin a gradual exercise program as the acute soft tissue injuries heal. Heat and massage along with judicious use of pharmacologic muscle relaxation provide relief of the muscle spasm, which may come and go for weeks to months. Active range of motion exercises performed on a regular basis provide the best long-term relief of muscle spasm. Patients should be encouraged to sleep with a single flat pillow and avoid long periods of hyperflexion of the neck. In our experience, the nonspecific dizziness associated with whiplash injuries improves as the local symptoms of muscle spasm and stiffness subside (assuming the medicolegal aspects can be resolved).

BELL'S PALSY

Bell's palsy has been considered a cranial mononeuropathy of unknown cause limited to the facial nerve. Some patients complain of dizziness, however, and testing may reveal evidence of auditory and vestibular impairment.[19, 26, 27] The dizziness is usually described as a sense of unsteadiness, but vertigo occurs in a small percentage of patients. Caloric testing reveals a vestibular paresis on the side of the facial paralysis in about 20 percent of cases, and occasionally responses are decreased bilaterally. Two likely possibilities to explain the associated auditory and vestibular findings in patients with Bell's palsy are (1) the same disease process involves the seventh and eighth nerves, or (2) the swollen facial nerve compresses the eighth nerve, which it closely accompanies in the internal auditory canal.

Pathophysiology

As in the case of vestibular neuritis, there is considerable circumstantial evidence suggesting a viral etiology for Bell's palsy.[2, 23] It frequently can occur in epidemics, it can be part of a cranial polyneuropathy, and there is often serologic evidence of a recent viral infection. However, efforts to culture a specific virus from the blood, pharynx, and CSF have been disappointing.

Adour and associates[2] proposed that Bell's palsy results from a reactivation of a latent *Herpes simplex* infection. Antibodies to *H. simplex* have been found in nearly all patients with Bell's palsy, exceeding the prevalence in age-matched controls. They further pointed out that cold drafts, which patients frequently report as an inciting factor, might be a nonspecific stresser that would trigger a reactivation of *H. sim-*

plex analogous to the situation with *H. labialis.*

Diagnosis

The key to the diagnosis of Bell's palsy is to rule out other likely causes of facial paralysis. Idiopathic Bell's palsy can come on abruptly, but it can progress for a few hours to as long as 10 days. By contrast, tumor-induced facial paralysis is nearly always gradual, progressing over weeks to months. When auditory and vestibular symptoms and signs are associated with Bell's palsy, they are usually mild and transient; progressing hearing loss or persistent vertigo should suggest a diagnosis other than Bell's palsy. Computerized tomography (CT) scan of the temporal bone should be conducted in any patient with atypical features; as suggested earlier, all infants who present with facial paralysis should have a CT scan performed (see Tumors of the Middle Ear and Temporal Bone, Chapter 13). As in the case with acoustic neuroma, a magnetic resonance (MR) scan is more sensitive for identifying soft tissue masses within the internal auditory canal and should be considered in a patient with atypical features even though the CT scan is negative.

Management

Before considering management of patients with Bell's palsy, one must have an understanding of the natural history of the disorder. Nearly all patients recover normal or nearly normal facial strength regardless of the form of treatment.[21] Many patients will recover within days to weeks, although there is a significant number who have a delayed recovery after 4 to 6 months. Patients who recover within the first 3 weeks probably have lesions that primarily produce a conduction block, whereas those who show no signs of recovery until the fifth month probably have near total degeneration of the nerve, and recovery must occur by axonal regeneration from the lesion site to the muscles.

Steroids have been advocated for the treatment of Bell's palsy to reduce inflammation within the facial canal and thus reduce the amount of nerve degeneration. Adour[1] recommends that any patient who is seen within 1 week of onset should receive prednisone, 1 mg per kg per day for 5 days. If, on return visit, the facial paralysis is incomplete or recovering, the steroids are rapidly tapered over 5 days. If the paralysis is complete on return visit, the patient is given another 10 days of high-dose prednisone for a total of 15 days, followed by tapering over the 16th to 20th days. Whether the benefits of this form of treatment outweigh potential complications (which are admittedly infrequent) has yet to be convincingly proven. Surgical decompression of the facial nerve for idiopathic Bell's palsy—although initially enthusiastically endorsed by some otolaryngologists—is now in disrepute; the risks and complications outweigh potential benefits.

REFERENCES

1. Adour, KK: Diagnosis and management of facial paralysis. N Engl J Med 307:348, 1982.
2. Adour, KK, Byl, FM, Hilsinger, RL, et al: The true nature of Bell's palsy: Analyses of 1000 consecutive patients. Laryngoscope 88:787, 1978.
3. Aschoff, JC, Conrad, B, and Kornhuber, HH: Acquired pendular nystagmus with oscillopsia in multiple sclerosis: A sign of cerebellar nuclei disease. J Neurol Neurosurg Psychiatr 37:570, 1974.
4. Barré, MJA: Sur un syndrome sympathique cervical postérieur et sa cause fréquente: L'árthrite cervicale. Rev Neurol I:1246, 1926.
5. Biemond, A: Further observations about the cervical form of positional nystagmus and its anatomical base. Proc K Ned Akad Wet 43:901, 1940.
6. Biemond, A: Nystagmus de position d'origine cervicale. Psychiatr Neurol Neuroclin 64:149, 1961.
7. Cogan, DG: Internuclear ophthalmoplegia typical and atypical. Arch Ophthalmol 84:583, 1970.
8. Compere, WE, Jr: Electronystagmographic findings in patients with "whiplash" injuries. Laryngoscope 78:1226, 1968.
9. Compston, A: Methylprednisolone and multiple sclerosis. Arch Neurol 45:669, 1988.
10. Coria, F, et al: Occipitoatlantal instability and vertebrobasilar ischemia: Case report. Neurology (NY) 32:305, 1982.
11. Dam, M, et al: Vestibular aberrations in multiple sclerosis. Acta Neurol Scand 52:407, 1975.
12. Daugherty, WT, et al: Hearing loss in multiple sclerosis. Arch Neurol 40:33, 1983.
13. DeJong, PTVM, et al: Ataxia and nystagmus induced by injection of local anesthetics in the neck. Ann Neurol 1:240, 1977.
14. Fields, WS: Arteriography in the differential diagnosis of vertigo. Arch Otolaryngol 85:111, 1967.
15. Grenman, R: Involvement of the audiovestibular system in multiple sclerosis: An otoneurologic and audiologic study. Acta Otolaryngol (Suppl) 420:9, 1985.
16. Hardin, CA, Williamson, WP, and Steegman, AT: Vertebral artery insufficiency produced by cervical osteoarthritis spurs. Neurology 10:855, 1960.
17. Jongkees, LBW: Whiplash examination. Laryngoscope 93:113, 1983.
18. Lukes, SA, et al: Nuclear magnetic resonance imaging in multiple sclerosis. Ann Neurol 13:592, 1983.
19. Mangabeira-Albernaz, PL and Gananca, MM: Vestibular function and facial nerve paralysis. In Fisch, U (ed): Facial Nerve Surgery. Aesculapius, Birmingham, 1977.
20. Mastaglia, FL, Black, JL, and Collins, DWK: Quantitative studies of saccadic and pursuit eye movements in multiple sclerosis. Brain 102:817, 1979.
21. May, M, Klein, SR, and Taylor, FH: Idiopathic (Bell's) facial palsy: Natural history defies steroid or surgical treatment. Laryngoscope 95:406, 1985.
22. McAlpine, D, Lumsden, CE, and Acheson, ED: Multiple sclerosis: A reappraisal. Churchill Livingstone, Edinburgh and London, 1972.
23. Nieuwmeyer, PA, Visser, SL, and Feenstra, L: Bell's palsy: A polyneuropathy. Am J Otol 6:250, 1985.
24. Noffsinger, D, et al: Auditory and vestibular aberrations in multiple sclerosis. Acta Otolaryngol (Suppl 303):7, 1972.
25. Penfield, W and Kristiansen, K: Epileptic seizure patterns: A study of the localizing value of initial phenomena in focal cortical seizures. Charles C Thomas, Springfield, IL, 1951.
26. Rauchback, E and Stroud, MH: Vestibular involvement in Bell's palsy. Laryngoscope 85:1396, 1975.
27. Rosenhall, V, Edström, S, Hanner, P, and Badr, G: Auditory brainstem response abnormalities in patients with Bell's palsy. Otolaryngol Head Neck Surg 91:412, 1983.
28. Smith, BH: Vestibular disturbances in epilepsy. Neurology 10:465, 1960.
29. Solingen, LD, et al: Subclinical eye movment disorders in patients with multiple sclerosis. Neurology 27:614, 1977.
30. Stockard, JJ, Stockard, JE, and Sharbrough, FW: Detection and localization of occult lesions with brainstem auditory responses. Mayo Clinic Proc 52:761, 1977.
31. Toglia, JU: Acute flexion-extension injury of the neck: Electronystagmographic study of 309 patients. Neurology 26:808, 1976.
32. Waxman, SG: The demyelinating diseases. In Rosenburg, RN (ed): The Clinical Neurosciences, Vol 1. Harper & Row, Philadelphia, 1983.

APPENDIX

CUPULAR DYNAMICS

The moment-to-moment fluid displacement during a constant angular acceleration stimulus follows an exponential time course which can be determined by a more detailed mathematical treatment of the equation of the pendulum model (equation 1, Chapter 2).[7, 14, 16] The complete cupular trajectory as a function of time (t) after the application of a constant angular acceleration α is given by

$$\Theta_c(t) = \alpha \frac{M}{K}(1 - e^{-t\frac{K}{C}}) \qquad 5$$

Accordingly, after a very long time, the exponential term vanishes ($e^{-\infty} \to 0$), and the cupular deviation becomes proportional to the magnitude of the acceleration α and to the coefficient $\frac{M}{K}$ (as shown in equation 4, Chapter 2). Considering the exponential term $e^{-t\frac{K}{C}}$, it can be appreciated that when t is equal to $\frac{C}{K}$, the value of the exponent is 1 and the exponential term has the value $e^{-1} \sim 0.37$. The term within the parentheses on the right-hand side of equation 5 is now equal to 0.63. Measuring the time at which the response is 63 percent of the total provides an estimate of the value of $\frac{C}{K}$. This value is referred to in vestibular physiology as T_1, the long time constant of the cupula. Another value, the so-called short time constant of the cupula or T_2, defines the high frequency sensitivity of the cupula. The product of $\frac{M}{K} \cdot \frac{K}{C}$ provides an estimate of T_2 $\left(T_2 = \frac{M}{C}\right)$.[16]

According to the pendulum model, not only is the deviation of the cupula driven by a constant acceleration stimulus dependent on the restraining elastic force of the cupula, but after the stimulus is terminated, the same force becomes a restoring drive and the cupula returns to the resting position. If the cupula was deviated an amount Θ_c, the return to the resting position takes place according to the following equation:

$$\Theta_c(t) = \Theta_c e^{-t\frac{K}{C}} \qquad 6$$

Thus the recovery process takes place with the same time constant $T_1 = \frac{C}{K}$ as that of the initial deviation. The deviation decays 63 percent for every interval of time (t) equal to T_1, as shown graphically in Figure 2–11a.

A more detailed assessment of cupular motion [or any physiologic response depending on cupular motion (e.g., subjective sensation of turning or the slow component velocity of nystagmus)] can be obtained with the application of the concept of a transfer function (T_f).[7] The mathematical manipulations of this function are greatly simplified by the use of Laplace transformations—a method commonly used in engineering to perform systems analysis.

In Laplace notation, the output $O(s)$ of a linear time-invariant system to an input $I(s)$ is given by a simple algebraic relationship:

$$O(s) = T_f(s) \cdot I(s)$$

In other words, the transfer function T_f describes the relationship between the input and the output, which often is referred to as the system gain:

$$T_f(s) = \frac{O(s)}{I(s)}$$

After dividing through by M, the pendulum equation (equation 1, Chapter 2) can be written in Laplace notation as

$$\ddot{\Theta}_h(s) = \Theta_c(s)s^2 + \Theta_c(s)\frac{C}{M}s + \Theta_c(s)\frac{K}{M}$$

where $\ddot{\Theta}_h(s)$ and $\Theta_c(s)$ are the Laplace expressions for head acceleration and cupular deviation. To form a transfer function, this equation can be rewritten as

$$\frac{\Theta_c}{\ddot{\Theta}_h}(s) = \frac{1}{s^2 + \frac{C}{M}s + \frac{K}{M}}$$

After simplification and factoring,

$$\frac{\Theta_c}{\ddot{\Theta}_h}(s) = \frac{M}{K}\frac{1}{\left(\frac{M}{C}s + 1\right)\left(\frac{C}{K}s + 1\right)}$$

Substituting the ratio of the coefficients by their simplified notations $\frac{M}{C} = T_2, \frac{C}{K} = T_1$ and $\frac{M}{K} = T_1 T_2$, we have

$$\frac{\Theta_c}{\ddot{\Theta}_h}(s) = \frac{T_1 T_2}{(T_1 s + 1)(T_2 s + 1)}$$

because in Laplace notation the head acceleration and head velocity are related by

$$\ddot{\Theta}_h(s) = s\dot{\Theta}_h(s)$$

The gain of the system (re head velocity) is

$$\frac{\Theta_c}{\dot{\Theta}_h}(s) = \frac{T_1 T_2 s}{(T_1 s + 1)(T_2 s + 1)} \qquad \textbf{7}$$

In the case that the stimulus is a sinusoidal function of angular frequency ω ($2\pi f$), equation 7 can be rewritten as[16]

$$\frac{\Theta_c(t)}{\dot{\Theta}_h(t)} = \frac{T_1 T_2 \omega}{(T_1 \omega + 1)(T_2 \omega + 1)}$$

This gain and phase relationship between the output and the input as a function of the frequency is commonly repre-

sented by a logrithmic plot called a Bode plot (Fig. A–1).

Some practical interpretations of the Bode plot for the equation of the pendulum model are as follows. For very low frequencies where $\omega << \frac{1}{T_1}$, the terms in the denominator of equation 7 approach 1 and the gain is determined by the product $T_1 T_2 \omega$. The gain, therefore, increases linearly as the frequency (ω) increases:

$$\frac{\Theta_c(t)}{\dot{\Theta}_h(t)} \approx T_1 T_2 \omega.$$

For middle frequencies, when $\frac{1}{T_1} < \omega < \frac{1}{T_2}$, the gain is controlled by the first term in the denominator

or

$$\frac{\Theta_c(t)}{\dot{\Theta}_h(t)} \approx \frac{T_1 T_2 \omega}{T_1 \omega}$$

$$\Theta_c(t) \approx T_2 \dot{\Theta}_h(t)$$

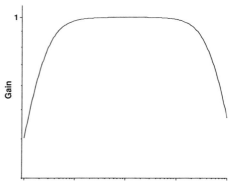

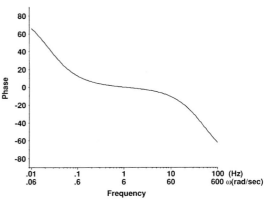

Figure A–1. Bode plots of normalized gain and phase values given by the equation of the pendulum model (equation 7). $T_1 = 7$ seconds, $T_2 = 0.003$ second.[16]

Cupular deviation, therefore, is proportional to the velocity of the stimulus in this frequency range.

Finally, for very high frequencies $\omega > \dfrac{1}{T_2}$ the gain decreases as a function of frequency:

$$\frac{\Theta_c(t)}{\dot{\Theta}_h(t)} \approx \frac{1}{\omega}$$

The phase relationship between the stimulus and response also varies with frequency (Fig. A–1, *bottom*). At low frequencies the response (Θ_c) leads the stimulus ($\dot{\Theta}_h$), reaching a maximum of 90 degrees or a quarter cycle at very low frequencies $\left(\omega << \dfrac{1}{T_1}\right)$. In the middle frequency region $\left(\dfrac{1}{T_1} < \omega < \dfrac{1}{T_2}\right)$, the response and the stimulus are in phase. For very high frequencies $\left(\omega > \dfrac{1}{T_2}\right)$, the response lags behind the stimulus, reaching a maximum phase delay equivalent to another quarter cycle.

THE CANAL-OCULAR REFLEX

With the initial development of the pendulum model, the dynamics of the canal-ocular reflex (COR) were assumed to reflect cupular dynamics with the central nervous system (CNS) simply transferring signals originating in the labyrinth to the oculomotor neurons. Within this simplified framework, clinicians referred to the results of rotational testing of the COR as "cupulometry" (see Psychophysical Studies, Chapter 3).[4] However, as quantitative measurements of the COR in normal subjects and patients with vestibular lesions became available, it was apparent that the CNS played a major role in determining the dynamics of the COR. For example, in normal subjects the gain and time constant of the COR could be modified by prior visual experience, and patients with deficits in the peripheral vestibular apparatus could have normal or nearly normal COR function. To be useful clinically, the model had to be expanded to include features of the central COR.

The anatomic connections graphically illustrated in Figure 3–4A provide the framework for the control systems model of the COR shown in Figure A–2. The key features of the anatomic diagram are a direct pathway from secondary vestibular neurons to the oculomotor neurons and a series of internuncial neurons providing positive feedback to the vestibular nuclei neurons.[5] Two main positive feedback loops are identified, one receiving input from ipsilateral secondary vestibular neurons $\left(\dfrac{K}{1+sT_b}\right)$ and the other from contralateral secondary neurons (C) via the commissural pathways. Although the contralateral neuron response is opposite in sign to the ipsilateral neuron response, the inhibitory interneuron converts it to a positive feedback loop. To simplify the presentation, the short time constant (T_2) of the pendulum model has been deleted and the peripheral dynamics are represented by a first-order system with a single dominant time constant (T_1). This is reasonable because, as shown in Figure A–1, T_2 becomes important only at very high frequencies (>10 Hz) beyond the range of clinical testing. The direct and feedback pathways each have variable gain elements that can be adjusted independently (D = direct, K = ipsilateral loop, C = commissural loop). Central velocity storage occurs via the ipsilateral feedback pathways represented in the model by a lag element with a time constant T_b. The minus 1 represents the crossing of the vestibular-oculomotor pathway. If we set $T_b = T_1$ (as per Robin-

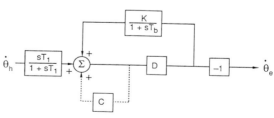

Figure A–2. Control systems model of the canal ocular reflex based on the anatomic pathways graphically illustrated in Chapter 3, Figure 3–4A. $\dot{\Theta}_h$, head velocity; $\dot{\Theta}_e$, eye velocity; T_1, long time constant of the cupula; T_b, time constant of brainstem positive feedback pathways; K, gain of positive feedback pathways; C, gain of commissural pathway (*dashed line* indicates contralateral input); D, gain of direct canal ocular pathway; -1 accounts for the reversal in direction of eye movements.

son[11]) and assume symmetry, the transfer function of the COR is given by

$$\frac{\dot{\Theta}_e}{\dot{\Theta}_h} = \frac{-s\,G_{COR}T_{COR}}{1 + s\,T_{COR}} \qquad \mathbf{8}$$

where $\qquad G_{COR} = \dfrac{D}{1-C}$ and

$$T_{COR} = \frac{T_1(1-C)}{1-C-DK}$$

Stated simply, the dominant cupular time constant (T_1) has been replaced by a system time constant (T_{COR}). Both the gain and time constant of the COR are sensitive to small changes in the central feedback loops. The relationship between T_{COR} and the gain and phase of the COR at different sinusoidal frequencies is graphically illustrated in Figure A–3. The net effect of increasing T_{COR} is to improve the low-frequency response of the COR. Lesions of the peripheral vestibular system (unilateral or bilateral) typically result in a shortening of T_{COR}, that is, a decrease in gain and an increase in phase lead at low frequencies[1] (see Fig. 7–4).

VISUAL-VESTIBULAR INTERACTION

As noted in Chapter 3 the pursuit and optokinetic systems are negative feedback systems (see Fig. 3–16). The effective stimulus for visual tracking is the retinal velocity error (r_e), the difference between the target velocity ($\dot{\Theta}_t$) and eye velocity ($\dot{\Theta}_e$). These systems operate as amplifiers receiving the error signal (r_e) and generating an appropriate eye velocity given by

$$\dot{\Theta}_e = V \cdot [\dot{\Theta}_t - \dot{\Theta}_e] \qquad \mathbf{9}$$

where V, a central processor, represents the multiplicity of connections between the retina and the oculomotor neurons (those illustrated in Fig. 3–19). Since $\dot{\Theta}_e$ and $\dot{\Theta}_t$ can be measured, equation 9 provides an estimate of V.

$$V = \frac{\dfrac{\dot{\Theta}_e}{\dot{\Theta}_t}}{1 - \dfrac{\dot{\Theta}_e}{\dot{\Theta}_t}} \text{ or } \frac{G_v}{1 - G_v} \qquad \mathbf{10}$$

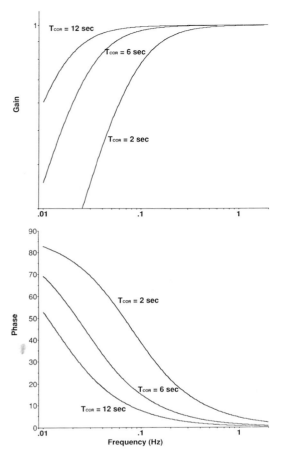

Figure A–3. Bode plots of normalized gain and phase lead values given by the equation of the canal ocular reflex (equation 8) assuming three different dominant time constants (T_{COR}). As T_{COR} decreases, the gain decreases and the phase lead increases at low frequencies.

where $\dfrac{\dot{\Theta}_e}{\dot{\Theta}_t} = G_v$, the gain of the closed-loop visuomotor system.

Note that G_v is relatively insensitive to changes in the value of V, a major advantage of a negative feedback system. For example, a change in V by an order of magnitude (99 to 9) results in a change in gain of only about 10 percent (0.99 to 0.90).

The control systems model in Figure A–4 combines the visuo-ocular and vestibulo-ocular reflexes as proposed by Cohen and colleagues[2, 15] (also see Fig. 3–20). The retinal velocity error is generated by subtracting head and eye velocity from target velocity (e.g., a surrounding optokinetic drum). The visual signal is divided into a direct

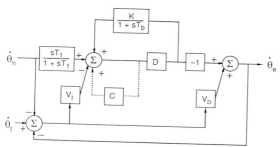

Figure A–4. Control systems model of visual-vestibular interaction as per Cohen et al.[2, 15] $\dot{\Theta}_t$, target velocity (e.g., surrounding optokinetic drum); V_I, gain of indirect visuomotor pathway; V_D, gain of direct visuomotor pathway. Other symbols as in Figure A–2.

and indirect pathway, the latter feeding into the velocity storage mechanism shared by the vestibular system. Thus, the dynamics of the indirect pathway are influenced by the same variables that influence the COR. The transfer functions of the direct and indirect pathways are represented by V_D and V_I, respectively. The direct pathway generates the rapid component of OKN, whereas the indirect pathway accounts for the slow build-up of OKN and for OKAN (see Fig. 3–15).

Analytic assessment of this model is simplified if one assumes that $V_D{>}{>}V_I$, a reasonable assumption in normal human subjects (see Organization of Visually Guided Tracking Eye Movements, Chapter 3). With this assumption, the eye velocity ($\dot{\Theta}_e$) is related to the head ($\dot{\Theta}_h$) and target ($\dot{\Theta}_t$) velocity by[6]

$$\dot{\Theta}_e = -\left(\frac{G_{COR}+V_D}{1+V_D}\right)\dot{\Theta}_h + \frac{V_D}{1+V_D}\dot{\Theta}_t \qquad \textbf{11}$$

where G_{COR} is the gain of the canal ocular reflex and V_D the transfer function of the direct visuomotor pathway. From equation 10, V_D can be estimated from the measured visuomotor gain (G_v) by

$$V_D = \frac{G_v}{1-G_v}$$

For example, a visual tracking gain of 0.95 corresponds to a V_D value of 19.

Equation 11 can be used to predict the results of visual-vestibular testing. If a subject is rotated with a stationary surrounding optokinetic drum (i.e., synergis-

tic visual-vestibular interaction, the Vis-VOR test), $\dot{\Theta}_t = 0$ and

$$\dot{\Theta}_e = -\left(\frac{G_{COR}+V_D}{1+V_D}\right)\dot{\Theta}_h$$

At low frequencies of rotation ($<$0.1 Hz) $V_D{>}{>}G_{COR}$, and

$$\dot{\Theta}_e/\dot{\Theta}_h \sim -1$$

in other words, at low frequencies at which the visuomotor gain is high ($>$0.9), the gain of the visuovestibulo-ocular reflex is near 1, regardless of the gain of the canal ocular reflex.

By contrast, at high frequencies ($>$2.0 Hz) $G_{COR}{>}{>}V_D$ and

$$\dot{\Theta}_e/\dot{\Theta}_h \sim -G_{COR}$$

the visuovestibulo-ocular reflex gain is essentially that of the canal-ocular reflex.

If the head velocity and target velocity are the same ($\dot{\Theta}_h = \dot{\Theta}_t$) such as when a subject is rotated with the chair and drum mechanically coupled (i.e., fixation suppression, the VOR-FIX test) then equation 11 becomes

$$\dot{\Theta}_e = -\left(\frac{G_{COR}}{1+V_D}\right)\dot{\Theta}_h$$

At low frequencies where $V_D{>}{>}G_{COR}$

$$\dot{\Theta}_e/\dot{\Theta}_h \sim 0$$

the subject will have complete suppression of eye movements. At high frequencies where $G_{COR}{>}{>}V_D$

$$\dot{\Theta}_e/\dot{\Theta}_h \sim G_{COR}$$

there is no suppression; the eye movement response is about the same as if the subject were rotated in the dark. These predictions are essentially the results observed in normal humans during visual-vestibular interaction testing (see Visual-Vestibular Interaction, Chapter 7).

FUTURE DIRECTIONS

Although useful for didactic purposes, the simple engineering models described in the prior sections are of limited value for understanding how the vestibular and visuomotor reflexes work at the cellular level. They assume an average response in a single dimension, whereas the sensorimotor transformations that they represent have a range of inputs occurring in multiple directions. For example, the canal ocular reflex transforms signals originating from six semicircular canals into motor commands for 12 eye muscles lying in different planes from the canals. As described in the text (see Semicircular Canal-Ocular Reflexes, Chapter 3), both dynamic and spatial transformations occur at each neuronal level within the reflex. The activity of a single neuron or group of neurons may deviate markedly from the dynamics of the overall reflex behavior. The problem becomes even more complex when dealing with visual-vestibular interaction. Signals originating in retinal and canal coordinates must be combined and transformed to eye muscle coordinates.

To deal with these problems, neuroscientists have begun to develop multidimensional models using matrices to mathematically represent the many parallel neuronal networks involved in the sensorimotor reflexes.[3, 12] Raphan and Cohen[10] expanded the model of visual-vestibular interaction shown in Figure A–4 to include a three-dimensional velocity storage element that received semicircular canal, otolith, and visual inputs to produce compensatory eye movements in all planes. The new model, the parameters of which were generalized to matrix and system operators, focused on the effect of gravity on the dynamic transformations of head and surround velocity signals to an eye velocity command. Pellionisz and Llinás[8] introduced tensor network theory to deal with the complex spatial transformations that occur within the sensorimotor reflexes. This theory assumes that the physical geometry of the organism determines the natural coordinate systems (usually nonorthogonal) that are intrinsic to the expression of their function, that is, "letting the brain speak in its own terms."[13] A "tensor model" of the vestibulocolic reflex in the cat showed how the transformation from sensory coordinates (the three semicircular canals) to a motor frame (the motoneu-

rons supplying the 30 major neck muscles) could be accomplished by a three-step tensorial scheme.[9] Furthermore, the model could be generalized to predict the neck motor responses to visual, somatosensory, or other inputs.

A major advantage of these more complicated multidimensional models is that they predict the neural signals at intermediate stages of the sensorimotor transformation; they can be modified to reflect the results of actual neural recordings. They will provide the framework for the design and interpretation of future experimental studies of sensorimotor integration within the CNS.

REFERENCES

1. Baloh, RW, Honrubia, V, Yee, RD, and Hess, K: Changes in the human vestibulo-ocular reflex after loss of peripheral sensitivity. Ann Neurol 16:222, 1984.
2. Cohen, B, Helwig, D, and Raphan, T: Baclofen and velocity storage: A model of the effects of the drug on the vestibulo-ocular reflex. J Physiol 393:703, 1987.
3. Cohen, B and Henn, V (eds): Representation of 3-Dimensional Space in the Vestibular, Oculomotor and Visual Systems. Ann NY Acad Sci 545:1, 1988.
4. Groen, JJ and Phil, M: Compulometry. Laryngoscope 67:894, 1957.
5. Honrubia, V, et al: Evaluation of rotatory vestibular tests in peripheral labyrinthine lesions. In Honrubia, V, Brazier, MAB (eds): Nystagmus and Vertigo: Clinical Approaches to the Patient with Dizziness. UCLA Forum in Medical Sciences, no. 24. Academic Press, New York, 1982, pp 57–77.
6. Lau, CGY, et al: Linear model for visual-vestibular interaction. Aviat Space Environ Med 49:880, 1978.
7. Milsum, JH: Biological Control Systems Analysis. McGraw-Hill, New York, 1966.
8. Pellionisz, A and Llinás, R: Tensorial approach to the geometry of brain function. Cerebellar coordination via a metric tensor. Neuroscience 5:1761, 1980.
9. Pellionisz, A and Peterson, BW: A tensorial model of neck motor activation. In Peterson, BW and Richmond, FJ (eds): Control of Head Movement. Oxford University Press, New York, 1988, pp 178–186.
10. Raphan, T and Cohen, B: Velocity storage and the ocular response to multidimensional vestibular stimuli. In Berthoz, A and Melvill Jones, G (eds): Adaptive Mechanisms in Gaze Control: Facts and Theories. Elsevier North Holland Press, Amsterdam, 1985, pp 123–143.
11. Robinson, DA: The use of control systems analy-

sis in the neurophysiology of eye movements. Ann Rev Neurosci 4:463, 1981.

12. Robinson, DA: The use of matrices in analyzing the three-dimensional behaviour of the vestibulo-ocular reflex. Biol Cybern 46:53, 1982.

13. Simpson, JI and Graf, W: The selection of reference frames by nature and its investigators. In Berthoz, A and Melvill Jones, G (eds): Adaptive Mechanisms in Gaze Control: Facts and Theories, Reviews of Oculomotor Research, Vol 1. Elsevier North Holland Press, Amsterdam, 1985, pp 3–20.

14. Van Egmond, AAJ, Groen, JJ, and Jongkees, LBW: The mechanics of the semicircular canal. J Physiol 110:1, 1949.

15. Waespe, W, Cohen, B, and Raphan, T: Role of the flocculus and paraflocculus in optokinetic nystagmus and visual-vestibular interactions: Effect of lesions. Exp Brain Res 50:9, 1983.

16. Wilson, VJ and Melvill Jones, G: Mammalian Vestibular Physiology. Plenum Press, New York, 1979.

INDEX

A page number in *italics* indicates a figure. A "t" following a page number indicates a table.